THE ROCKET THAT
FELL TO EARTH

Also by Jeff Pearlman

The Bad Guys Won!
Love Me, Hate Me
Boys Will Be Boys

THE ROCKET THAT FELL TO EARTH

ROGER CLEMENS

and the

RAGE

for

BASEBALL IMMORTALITY

Jeff Pearlman

HARPER

An Imprint of HarperCollins*Publishers*

HarperCollins books may be purchased for educational, business, or sales promotional use. For information, please write: Special Markets Department, Harper-Collins Publishers, 10 East 53rd Street, New York, NY 10022.

FIRST EDITION

Library of Congress Cataloging-in-Publication Data is available upon request.

ISBN: 978-0-06-172475-6

09   10   11   12   13   OV/RRD   10 9 8 7 6 5 4 3 2 1

For my beloved sisters,
Leah Guggenheimer and Jessica Guggenheimer
Long live Kelsey Crouch and The Doctor . . .

"What would I be without baseball? I could think of nothing."
—Pat Jordan, *A False Spring*

CONTENTS

THE ROCKET THAT FELL TO EARTH

CHAPTER

High Heat

The candle is lit. It shouldn't be, but it is.

We are, after all, human. We walk out of the supermarket without remembering to pay for a mango. We jaywalk and run reds and bum cigarettes when we're six months into quitting.

We forget to extinguish candles.

It happens. In fact, it's literally happening, right here by the bedside of Jonathan Benoit, a 14-year-old Seekonk, Massachusets, resident and one of the world's biggest Red Sox fans. It is a warm May night in 1996, and as he drifts off to sleep, young Jonathan takes one last glance at the walls covered with images of his hero, Roger Clemens. Along with a few pictures of a half-naked Pamela Anderson, there are eight full-sized posters of Clemens—each one depicting the Boston ace in a different phase of his windup and release. You can't count the ways this boy loves Roger Clemens. His snarl. His intensity. His blue Red Sox cap pulled down over his eyes just so. His 97-mph fastball that causes opposing hitters to instinctively flinch. Clemens is the reason Jonathan wears uniform number 21 in youth ball, the reason he relishes brushing batters back. "The Rocket," he tells anyone who will listen, "is the man."

As the boy's eyelids grow heavy, the candle falls onto his blanket, and fire and smoke engulf Jonathan and those eight Roger Clemens posters. Jonathan's door is shut, so his parents don't hear the crackling of wood. But his dog, a husky named Tasha, wakes everyone up. As Jonathan's father rushes for the nearest fire extinguisher, his mother begs for the boy to stay alive. "I don't want to die!" he screams. "I don't want to die!"

He never loses consciousness, even though burns cover more than 60 percent of his body. The paramedics arrive and strap him to a stretcher. Tasha barks wildly. His parents clasp hands. His walls, once covered by images of his idol, are now black.

"I eventually returned to my body," Jonathan says, "and fought to live."

WHEN THE EIGHTH-GRADERS AT Seekonk Intermediate School learned of their classmate's accident, they were devastated. The details were sketchy: Jonathan was in a fire. Jonathan had been taken to the Shriners Burns Institute. Jonathan might live. Jonathan might die. "It was very hard," says Kathryn Dunlap, Jonathan's teacher. "As an educator, you're fairly powerless in that situation. But we came up with a plan."

One hundred and sixty-three of Jonathan's classmates wrote to Roger Clemens, telling him that his biggest fan was on the verge of death. "To be honest," says Dunlap, "I had no expectations. It was just something to do. I hoped he would see them." Two weeks after the fire, Clemens saw them. The Red Sox were in Seattle to play the Mariners when, before the fourth game of the series, a thick FedEx bundle was placed atop his clubhouse chair. In the midst of recovering from a knockout fever that sapped most of his strength, Clemens leaned back on a table in the trainer's room and started to read. Tears streamed down his cheeks. The man known as a cold, heartless baseball killer was speechless.

Within a month, Clemens was standing in the auditorium at Seekonk Intermediate School, addressing the eighth-graders as their classmate was swaddled in bandages, lying in a hospital bed. The baseball star insisted that no media be admitted, so the next day's newspapers carried no stories. "When Jon recovers—and he *will* recover—he'll need your love and strength and support," Clemens told the children. "There's nothing more powerful than friendship. Use that power."

Five weeks later, Clemens walked into Room 325 at Shriners Burns Institute wearing a blue Boston Red Sox jersey and cap and white pants, and armed with a slew of autographed items. It was Jonathan's 54th day in the hospital, and his hope had long ago been replaced by despair. Yet when Clemens arrived, everything changed. "I knew at that very moment that I would be OK," says Jonathan. "He represented something very powerful to me."

The pitcher took a long look at his young fan—arms layered in bandages, hands wrapped in blue gauze, neck coated with reddened scabs and scars—and asked that everyone leave the room. For the next one and a half hours, Clemens forcefully told Jonathan he would again wear number 21 and throw inside fastballs. "We all face obstacles in life—some harder than others," he said. "This is your big one."

One year to the day after the fire, Jonathan was back on the baseball field. He would go on to play two years of junior varsity baseball at Seekonk High before—late in his junior year—being called up to varsity. "That was a big day for me," he says. "Most of the people I knew thought I'd never play again, and I made it. I owed that to a lot of friends—beginning with Roger Clemens. He had a fan for life."

●   ●   ●

THE YEARS HAVE PASSED. The photographs and memories have faded. The Roger Clemens who visited Jonathan Benoit on that July afternoon was a 33-year-old 185-game winner who hoped to finish his career with the Boston Red Sox. The Roger Clemens who exists today is a 46-year-old 354-game winner who turned himself into a baseball mercenary. The Roger Clemens who visited Shriners Burns Institute that day was known as a happily married father of three who refused to go more than a handful of days without seeing his wife, Debbie. The Roger Clemens who exists today is still battling bad press over his 10-year affair with a country singer named Mindy McCready—a woman he allegedly first had sex with when she was 17. She was only one of many women with whom he committed adultery over the past 15 years.

The Roger Clemens who motivated Jonathan that day was baseball's hardest worker—one of the first pitchers to regularly lift weights, to run outfield sprints between spring training innings and to conduct rigorous offseason regimens that would cause some Green Berets to vomit. "I've never met anybody who was driven like Roger," says Mike Greenwell, the longtime Red Sox outfielder. "When they told him not to lift weights, he did it anyway. When they told him not to run, he said, 'Screw you,' and went running. The man would throw nine innings, come in early the next morning, toss on his running shoes and spend an hour running the streets of Boston. There was nobody like him."

The Roger Clemens who exists today is scorned by many as a cheater who used performance-enhancing drugs, broke the law to do so and then lied about it before Congress. He is a man who lives in shame.

Like his hero, Jonathan Benoit has changed, too. Now 26 years old, married and the father of two boys, he works distributing electronic components near his home in Kingstown, Rhode Island. To this day, Jonathan thinks of Clemens nearly every time he rubs his fingers over the scars he bears from that fiery night. He recalls the baseball player who, in a sense, helped bring him back to life. "I've been defending Roger for years," he says. "If you come to the office in my house, you'll see his jersey, his hat, the signed baseball cards and the signed pictures. The man is an idol to me, and when I needed him—when I really needed him—he was there. He stepped up."

Yet, something has changed for Jonathan. Of all the bromides Clemens spouted that day at the Shriners Burns Institute, the one that stuck with that young boy lying in the hospital bed was to do things the right way. You bust your tail. You maintain conviction. You tell the truth. *You always tell the truth.*

"I still love Roger, and the 14-year-old inside of me still defends Roger," Jonathan says. "But I can assure you there are hundreds of little kids, just like me, who believed in everything Roger Clemens stood for. When he told me not to do drugs, he looked me in the eyes and said it with conviction. When he told me to live the right way, he meant it. He really, really meant it."

He pauses.

"I've learned a hard lesson. Our heroes aren't always heroes after all."

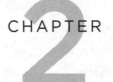

CHAPTER

2

Fat Boy from Ohio

He is out there.

Somewhere, the former cocaine addict exists, living a life of—well, uh . . . nobody seems quite sure. Through the years, he has bounced around like one of those pink Spaldeen balls, moving from Troy, Ohio, to Houston to Katy, Texas, to Georgetown, Texas. If he has an e-mail address, no one knows it. If he has a phone number, it is hard to come by. Friends shrug their shoulders. Relatives plead ignorance. After his ex-wife was murdered by drug dealers, he vanished. Moved to Louisiana to work as a chef. Dwelled under a bridge in Jackson, Mississippi, trolling for that next hit. "Randy Clemens?" says Larry South, once his closest friend. "Randy is a ghost."

But he is out there.

He is definitely out there.

When it comes to the revisionist history that William Roger Clemens often tells of his long road from the Houston suburbs to seventime Cy Young Award winner, there are plot points that flow with a too-good-to-be-true ease.

Roger Clemens never knew his deadbeat father.

Roger Clemens was raised by a tough single mother and a tough single grandmother.

Roger Clemens was born to play baseball.

Roger Clemens is a rugged, snarling Texan.

The truth, like Clemens' nasty split-fingered fastball, often seems to be right in front of us, only to drop off the table at the last possible second.

One thing, however, is indisputable: It all comes back to the broken older brother. To the ghost.

His name is Gary Randall Clemens, and while Roger usually praises his mother, Bess, and his grandmother Myrtle Lee, it was Randy—nine years Roger's senior—whom he strove to emulate. Roger did not merely admire Randy—he wanted to *be* Randy.

To tell Roger's story, a few lies need to be pushed aside. For example, despite decades of selling the world a different tale, Roger Clemens wasn't born in Texas, wasn't raised in Texas, wasn't taught how to grip a baseball in Texas. No, the story of the Rocket begins in Dayton, Ohio, where he was born on the afternoon of August 4, 1962, the youngest of Bill and Bess Clemens' five children. Through the years, Clemens has told various magazine and newspaper writers just enough about his parents to make certain everyone loathes the father and loves the mother. Bill Clemens, according to his son, was a loser. "He was anti-sports and discouraged my oldest brother, Rick, from playing basketball, which he loved," Clemens wrote in his 1987 autobiography, *Rocket Man*. "I was three and a half months old when my mother picked up and left him. And as usual, she made the right decision."

Bill Clemens, who died in 1981, is no longer here to defend himself. A blue-collar Ohioan without much of an education or family life as a child, Bill enlisted in the U.S. Navy on January 12, 1942, and served as a coxswain during World War II. Before his honorable discharge in 1946, he was awarded the prestigious Asiatic Pacific Area Campaign and American Area Campaign medals. When at age 24 he married 17-year-old Bess Lee in 1947, he was working as a truck driver for a chemical plant, on the road for weeks as his wife raised the children. Though Bill was, by all accounts, an absentee parent, it was conceivably not by choice.

In fact, though Roger Clemens has publicly blamed his father for ditching the family, it was Bess who packed up her children and left Bill while he was on a lengthy road trip. They had been married for 15 years. "It was one of those impossible things," Bess once said of her marriage. "You couldn't live with him." In the ensuing years she rarely mentioned Bill to the children, though Roger occasionally tells the story of the one subsequent conversation he had with Bill, when he was 10. "My father had called my mother and was irritating her," he said. "So I got on the phone and said, 'There is no need for you to call here anymore.'"

The two never spoke again.

Less than two years after Bill Clemens vanished, an embarrassed Bess informed her family that she was pregnant with the child of the lumpy, wrinkled, gray-haired 48-year-old mechanic who serviced her car. When Elwood "Woody" Booher learned of his impending fatherhood, he let out a euphoric *"Whooo-hoo!"* and immediately proposed to Bess. For the next six years, Roger, his two brothers (Richard and Randy) and his three sisters (Brenda, Janet, and Bonnie, the new baby) were embraced by a man who, upon popping the question, told Bess, "I love you, but I'll always look after your children first, you second. They're my priority."

Booher moved Bess and her offspring to his hometown, Butler Township, a tiny suburb (population: 8,212) 10 miles outside Dayton known—if at all—as the onetime home of the Grand American Trapshoot Championship. Butler Township featured the usual small-town clichés: safe streets, grassy fields, unlocked doors and trustworthy neighbors. The town had one traffic light, a handful of police officers, a gas station and "The Little Store" that sold ice pops, Coca-Cola and three pieces of Bazooka gum for a quarter. Booher installed his new family in a small brick house near the corner of Little York Road and Peters Pike with a miniature basketball court in the driveway. As her husband worked long hours for minimal pay as a tool-and-die man, Bess spent her days as a janitor at a nearby hospital, cleaning beds, sweeping hallways, counting the hours until she could rush home to prepare dinner. A smallish woman with curly brown hair and a room-filling cackle, Bess smoked two packs of cigarettes per day and often had the sagging cheeks and wrinkled forehead of someone twice her age. "Bess was the type of woman who would do anything for anybody," says South, Randy Clemens' longtime friend. "She sacrificed her life for those kids without ever thinking twice about doing so. You'd never hear her complain about her place in the world."

Though the family was poor, with the thrift-store shirts and patch-sealed dungarees to prove it, the children never noticed. They played tag and kick the can in the street, rode bicycles to their friends' houses, somehow always had plenty of presents beneath the Christmas trees. "I had a tremendous amount of fun playing sports," Clemens once said. "My mother made sure I had all the right equipment and plenty of it. People would be having a little softball game in their yards a few streets down and next thing you know, me and my friends, we'd be in the game." Woody would take Roger on long rides on his black BMW motorcycle, let the boy help him repair broken appliances, tuck him in at night and wake him in the morning. When Roger was upset, Woody would sing to him, croaking out old country-and-western tunes that would quickly have his stepson laughing. He would bring home a gallon of Blue Bell ice cream after work, inviting all the kids to grab a spoon and dig in. Woody was an even-tempered man who refused to raise his voice even when Brenda decided to light a fire on a frigid winter day and wound up burning down the garage. "We would watch *Bonanza* on TV every week, just me and him," Clemens said.

"He really enjoyed that show. I remember, during commercials, he'd hold me down and tickle me with his whiskers."

Everything changed for the Clemens-Booher family on the evening of October 4, 1970. With Bess at work, Woody cooked up steak and potatoes and sat down at the kitchen table with five of the children, Randy, Roger, Brenda, Janet and Bonnie (Richard, the oldest, was a member of the U.S. Army and serving in Vietnam), as well as Randy's friend Larry South. Midway through the meal, Woody excused himself. He was breathing awkwardly and grimacing.

Upon reaching the bathroom, Woody—who was overweight and a heavy smoker—clutched his heart and collapsed into the bathtub with a thud. Randy ran toward his stepfather, screaming for someone to call an ambulance. South, meanwhile, ushered the younger kids to the basement bedroom Woody had recently built for Randy.

As the ambulance pulled into the driveway. Roger climbed atop a milk crate and peered through the basement window; he saw the man he considered to be his real father loaded into the back of the ambulance. Woody's arms and legs were motionless. An oxygen mask covered his face.

Roughly 45 minutes later, the phone rang in the Clemens household. Bess, who had rushed home to be with her children, answered.

Woody Booher, age 54, was dead of a heart attack.

Roger Clemens had lost his second dad.

YOU ARE EIGHT YEARS OLD.

You have gone through not one but two fathers.

Your family is poor and about to become significantly poorer.

What do you do?

In the case of Roger Clemens, you look for someone new to lead the way.

You look for Randy Clemens.

With Woody's sudden passing, where else was there for young Roger to turn than to his 17-year-old brother? "I'm a Christian," Clemens once said. "As a boy we were solid churchgoers. After my stepfather died I had doubts that God was fair. Why did God take him away? Why?"

If we are to go back in time and pinpoint the exact moment when Roger Clemens began to become, well, *the* Roger Clemens, it is here, in the aftermath of Woody's death, when the older brother emerged as the father. Or at least the father figure. Not that Randy wasn't up to the task. In the smallish world of Butler Township, where everyone knew everyone, Randy Clemens was as admired and revered as Benjamin Wilhelm, the town's first mayor. Maybe even more so.

At Vandalia-Butler High School, where he was a senior, Randy cruised the hallways with the regal elegance of a kid who knew where he was headed. He was handsome, with a Robert Redford grin and a confidence that announced itself with each step. He was the short-stop on varsity baseball and the star shooting guard for the varsity basketball team, a fearless slasher nicknamed "Radar" by Coach Ray Zawadzki for his ability to nail long jumpers. With the five-foot-ten, 180-pound Randy Clemens guiding the way and averaging 20 points per game, the Aviators went 18-2 his senior year. Joe B. Hall, the legendary Kentucky coach, sent a recruiter to see him play. "Randy wasn't on our football team, but I remember one day he came out to one of our practices, just goofing around," recalls George Toman, a classmate. "He picked up the ball and just started launching it as far as humanly possible. It all came so naturally to him."

In a class of 280 students, Randy was voted king of the "Southern Nights"–themed senior prom. The queen was his girlfriend, Kathy Huston, who was—naturally—captain of the cheerleading squad. "Randy just had it all going on," says Mark Vennerholm, Roger's child-hood friend. "He was good-looking, smart, a great athlete, well known, popular. If you were Roger, you couldn't help but watch him across the dinner table and think, 'I want to be just like him.' And Roger did. He absolutely idolized his brother."

If Randy was a new Jaguar XJ6, sleek and smooth and powerful, Roger was a Dodge Dart with some chipped paint and a dangling muffler. In the years leading up to puberty, Roger was—physically and athletically—unremarkable. He had a double-chinned, doughy face, with a pear-shaped body and a way of walking that reminded one of a slug. He even struggled with occasional asthma attacks and a bowl-styled haircut straight out of *My Three Sons*. "Roger was short and fat," says Walter Peck, who coached him in Little League. "I had him on an all-star team, and he didn't even start. He simply wasn't good enough."

"Roger wasn't a great hitter, and he didn't throw very hard," says Glen Burchfield, his closest childhood pal. "And he wasn't fast afoot. But he tried really hard."

With Woody's passing, Bess had to work two and three jobs to keep the family afloat. She cleaned offices in a nearby building at night and picked up extra shifts at a local dive. Thanks to some funds Woody had left in a trust, Bess was able to move the family—first to a larger home on Little York Road with a pool in the backyard, then to an even nicer four-bedroom spread in the nearby Imperial Hills subdivision. "They were not well off," says Jean Crutcher, a family friend. "But Bess was committed to treating her children well."

With his mother usually at work, Roger spent a lot of the time with his grandmother Myrtle Lee, who considered the boy to be her own son. "I can remember [Grandma] twisting off a chicken's neck," Roger recalled. "I didn't know it was dying as it ran after me. I cut left, it cut left. A chicken can run for two or three minutes with its head off. My grandfather was watching, laughing, calling me 'Rooster Peck.' They were very tough on us. That's why I am the way I am."

When he wasn't with family, Roger could usually be located down the street at the Burchfields' house, where he and Glen would while away the afternoons and evenings. The boys shared a passion for chocolate ice cream, the James Caan film *Rollerball* and sports. Alongside other neighborhood kids, Roger and Glen competed in backyard home-run derbies, smear the queer, and dunk contests. Roger would often eat dinner with Glen's family, then be dropped off at home come 9 P.M. Sometimes his mother would be there. Oftentimes she wouldn't. "He was a normal little boy in a tough situation," says Emily Burchfield, Glen's mother. "If he didn't have a way to or from a ball game, we took care of it. One thing I recall is that Roger was always very proud of his house. He'd say, 'Come in! Come see my house!' It meant a lot to him."

Roger found sports to be the perfect balm for an imperfect life. Millie Donathan, a secretary at John E. Smith Junior High, recalls a roly-poly boy with a hangdog expression who would arrive to school in hand-me-downs. "Every time he'd come into the office, he'd have a snotty nose," says Donathan. "I mean, every time. And I'd say, 'Roger, get around here and blow that nose right now!' He'd come in and say, 'Ms. Donathan, I forgot my lunch money again,' and I'd take him back to the cafeteria and tell the girls to give him his lunch. They probably could have qualified for free lunches, but Bessie refused to fill out the form. She was just that proud."

With the family's struggles, Randy deemed it his duty to instill in his brother a simple philosophy: Either you're a winner or you're a failure. That was Randy's approach to sports, one that resulted in on-court tantrums and browbeatings of opponents and referees. Basketball teammates still speak of the game against Brookville when Randy pushed an official and was placed on probation by the school. Roger, who served as a batboy for the high school baseball team and attended nearly all his brother's home basketball games, watched closely. He even wore the same uniform number as his brother: 21. "Randy was very arrogant, very pushy, very abrasive," recalls Mike Lawson, Randy's former basketball teammate. "He wanted to play every minute of every game, and he wouldn't let you forget it. He lacked a certain perspective; an acknowledgment that, at the end of the day, it's just a game."

Before long, Roger came to lack this perspective, too. Although Randy was no longer living at home, having graduated from high school in 1971 and accepted a basketball scholarship to Division III Bethel College in Mishawaka, Indiana, his influence on his brother remained profound. As he advanced from elementary school to junior high to high school, Roger turned increasingly combative. Though he was still a chunky kid through his early teens, on the courts and fields Roger carried himself like a scowling, trash-talking 20-game winner. He even promised those around him that one day he would start the All-Star Game, win the final game of the World Series and wind up on the cover of *Sports Illustrated*. In football he was a stout defensive and offensive lineman. In basketball, he was a physical power forward and center. And in baseball he was a gap-hitting third baseman and a soft-tossing control artist.

Yes, Roger Clemens was a soft-tossing control artist.

Though Roger was usually one of the better pitchers in the various leagues in which he participated, intimidation was not his game. While playing in the Vandalia Recreational League as a 12-year-old, an opposing pitcher named Ken Mann told Roger he was going to plunk him with a pitch in order to have him leave the game. "That's fine," Roger replied. "But if you hit me, I hit you."

Just moments later, Mann—knowing full well there would be retribution—nailed Clemens in the shoulder. Shortly thereafter, the favor was returned. Clemens wound up, unleashed his best fastball and—*poof!*—watched as Mann barely flinched as the ball brushed against his leg. "Roger was a big kid, but he didn't throw hard," says Mann. "So I wasn't too scared."

If one person in particular felt the brunt of the bullying attitude Randy had instilled in his younger brother, it was Kelly Krzan, Roger's teammate on the Murlin Heights Class E Little League baseball team in 1977.

Four years earlier, to much ridicule and a *Dayton Daily News* feature titled "Cute Batter Up," Krzan had been the first girl in the state of Ohio to participate in boys' Little League, going 1-for-2 for the Lions Club at Vandalia's Edgewood Field. Now well established as a local baseball phenom, Krzan joined the Murlin Heights team and found herself part of Coach Mike Kessler's fascinating two-person pitching rotation—the fat kid and the girl. "I don't want to say anything bad about Roger, because he had a good side to him," says Krzan. "But when push came to shove, Roger was very arrogant when he pitched. He had to be the star, and if we lost it was always somebody else's fault. He was the kid who'd yell, 'Catch the ball!' and 'You blew it for us!'"

Clemens dreaded splitting starts with a girl. "Whenever Kelly was pitching, Roger made it real clear that he disapproved," says Patricia Krzan, Kelly's mother. "He'd get mad and throw things. He'd stomp around and tell people that a girl shouldn't be pitching. It hurt me to watch, because that was my daughter. She deserved more respect than that."

Behind the Clemens-Krzan one-two punch ("Actually," says Tony Kessler, the team's assistant coach, "they were equal pitchers. Roger was no better than Kelly"), Murlin Heights went 13-0 and won the league championship. But for most involved, it was a relatively joyless experience. Clemens, who fancied himself as Randy's heir to athletic greatness, was humiliated by having to split time with a kid in pigtails. And Krzan heard the jeers of parents urging Kessler to "get that girl out of there," as well as the taunts from opposing players.

"When I got up to bat, I learned to duck quite often," she says. "I loved the game, but, to be honest, after a while I got tired of the attitudes."

Come season's end, Krzan hung up her cleats. She never played organized baseball again.

*   *   *

FROM AFAR, RANDY CLEMENS kept tabs on his brother, urging him to work harder, to accept nothing less than excellence, to ignore those not named Gary Randall Clemens who tried to guide his athletic career.

Yet if anyone was in need of guidance, it was Randy Clemens.

Though he was known in Butler Township as a relatively clean-living kid, his two years at Bethel College had brought a disconcerting metamorphosis. No longer the prep superstar, Randy struggled to adjust to being merely another good college basketball player performing in a gymnasium, Goodman Auditorium, that seated a mere 1,200 spectators. "Back in the 1970s, the high school athletes in Ohio were held up as role models for the community," says Jon LeCrone, Randy's prep teammate. "We were the hope for the generation, because we all appeared to be polite, clean-cut, athletic, hardworking. The community invested in us. They came to our football games, to our basketball games, to our baseball games. It was a source of pride for the town, and there was the expectation we'd go on and do great things. Nobody exemplified that more at our school than Randy Clemens. And clearly he had some demons nobody cared to notice." It was the all-too-familiar tale of a local phenom coming to the realization that he is not so phenomenal after all. It was also the all-too-familiar tale of a kid who spent 18 years trying to do everything absolutely right finally being set free to indulge. He no longer had to look after his brothers and sisters, no longer had to concern himself with his mother's work schedule.

"Randy changed," says Lawson. "He went to Bethel and never adjusted. I think we were all naive in high school when it came to drugs. But Randy went away and started smoking marijuana at Bethel. For those of us who had played with him in Ohio, it was very surprising news."

Despite Randy's troubles, he was a solid guard who could handle the ball and shoot from long range. When Bethel coach Doug Hines was hired by Division II Mississippi College before the 1973–74 season, he took four of his players along with him to Clinton, Mississippi—including Randy. In his two years at the small Baptist school, Randy performed well, notching a school record that still stands, with 17 assists in a game against Troy State. "You had to be a little cocky to be a point guard, and Randy was certainly confident," says Buck French, Mississippi College's starting shooting guard. "But he was a good guy. We liked him."

Unfortunately, the drug usage that began at Bethel only increased in Mississippi. As a senior Randy was caught with marijuana on a road trip, and Hines—who had great affection for his court leader—had to kick him off the team. Randy told friends back home that he had been set up. "I loved Randy," says South, "but I found that unbelievable."

Over the next two years, Randy struggled to overcome the humiliation of his fall from grace. There was a failed tryout with the fledgling American Basketball Association, a gig with a lawn service company, a brief tenure as an assistant coach at Houston Baptist College, and finally a return to Mississippi College, where Hines agreed to take Randy on as an assistant so that he could earn his degree.

On December 21, 1975, Randy married Kathy Huston, his high school girlfriend and prom queen, in a ceremony at St. Rita's Church in Dayton. In Butler Township, the union was hailed as two high school sweethearts meant to be together. To Roger, who looked to Kathy as a big sister–mother, it meant the addition of a beloved family member. To Bess Clemens, it meant the addition of the daughter-in-law she always wanted. Kathy was smart, pretty, savvy—an elementary school teacher with a joyful disposition.

Kathy's family, however, viewed the union with skepticism. Her parents and two siblings looked at Randy and saw a used-car salesman. He would pour on the charm in their presence, then talk trash as soon as everyone was out of earshot. There was a lot of Eddie Haskell in the kid.

"Randy was involved in this secret world—that much we knew," says Carolyn Gray, Kathy's older sister. "I knew he was delving into a bunch of drugs; at least I started getting that feeling. But Kathy was very protective of Randy. If she was fully aware of how bad he was, she wasn't saying."

Shortly after the wedding, Randy and Kathy moved to Houston, where he worked with his older brother, Richard, in the tool-and-die industry, and she found employment as an elementary school teacher. Randy continued to play an important role in the life of Roger, who in the fall of 1976 made his debut with the freshman baseball team at Smith Junior High. Roger didn't exactly stand out. Alongside his picture on page 13 of the 1976–77 school yearbook, he is identified as "Roger Clemmens." The football team went 4-2-1 with Clemens contributing as a defensive lineman, and basketball compiled an 0-6 mark before, according to the yearbook, "the freshman team was unable to complete its season due to the energy shut down." A stiff, burly post player, Clemens averaged around eight points per contest.

Unlike Randy, who had all but emerged from the womb bursting with athleticism, Roger struggled. Even as a freshman, by which time most boys have traded in their baby fat, Roger's body was similarly proportioned to that of a popular childhood toy from the time period, the Weeble. He was now six feet tall but lumpy. Away from the fields, his confidence befitted his frame. Shy and awkward, through his freshman year Clemens had neither kissed a girl nor taken one on a date. "Roger was a nice kid," says Bob Costello, the Vandalia-Butler High junior varsity baseball coach. "But there was nothing to make you think he'd be anything more than above average."

From his home in Houston, Randy Clemens couldn't believe what he was hearing. How could his brother, blessed with the same blood and DNA, be so forgettable? Why wasn't he the hottest young ballplayer in town? Why weren't the girls swooning at his side? Maybe Roger would never be as good as his older brother, but he certainly could do better than . . . *this.*

Early in Roger's sophomore year at Vandalia-Butler High School, Randy convinced Bess that it would be in the boy's best interest to relocate to Houston and live with him and Kathy. They would feed him, nurture him, mold him into the athlete he could—*and should*—become. Living 1,120 miles away from her second-oldest son, Bess knew nothing of the drugs that had seeped into his life. "OK," Bess said, finally relenting. "But take good care of him."

Roger played JV football and basketball, then one day informed his close friend Glen Burchfield that he would be leaving for Texas. "I thought it would be sort of gradual," says Burchfield. "Well, it was right after basketball season had ended. Roger told us he'd be moving soon, and one day he didn't make baseball practice. That's how I found out my friend had left—he just never showed up. We had a lot of history with Roger—my family and I. I never understood how he could just vanish like that.

"But," adds Burchfield, "that's exactly what he did. He just vanished."

Houston Bound

For the typical American tenth-grader, a mid–high school relocation can elicit varying emotions: Anger for being dragged away from longtime friends. Fear for having to face a new situation. Despair for the shedding of comfort and the headfirst plunge into the unknown.

For Roger Clemens, age 15, it was a cause for joy.

As Clemens later told the *Dayton Daily News,* his favorite part of growing up in Ohio was "seeing it in my rearview mirror." For the many friends and neighbors who took offense at the remark (and, indeed, *many* took offense), an important bit of context is missed. When Clemens reflected upon his one and a half decades in Ohio, he didn't think about riding his bicycle through warm summer breezes or pretending to be Dr. J outside the Burchfields' house. No, to Clemens, Ohio was the place where he had lost both his fathers, where he had lived in relative poverty, where his mom had worked three jobs to pay the bills and where he had been the dumpy fat kid who never kissed a girl.

Ohio? To bleeping hell with Ohio.

On February 25, 1978, Roger arrived for his first day as a sophomore at Dulles High School. With a student body of approximately 4,500 students, Dulles was the state's largest high school—a place in which a newcomer could easily lose himself. Yet young Roger understood exactly where to go. Because of state transfer rules, he was ineligible to play varsity baseball for the Vikings. So immediately following his first full day of classes, Roger donned sweat pants and a T-shirt, grabbed his beige Rawlings glove and headed out to a side field, where Coach Gary Thiebaud was holding junior varsity tryouts.

At Vandalia-Butler, 30 kids might turn out for baseball; here more than 70 freshmen and sophomores lined the field, stretching and tossing before the workout began. Roger found himself paired with Brett Bozeman, the team's third baseman. "It was a windy, cold day, and Roger told me he was a pitcher," recalls Bozeman. "So I found a mitt, squatted down and caught some of his stuff." Two things grabbed Bozeman's attention. First, Clemens' fastball wouldn't snap a saltine cracker. And second, "I didn't have to move my mitt more than an inch or two. Everything he threw was precise and right to the spot."

Clemens made the Vikings JV, joining the rotation as the number three starter. The ace, a hard-throwing right-hander named Johnny Jones, dazzled teammates with a fastball that reached the low 80s. The number two starter, Scott Wooley, possessed equal velocity, but his lanky frame broke down in a matter of weeks. "Both those guys threw significantly harder than Roger," says Bozeman. "But, man, could he locate his pitches."

As was often the case in Ohio, Clemens was initially dismissed by teammates as the fat kid. Then people saw that the fat kid could pitch a little. Clemens went 12-1 with an ERA below 3.00 as Dulles High finished 18-3 and captured the district title over archrival Galveston. In the championship game, he pitched six scoreless innings before encountering trouble in the bottom of the seventh. With Dulles leading 2-0, Clemens allowed a single, followed by two walks. "The bases were loaded, and we had a problem," recalls Thiebaud. "And that's when Roger did something truly incredible." First Clemens picked the runner off third. Then he picked the runner off second. Then he picked the runner off first. Game over—Dulles High wins. "Was Roger the most impressive athlete on that team?" says Thiebaud. "No, he wasn't. But he struck me as special because he had this fire and that strong need to win."

Throughout Dulles' season, two figures could be counted on to attend many of the games. There was Bess, now living in Sugar Land with her children, who would sit nervously in the stands, shouting encouragement while taking drags from one cigarette after another. And there was Randy, who watched Dulles' games with a disapproving eye. As far as Randy was concerned, Dulles' program was a joke. The talent surrounding Roger was, at best, mediocre, with baseball facilities to match. If Roger was going to pitch at the next level, he needed a better high school to develop his skills. "I was dazzling [at Dulles]," Clemens said. "I thought I was Lord K, or whatever they say. And Randy said . . . the decision where we were gonna live [the following year] would be based on where I could get the best competition."

Toward the end of the season, Randy took Roger to observe a regional tournament meeting between two Texas baseball powerhouses, Bellaire and Spring Woods. "We'll watch this seven-inning game, and when it's over I want you to tell me which school you want to go to next year," Randy said.

Bellaire won, 4-2.

"So," Randy said, "you're picking Bellaire?"

Roger had paid close attention to the game. Though Bellaire prevailed, something about Spring Woods had caught his eye. The players were crisp, disciplined and uncommonly professional. While they weren't as talented as the opposition, they were significantly more impressive.

"No," Roger replied, "I'm gonna go to Spring Woods."

Slowly, surely, Randy was turning Roger into the second coming *of himself.* Whereas other kids his age were chasing girls and watching *Starsky & Hutch,* Randy demanded that his brother fully devote himself to athletic excellence. "Roger was driven," says Bozeman. "We were all concerned about having fun, and Roger was starting his weight-training regimen and running before and after practices. I mean, who did weight training for baseball? More than a few of us thought that was a bit odd."

Under Randy's watch, Roger morphed into a caged animal. Kathy would hover over Roger as he completed his homework, but nothing trumped athletics. Randy wanted Roger to be tougher, to be meaner, to be more ruthless, to see opposing hitters as arrogant SOBs trying to take what was rightly his.

Never an especially skilled student (he scored mostly low B's and high C's throughout his academic career), Roger spent the month following his sophomore year taking summer school algebra. He also played for a Babe Ruth League team of 14-, 15- and 16-year-olds, the White Sox, in nearby Missouri City, Texas. Deral Castle, a local health educator, volunteered to coach because his son Randy was one of the outfielders. Castle loved youth baseball—the learning, the excitement, the fun. He was, however, less than enamored with the chubby right-hander. "Roger was a real pain to deal with," recalls Castle. "He was probably our best pitcher, but you'd tell him what to throw and he would refuse to listen. You'd give him the sign to bunt and he wouldn't bunt. In his head he thought he was the best hitter, but it just wasn't true." Roger taunted opposing batters and relished beaning those he deemed annoying or disrespectful. "There was one pickoff play while Roger was on the mound, and instead of throwing it to the first baseman he heaved the ball over the guy's head and into the opposing team's dugout," says Steve Dzierwa, a White Sox pitcher. "Just to shut them up."

To those who knew Roger away from the diamond, there was a profound sadness to the boy. The same kid who fancied himself another Don Drysdale on the mound carried himself with slumped shoulders and a tucked-in chin. Roger longed for a father figure, dreamed of Woody Booher returning to tickle him with the whiskers covering his face. Instead, he was stuck with Randy, whose demands of 100 percent athletic devotion hardly boosted Roger's sense of self-worth.

The rock in Roger's life was Kathy, who—with Bess working 15-hour days—served as a second mother. Unlike Randy, Kathy embraced Roger's vulnerabilities. She helped teach Roger to swim; went through his homework, word by word. "He always gave a lot of credit to Kathy," says Carolyn Gray, Kathy's sister. "She really cared about him. She wanted him to turn out well."

WHEN ROGER CLEMENS DECIDED that Spring Woods High would be his third school in as many years, there was no press conference. No trumpets sounded, no red carpet was rolled toward the curb, no ROCKET TO SPRING WOODS headline graced the *Houston Post*.

Nothing.

In fact, on the day Roger took his mother to visit the school's campus, he sought out Charlie Maiorana, Spring Woods' legendary 27th-year head baseball coach. "My name is Roger Clemens," he said to the short, wrinkly man. "I'm transferring to your school next year, and I'm going to play on your team."

Was that so? "I'd never heard of Roger," said Maiorana. "But I remember him showing so much confidence that day in my office. Most kids that age are shy."

To allow her son to attend the school of his choice, Bess took a job as a bookkeeper for a national rug chain and relocated to Beekman Point, an apartment complex on Long Point Road in Spring Branch, Texas. She rented a two-bedroom town house that was divided into two floors and featured beige carpet, relatively clean white walls and enough comforts to make Roger—no longer under the watch of Randy and Kathy—feel at home. "It was a blue-collar, lower-middle-class sort of place," says Robert Hooper, a Spring Woods classmate. "It was nothing to write home about."

When the White Sox wrapped up their season, Clemens joined Spring Woods High's entry into American Legion ball. For Maiorana, the games were a chance to evaluate his talent. For Clemens, it served as a major eye-opener. If Randy thought his brother would simply don a Spring Woods baseball uniform and blow away the competition, he was badly mistaken. Not only had Roger opted to play for an elite baseball program, he had done so at a time when Maiorana's top two pitchers, right-hander Rick Luecken and left-hander Rayner Noble, formed the best one-two starting punch in the country. "That summer, when Roger arrived, I'm sure he planned on doing a lot of pitching," says Maiorana. "Well, we didn't know anything about him, and we had two guys who would be drafted out of high school. Needless to say, he didn't touch the mound all that often."

In what remains one of the most frustrating stretches of his life, Clemens pitched six games for the Spring Woods varsity as a junior in 1979. Behind their backs, Clemens would rip Luecken and Noble, complaining that he was every bit as talented. "Roger only threw in the low 80s, yet he let it be known to all of us that he would one day be a big-league pitcher," says Noble. "We all snickered at that." Neither Luecken nor Noble showed much interest in the ornery kid with so-so stuff. He was the third wheel on a motorcycle.

And yet . . .

"Roger worked his ass off—I mean, he worked and worked and worked and worked like nobody else on that team," says Rex Willis, a Spring Woods infielder. "When Coach made us run sprints around the outfield, we'd get to the center field fence where he couldn't see us, and we'd all slow up. Well, there goes this young guy, Roger, just flying by us. We'd be yelling, 'Slow up! Slow up!' but Roger didn't listen. We all thought we were big studs, being seniors on a top team, and his work ethic didn't fit into that coolness."

Among the seniors, Clemens was mocked. *An ass-kisser. Too driven. Too eager. Who was this fat kid, trying to show up the stars?* Unlike his time at Vandalia-Butler Township and Dulles, where the team fitness programs had been limited to stretching and long-tossing, Maiorana had a structured plan designed to develop multiple muscle groups. There were distance running and sprints, upper-body and lower-body weight programs. Though his teammates blew off many of the coach's requirements, Clemens upped the intensity.

Everywhere he went—school, the grocery store, the bathroom— Clemens gripped a tennis ball in his right hand, squeezing life *out of* the fuzzy green Wilson and squeezing life *into* his increasingly steel-like fingers. Because he often had no way of getting home from practices, Clemens would run the one mile from Spring Woods High to his town house, backpack slung over his shoulders. Sprinting down Gessner Road, Clemens would pass Andy Granatelli's Tune-up Shop, Porky's Pub, Kentucky Fried Chicken. Never would he stop to take a breather or sit down for a meal.

A prolific list maker, Maiorana compiled something called "The Pitcher's Checklist," which he presented to his players at the front of a notebook. Most read it once or twice and relegated it to the bottom of their lockers. Clemens taped it to his wall until the points—all 32 of them—were memorized.

1. Hitters do not own the plate.
2. Throw inside.
3. Don't let them dig in.
4. Let it rip.
5. Bow your neck.
6. Pull the string.

7. Make them chase.
8. When they're looking inside, throw outside. When they're looking outside, throw inside.
9. Get ahead.
10. Location, location, location.

And so on . . .

"Roger took that to heart," says Maiorana, a disciplinarian who required his players wear sport jackets and ties on road trips. "And even though he wasn't going to see much action as a junior, you could see something take hold. He wasn't playing, but—mentally and physically—he was developing."

Clemens felt more at ease than ever before. He was living with his mother, with his beloved (if troubled) brother and sister-in-law nearby. He quickly came to embrace Spring Woods—the diminutive baseball coach who drove him, the casual friendliness of the teachers, the lack of judgment regarding his less-than-glamorous clothes and lifestyle.

Equally important, there was a devotion to sports that had never existed at Butler Township or Dulles. The football team played on Astroturf before thousands of fans. The weights were clean. Sure, Spring Woods coaches were teachers by day, but when push came to shove, athletics was the priority. Though far from a star, Roger participated in the holy trinity of scholastic sports (he was a defensive lineman for the football team and a center in basketball), easily fitting in with the athletes who ruled the school. Suddenly Clemens was popular. He kissed a few girls (recalls a classmate named Becky Chen, "Roger dated a friend of mine for a little while. He was pretty good to her until he got really popular. Then he turned into a jerk"), hung out in the 7-Eleven parking lot, knocked back a beer or two. "If you were a jock at Spring Woods back then, you could pretty much get away with anything," says Bear Joubert, Clemens' classmate and a member of the baseball team. "There was that convenience store across from the high school, and the coaches would come in there Friday and Saturday evenings and see us downing beers on the hoods of our trucks. They'd just say, 'Take it easy' and drive off."

Although Roger's contributions were limited (in his one flash of brilliance, he set a school record by striking out 18 in a tournament at New Braunfels High School), his stature grew as the baseball team skyrocketed to a number two national ranking. So what if he threw no more than 300 pitches? He was a player.

That the Tigers ended a 31-4 dream season by losing two of three games to Baytown Sterling in the regionals stung but hardly deterred Clemens. With Noble about to leave for the University of Houston and Luecken off to Texas A&M, Spring Woods was in dire need of a number one starter.

EVEN THOUGH HE WAS but 16 at the start of his senior year of high school, Roger Clemens knew exactly what he wanted. As other classmates dreamed of mechanical engineering at MIT or journalism at Southern Methodist or accounting at Oklahoma State, Roger possessed a single goal: Major League Baseball.

Not that it was even remotely realistic.

Here was a little-known number three starter who possessed one decent pitch—an 82-mph fastball. Clemens' curveball was loopy yet hittable, and his splitter, *the* pitch of the 1990s, did not yet exist. In the summer of 1979, Clemens again participated in American Legion ball, and again he was an afterthought, playing first base and pitching sporadically. In the championship series against Periland, Roger started and was rocked, allowing five runs in two innings. Any scouts on hand surely looked at Clemens and—*scratch that*. No scouts were looking at Roger Clemens. "He was an above-average high school pitcher," says Noble. "That's it."

Clemens' senior year began well, as he started at defensive end for coach Ben Bloomer's varsity football team. Though the Tigers pro-gram never earned much respect in a state entranced by fall Friday nights, Clemens was a key player on back-to-back 6-3-1 squads. Now topping out at six-feet-four, with a sturdy 220-pound frame, he took great pleasure in strutting through Spring Woods' hallways on the Fri-days before games, slapping hands with teammates, flirting with the cheerleaders, talking trash about Lufkin or Jersey Village or whoever was next up on the schedule. Never a thinking man's athlete, Clemens relished the pure physicality of football. See quarterback, rush quar-terback, hit quarterback. "Roger wasn't Division I caliber, but he could certainly compete," says Kurt Poole, an assistant coach. "He was gifted with big size, and that never hurts on the line."

For the first time in his life, Clemens decided not to play basketball, following Randy's advice that he could best enhance his baseball pos-sibilities by devoting the winter to running and weight training. By the time spring arrived, he was ready.

On a team that overcame mediocre talent to finish 17-10, Clemens was a godsend, posting a 10-5 record with a 1.10 ERA. He even tied his own school mark by striking out 18 against Gonzalez High. But the scouts who happened to see him pitch did so only because they were checking out other players. Clemens still topped out at 84 mph.

As the Tigers' season crawled to a close, Clemens—frustrated by the lack of interest from professional and college teams—met with Maiorana to explore his options. In his autobiography, *Rocket Man*, Clemens writes that he was offered dual football-baseball scholarships by North Texas State, Northeastern Louisiana and the University of Georgia. This is not true. He also tells the story of a scout with the Minnesota Twins coming to his house after the team selected him with their 22nd-round pick. Not only was he not drafted by Minnesota in the 22nd round (that honor belongs to Reggie Wyatt of Santa Monica Community College)—he wasn't drafted at all. According to Clem-ens, the scout said, "If you don't sign now, you'll never get the chance to play." Wrote Clemens, "My mother threw him out of the house and told him, 'Don't let the door hit you in the behind on the way out.'" Though the tale makes for good reading, it is also likely fiction.

Truth be told, as Maiorana and his ace sat down and talked baseball, Clemens received neither the answers nor the reassurance he was seeking. "You've been a great high school player," Maiorana told him. "But unless you want to go local, I'm not sure whether there's a Division I baseball scholarship out there for you."

Clemens was devastated. Shortly after Spring Woods held its graduation ceremony for the Class of 1980, he and a teammate, pitcher Steve Calderone, packed up a Chevrolet Chevette and hit the road, driving from one free-agent tryout camp to another. They stopped at San Jacinto Junior College outside Houston, where the Cincinnati Reds were holding auditions. They went to Blinn College in Brenham and played in front of Los Angeles Dodger bird dogs. "We were going places, meeting people, looking for something that wasn't there for us," says Calderone. "We knew we could play at a higher level, it was just a matter of getting noticed. Both of us dreamed of playing for the University of Texas. But that was a long way away."

As high school seniors throughout the state signed with this college or that major league team, Clemens fumed. He knew he could pitch at a higher level. He just *knew* it. Finally, midway through the summer, Maiorana contacted Leroy Dreyer, a close friend and Blinn's head baseball coach. "Look, will you do me a favor," Maiorana pleaded. "Just give Roger a look." Clemens arrived the next day at Blinn's campus, threw for Dreyer and left a less-than-profound impression: "He was a fat boy, and who wants fat boys?" says Dreyer. "I thought he was gonna have a soft middle and no shelf life. But Charlie's a good man, so I presented Roger with a half scholarship—books, tuition and fees."

Clemens considered accepting Dreyer's offer but hoped he could do better. Maiorana placed another phone call, this one to Wayne Graham, the new head baseball coach at San Jacinto. Graham just served as the coach at Spring Branch High (a Spring Woods rival) and knew Clemens well. Like everyone else, he was uninspired. "Wayne," said Maiorana, "Roger really has his heart set on pitching for the University of Texas. Is there anyone over there you can call?"

Graham contacted Longhorns coach Cliff Gustafson, who laughed. "Kid doesn't throw hard enough," he said. "No chance."

Having been named San Jacinto's coach midway through June, Graham had missed out on nearly every high school senior with a modicum of talent. What remained were the crumbs—slow outfielders, lazy catchers, fat pitchers with so-so velocity. "I'd seen Roger pitch twice versus us at Spring Branch, and I sort of kind of liked him," Graham says. "He had good size, great mechanics and he threw strikes. I thought that maybe he could one day develop into a solid college pitcher, so I offered him a spot."

The school provided tuition, textbooks, fees and $70 per month in living expenses. "That was all we could give Roger," says Graham. "It was take it or leave it."

Roger Clemens took it.

CHAPTER

College

oward the end of the summer of 1980, Roger Clemens seemed comfortable with the idea of attending San Jacinto College. Sure, he'd be sharing a two-bedroom pad with teammates in the shoddy Woodforest Apartment Complex near the school's north campus in desolate Pasadena, Texas. And sure, junior college was a *long* way from the University of Texas, where Clemens dreamed of donning a burnt orange-and-white uniform and pitching for the Longhorns. And sure, he couldn't have told you San Jac's nickname (Gators) or the name of its stadium (trick question—it was known simply as "the North Campus field").

But Clemens had convinced himself that this was still the big time. Armed with golden stuff and unrivaled drive, he would bring some magic to the ol' diamond—*whatever its official name might be.* This was the start of something unique. Great. Spectacular.

What Clemens quickly discovered, however, was that a junior college is, at its core, a place where students lacking passion and interest shuffle about their lives. Although San Jacinto fielded teams in 16 sports, the stands were filled mostly with ants and wayward dust particles. Nothing represented the general malaise better than the college newspaper, the *North Star,* which ran front-page stories such as "San Jac Offering Underwater Welding" and "Maroon Spots Plague Woman Who Wants Some Answers" ("The people at work have gotten used to me," Sharon Flowers said with a smile. "They call me 'Spot' ").

Though San Jacinto was largely a dead zone, to Clemens it was a golden opportunity—whether he knew so or not. Had he attended Texas straight out of high school, Clemens would have been buried beneath 10 . . . 12 . . . 15 pitchers with better stuff, higher ceilings, more impressive pedigrees. The coaching staff would have given up on his fastball in a week, either transferring him to another position or encouraging him to pursue a different line of work (such as, say, intramural softball).

San Jacinto, on the other hand, was all about player development. With little in the way of a social life and a relatively light academic schedule (he took three classes his first semester), Clemens devoted his time to the singular task of becoming a Division I pitcher. "His work ethic was unlike anything I'd ever seen," says Trey South, San Jacinto's first baseman. "We all lived in the same apartment complex, and at night he'd lift weights in his room, then go out into the parking lot and run sprints. When he first got there a bunch of us nicknamed him 'Baby Huey,' because he had all this baby fat. But he changed our opinions of him awfully quickly." Before long, the fat had melted from his body, replaced by a barrel chest and tree trunks for legs.

In Wayne Graham, Clemens was blessed with the perfect coach at the perfect time. A 44-year-old Yoakum, Texas, native, Graham had spent 10 years as a minor league third baseman, jumping from town to town and class to class in what often felt like a fruitless search for baseball salvation. When he finally reached the big show, appearing in 10 games with the 1963 Philadelphia Phillies, he failed miserably, batting .182. The following year was even worse—an .091 average in 20 games with the New York Mets. He never got back to the majors.

Yet through his winding journey, Graham gained perspective. Like thousands of his baseball-playing brethren, Graham was the once-upon-a-time high school hotshot who had believed himself destined for stardom. Now, after years of coaching, he knew that talent, though important, wasn't everything. Drive, determination, steeliness—those were the virtues that could transform the average ballplayer into something special. "The mental aspect means a great deal," Graham said. "I got into Major League Baseball with the tools I had and was lucky to play as long as I did. There were some players who had the tools I had and they played longer. It's all mental. Character is something you have to develop also. It's not something you have or don't have. It has to be developed as far as baseball is concerned."

Was Clemens capable of making such a transformation? Graham wasn't sure. The Gators kicked off their fall season with a 3-2 exhibition win over Alvin Community College, and though the coaching staff was euphoric over the team's pitching, that pitching *did not* include Clemens. Through its regular September, October, November and December baseball coverage, the *North Star* referred to Clemens all of four times—and never mentioned his first name. "I still remember my assistant coach, Paul Miller, turning to me one day and asking, 'Why did you recruit this fat boy?'" says Graham. "These junior college hitters were advanced, and they battered him pretty good."

Graham, however, saw *something*. With unparalleled lower-body strength and a near-perfect delivery, Clemens should have been hitting 90, 91 mph on the radar gun. "But he didn't finish," says Graham. "He looked like he was throwing batting practice, as far as the effort. I kept saying to him, 'Roger, finish! Roger, finish! Roger, finish!'"

Clemens, who fancied himself a pitching guru, was baffled.

Throughout his life, his brother had insisted that a pitcher's body does all the work, that the arm merely needs to come along for the ride. Having worshiped Randy, Roger had never questioned the wisdom. "Roger, I know your dream is to pitch in the big leagues," Graham told him. "But if you don't start finishing hard . . . if you don't really let it rip, you have no chance. I can't promise you that your arm won't fall off of your body. But as it stands right now, you have no chance of reaching the major leagues. None whatsoever."

The words were a punch to Clemens' gut. *None whatsoever?* Over the coming days, Clemens' sole focus was on following through with his arm. He would stand in front of a mirror and tinker with his motion. *More arm. More arm. More arm.* Within two weeks of Graham's lecture, his fastball jumped from 83 mph to 88 mph. Within a month, he was hitting 90. By season's end, he was throwing 91! Ninety-two! Ninety-three! "He already had genius-level control," Graham says. "He just needed some adjustments."

The new Roger Clemens made his spring debut with a 4-2 triumph over McClennan College on March 3, then followed that up with an 11-0, one-hit triumph over San Antonio College. In his first fourteen and a third innings as a Gator, Clemens had 12 strikeouts and a 1.25 ERA. Even when he didn't pitch well, he pitched well. Against Wharton on March 18, Clemens held the Pioneers to two runs in a 4-2 triumph. He went six innings, struck out nine and earned high grades from all around—save for his coach. "He's capable of pitching better than that," Graham told the *Pasadena Citizen*. "He was erratic and in trouble all the time. He had a lot of strikeouts which makes him look a little better than he was, but he was struggling." Other Gators would have heard Graham's words and crumbled. But Clemens, having spent a lifetime enduring Randy's critiques, swallowed hard. What good was the win if it weren't earned?

On the morning of March 24, the Gators were taking their bus to nearby Beeville, Texas, for a doubleheader against Bee County College. En route, Clemens and teammates Alan Brown and Mark Massey engaged in overheated horseplay, shouting aloud, slapping each other's heads. "Just young nonsense," says Don Spivey, a San Jac pitcher. "Stupid stuff." An enraged Graham spun around and screamed, "Stop the bus! Stop the damn bus!" He pointed toward the three players. "Clemens! Brown! Massey! You're walking! Get the hell off!" There was a lengthy pause. "You think I'm kidding?" Graham said. "Get the hell off the bus!"

The three exited the vehicle and watched as it pulled away. From up ahead they spotted some lights peeking above a cluster of trees. "Well," said Clemens, "that must be the field up there. Not too bad of a walk." He was wrong. The visible lights were on a farm. Bee County's Joe Hunter Field was four miles away down hilly, winding Interstate 59. The temperature was probably 90 degrees. "When they finally showed up it was two hours later, and they were melting," says Spivey. "We were all cracking up. But Coach didn't think it was especially funny."

Determined to score a Division I scholarship, Clemens viewed each of his starts as a potential get-out-of-jail-free card. How could Texas or Baylor or Oklahoma State turn down a kid who went 12-0 . . . 13-0 . . . 14-0, even if it was at the junior college level? As Randy used to say, "Give them a reason to want you. *Make* them want you." That's what Clemens was trying to do—and walking four miles immediately before a start hardly aided his cause. Coated in sweat, he stepped onto the mound, sucked in a deep breath . . . and fired. One angry fastball after another. Ninety-two mph—click. Ninety-three mph—click. Ninety-four mph—click. Perspiration blanketed his forehead; fatigue weighed down his legs. Clemens was a battered, wiped-out ballplayer—and he was untouchable. For five and two-thirds innings, Bee County's mighty Cougars managed nary a hit. When the afternoon ended, Clemens walked off the mound with a complete-game, one-hit, 2-0 masterpiece.

The performance was everything Randy had ever demanded of his little brother. No surrender, no pain, no forgiveness. Clemens *hated* Graham for having made him walk; *hated* Brown for messing with him; *hated* Bee County's overmatched hitters for daring to swing at his pitches. By late April, Clemens was 8-0 and arguably the nation's best junior college pitcher. Teammates nicknamed him "Goose," after Richard "Goose" Gossage, the feared New York Yankees closer. "There was a switch that needed to be turned on with Roger," says Graham. "That happened in his year with us."

A team featuring a first-year head coach and 13 new players was ranked number two in the nation. Yet with the success, something in Clemens seemed to change. The quiet kid who had arrived on campus carrying his own bags was quickly morphing into a room service type of guy. "I hate to say Roger wasn't likable, but he became pretty selfish," says Tim Englund, Clemens' co–number one starter on the Gators. "Quite honestly, Roger was more concerned with his own performance and how he did and how he prepared than he was with the overall success of the team. If he had a rough outing, you wouldn't find him in the dugout during the second game cheering the team on. He'd be alone somewhere, trying to figure out what he didn't do right." One afternoon, Clemens pitched poorly in the first game of a doubleheader at Wharton College, allowing six runs in five innings in a 6-5 defeat. When the game ended, he retreated to the team's van, remaining there the entire second game. "We were 18-, 19-year-old kids, and we were supposed to be a team," says Englund. "Believe me, the behavior was noticed."

"I considered most of the guys on the team to be good friends," says John Bermea, a catcher. "But Roger was his own man. He didn't have much to do with us."

Although he spent most of his free time either preparing for that next start or hanging with his girlfriend, a San Jacinto freshman named Christine McPherson, Clemens occasionally flashed a mischievous sense of humor. On one road trip to a junior college baseball tournament in Lufkin, Texas, Clemens and his teammates stayed the night at the Holiday Inn. As they pulled up to the hotel, the Gators were greeted by a marquee—approximately eight feet off the ground—that read WELCOME ALL JUNIOR COLLEGE BASEBALL PLAYERS.

"You know what we should do?" said Spivey, turning toward Clemens.

The pitcher nodded devilishly.

Later that night, while their teammates slept, Clemens and Spivey found a ladder in the hotel's maintenance closet and carried it toward the sign. With Roger holding the base, Spivey climbed to the top and began rearranging the letters to read SAN JAC RULES.

"Hey! Hey!" someone yelled. "What are you kids doing!"

It was the hotel manager.

"Fuck!" screamed Clemens. "Fuck!" With that, the San Jacinto ace took off, forgetting that the ladder he was holding needed his support to remain upright.

"Man, I fell off that ladder *hard*," says Spivey. "But Roger got the worst of it." As he ran away, Clemens stepped into a hole and—*pop!*—twisted his right ankle. He spent much of the night with his foot submerged in a bucket of freezing-cold water, then wrapped the ankle and tried to pretend nothing had happened.

Miller, the San Jacinto assistant, spotted Spivey and Clemens in the lobby the following morning. "Don," Miller said, "why the hell is Roger limping?"

"Uh . . . what?" Spivey replied.

Later that day, with his grapefruit-sized ankle cocooned in athletic tape, Clemens went five innings, allowing one run in a romp of Blinn College.

"It was," says Spivey, "an absolutely amazing performance."

Thanks to the emergence of Clemens and a roster with more than a dozen players who would earn Division I scholarships, the Gators posted the best season in school history, winning the Texas Junior

College Athletic Association championship while compiling a 43-7 record. Once overlooked, Clemens could now point to a statistical line that read: 9-2. 82 strikeouts. 38 walks. 85⅔ innings pitched.

"Roger began the year as one of the guys," says Graham, "and he ended it as an ace."

IN THE MAY 30, 1981, edition of the *Pasadena Citizen,* Wayne Graham spoke optimistically of the upcoming seasson. Somewhat naive to the transient ways of junior college baseball, the coach was counting on the return of nearly all of his 13 freshmen and fielding a team that would surely compete for a national title. "On the junior college level," he said, "you have to make sure all your guys are signed and then keep them eligible."

Clemens, he believed, wasn't going anywhere.

This was reinforced in the following weeks, after the New York Mets used their 12th-round pick in baseball's amateur draft to select Graham's prized pupil. It was no secret within San Jacinto's athletic department that *somebody* would likely take a shot on Clemens. Yet as the rounds passed, the odds of Clemens' return increased dramatically. The Mets selected Clemens only after Jim Terrell, a newly hired scout with an iffy track record, all but begged the franchise to do so. "Jim was a guy who had retired from working for the power and light company in Detroit, and he loved scouting," recalls Lou Gorman, the Mets assistant general manager. "We needed someone in Texas, so we rented him an apartment, gave him a two-year contract and hoped for the best."

The Mets begrudgingly agreed to select Clemens, but only after the team had drafted five other pitchers—Dave Cochrane, Jeff Keeler, Rich Webster, Albert Candelaria and Steve Walker. New York initially offered Clemens $7,500, then increased it to just $15,000. When the Mets traveled to Houston to face the Astros shortly after the draft, they asked Clemens to drive to the Astrodome and throw for manager Joe Torre and his pitching coach Bob Gibson.

Having attended numerous Astros games as a high-schooler, Clemens was thrilled. He had fond memories of watching Nolan Ryan warm up in the bullpen before his starts, drilling one blazing fastball after another into the catcher's mitt. Now it was his turn.

Upon arriving at the stadium, Clemens was presented with a blue Mets road jersey. He trotted out to the visitors' bullpen and stood alongside Tim Leary, New York's latest young pitching phenom. With Torre and Gibson lingering to the side, Clemens asked the bullpen catcher to make his balls sound harder by catching them in the pocket of his glove, then proceeded to throw 30 pitches.

A legendary pitcher, Gibson had recently been voted into the Hall of Fame on the strength of 251 career victories and two Cy Young trophies. Yet he was a horrific judge of talent. Gibson observed Clemens, shrugged, walked away without saying a word and later urged the Mets to save their money. "Nothing special" was his brief scouting report. "OK stuff."

Although the Mets increased their offer to $20,000, Clemens refused to budge unless the team also agreed to pay for the completion of his education. It was a no-go. "I've often thought about that," says Gorman. "Not one of the finest moments in Mets history. But to be honest, we always sort of felt Roger had his heart set on pitching Division I college ball."

Indeed, in the days leading up to the draft, Clemens had been contacted by Cliff Gustafson, the University of Texas' 14th-year baseball coach. In a preseason exhibition game between the Gators and Longhorns, Clemens had made Gustafson's hitters look foolish, holding them to two hits and no runs over four and two-thirds innings. Now, ignoring every protocol in collegiate baseball, Gustafson went behind Graham's back and called Clemens to gauge his interest in becoming a Longhorn. It wasn't an especially hard sell.

Clemens loved everything about Texas baseball: the tradition, the atmosphere, the dozens of players who wound up in the major leagues. From Burt Hooton and Pinky Higgins to Keith Moreland and Grady Hatton, UT had established itself as a baseball factory. As Clemens toured the magnificent facilities—the Grand Canyon–sized weight room and the spotless carpeted clubhouse—he was mesmerized.

Toward the end of the day, Gustafson sat Clemens down in his office and presented a typed-up scholarship offer. Clemens said he'd have to consult with his family first.

"OK," said Gustafson. "If you're leaving at 6 P.M., you'll be home in Houston by 8:30. I'll expect a call at 8:40 with a decision."

Later that night, Bess Clemens' phone rang. It was Gustafson, demanding an answer.

"Well, Coach," Clemens told him, "everybody wants to be a Longhorn."

Gustafson laughed. It was a glorious moment. A wonderful moment. A triumphant moment.

A *sleazy* moment.

At the same time Clemens was canoodling with Gustafson, Wayne Graham, the man who had taken a doughy 84-mph nobody and turned him into a rock-solid, highly coveted flamethrower, was spending the summer managing the Medicine Hat Blue Jays of the Pioneer League. Graham had last spoken with Clemens shortly after the Mets workout and was convinced his ace would either return to San Jacinto or turn pro. "I certainly didn't think he'd leave for Texas," says Graham. "I didn't see that coming."

"Leave," adds Roy Waldrep, San Jacinto's sports information director, "is being kind. Roger didn't leave—he snuck off when nobody was looking."

Clemens never called or wrote Graham to inform him of the decision. "I felt he owed me more than that," Graham says. "He didn't owe it to me to stay. But he at least owed it to me to tell me what he was doing, man to man. That caused a wedge between us that lasted for several years. It stung."

Graham could not have known that someone else was pulling the strings controlling Roger Clemens' thoughts and actions. Long before Gustafson came calling, long before the Mets used a draft pick, Randy Clemens had all but mapped out his brother's future: Roger would go to Texas. He would dominate. He would make the majors.

He would stomp anyone who dared stand in his way.

CHAPTER 5

A Legendary Longhorn

For the first time in their lives, Randy and Roger Clemens were simultaneously living their dreams.

As Roger was heading off to Austin to become a University of Texas Longhorn, Randy, along with his wife, Kathy, was returning to Ohio to begin what, he believed, was a path toward his rightful destiny.

Thanks to a good word from Ray Zawadzki, his coach back at Vandalia-Butler High, Randy had been offered the boys' basketball head coaching job at Troy High School in nearby Troy, Ohio. Ever since he'd left Butler Township for Bethel College, Randy had dreamed of prowling the sidelines of a high school or college gymnasium, a tie dangling from his neck, a rolled-up program in his right hand. Randy craved the smell of a gym, the sound of a whistle reverberating against the high ceiling and rubberized walls. He would longingly speak with Larry South, his childhood friend, of one day becoming the next John Wooden. "I understand this game as well as anyone," he would say. "I know I can do this."

When it came to *X*'s and *O*'s, few could match Randy, who was as quick with a chalkboard as he had once been with a crossover dribble. But within weeks of his arrival at the 1,500-student school, members of the Troy faculty began to express concern over their new hire. Whereas most educators believed in reaching students through compassion, Randy was a pit bull on speed. His practices were fast-paced and harsh, with curses flying like bullets from a machine gun. Randy never hesitated to berate players, forgetting that the 16-year-old boy he was calling a "no-good piece of shit" had pimples covering his face and an upcoming algebra exam. To Randy, basketball was a business, and if you didn't agree with his philosophy, well, go screw yourself. "He wasn't tactful, and he didn't stop and think about his actions often enough," says South, who would later join Randy as an assistant coach. "He just charged ahead, unsympathetic to others. But you have to remember, there were other factors involved."

By "other factors," South is referring to the chemical dependency problems that had plagued Randy since his early college days. Though it remains unclear whether Randy was coaching under the influence of drugs or merely struggling to stay clean, he was a far different person from the All-American boy who had graduated from high school 11 years earlier. "The change from the 17-, 18-year-old kid to the 28-, 29-year-old man was drastic," says Zawadzki. "I was still coaching at Vandalia-Butler, and we'd play Troy. I'd have officials come up to me and say, very bluntly, 'Ray, you need to talk to your boy and calm him down.' I'd say, 'I'm sorry, but my boy is my son, and he's in eighth grade.'"

Those well versed in Dayton-area prep hoops still recall the afternoon Troy visited Vandalia-Butler High for the first time with Randy at the helm. "You would think the fans here would have cheered for Randy, him being a local hero," says Bob Costello, Vandalia-Butler's former JV basketball coach. "But the people were really hard on him, booing him nonstop." Troy won on a last-second overtime shot, and afterward Zawadzki reached out to shake Randy's hand. "But Randy acted like a complete jerk," says Mike Lawson, a former classmate. "Instead of being gracious, he stuck his tongue out at our coach and started wiggling it at him. It was classless. You had to ask yourself what was wrong with this guy."

Although Troy finished 1-20 in Randy's first season, he quickly turned a long-dormant program around, going 15-13 in his second season and 21-3 the third. Yet something was clearly amiss. Friends and family members became increasingly concerned for Kathy, who seemed to shudder at the mere mention of her husband. They watched Randy's erratic behavior—giddy one moment, furious the next; detached from reality; bombastic; biting—and wondered where he was going; what he was becoming; who, exactly, he was.

"I won't speak for Roger," says one family friend, "but I've always believed he was very lucky Randy was in Ohio while he was at Texas. The last thing he needed was to deal with that train wreck."

By the time Roger arrived in Austin for his first day as a sophomore at the University of Texas, he was a confident, cocksure 18-year-old. Yet for all the projected bravado (before signing with Gustafson, Clemens made the coach promise he would start the Longhorns' home *and* road openers), Clemens questioned whether he was cut out for the big time. He was intimidated by his new environs and awed by the large sign hanging in the clubhouse at Disch-Faulk Field—the one that read THE UNIVERSITY OF TEXAS TRADITION WILL NOT BE ENTRUSTED TO THE TIMID OR THE WEAK. *Was he timid? Was he weak?* "It was so intimidating, so overwhelming," he later said. "I felt I could get lost in there." For his first two months of college, Clemens, a business and finance major, made the 185-mile drive back home to Houston every weekend in his battered olive green AMC Gremlin.

The primary cause of Clemens' early insecurities was his new coach, Cliff Gustafson. A narrow-faced man with a heavily creased forehead, light brown eyes and a smile that—on the rare occasion it bloomed—projected more scorn than joy, Gustafson had been raised on a farm in the rural outpost of Kenedy, Texas. His father had died when he was just five, so Cliff and his older brother, Marvin, were left to pick the family's entire cotton crop. "Money was always a problem," Gustafson said. "When I think about my dad's death, the thing that always comes to mind is the fact that he had been able to borrow enough money from the bank to buy a tractor just before he died. Life could have been so much easier for him if he had lived to use that tractor instead of plowing with that team of no-good mules."

By the time he was an early teen, Gustafson's mother, Wendla, moved with her boys to San Antonio, where Cliff was introduced to an odd new sport played with a wood stick and a ball ("Hardball," he called it). On October 1, 1941, he listened to his first baseball broadcast—the World Series clash between the New York Yankees and the Brooklyn Dodgers. Cliff Gustafson was in love.

Through the years, as he played baseball first at Harlandale High School, then at the University of Texas and later with the Plainview Ponies of the long-defunct West Texas–New Mexico League, Gustafson could never shed the pain of losing his father. Relying on equal helpings of stoicism and detachment, he became a highly successful high school coach, guiding South San Antonio High's varsity team to a 344-85 record and 7 state titles over 13 seasons. To his players, the taciturn Gustafson was as intimidating as a European dictator. He rarely yelled, instead relying on an expression of grave disappointment—eyes cast downward, lip slightly quivering—that could make an 18-year-old kid sob.

Before the 1967–68 academic year, Darrell Royal, the University of Texas athletic director, asked him to take over the Longhorns. "I was not presumptuous enough to believe they would offer that job to a high school coach," he said. "I never even daydreamed that I'd coach at Texas."

By the time Roger Clemens arrived in Austin, Gustafson had transformed the Longhorns into a powerhouse. Over 14 years, he had a 669-141-1 record, 12 Southwest Conference titles and 1 national championship. Sixty of his players had been drafted, and entering the 1982 major league season, 32 were active. Wrote Roger Campbell of the *Daily Texan,* the university's student newspaper: "If football has the Bear and basketball has the Wizard of Westwood, then—right in your own backyard—baseball has Gus."

Yet for all the accomplishments, Gustafson was hardly beloved. Players tiptoed around their coach, hoping to avoid his ire. Gustafson saw little value in anything short of victory. The team's official slogan for the upcoming season was vintage Gus: "Winners will find a way to win, losers will find a way to lose."

Clemens had never played for a man like Gustafson. For more than 20 years, the coach had eaten the same lunch *every . . . single . . . day:* peanut butter and honey, a bag of chips and iced tea with lemon. His obsessive nature was similar to Randy's, except that Gustafson provided stability. "In a way, Texas was a very negative atmosphere," says David Denny, a Longhorns outfielder–third baseman. "There was no pleasing Gus. We could win 10-0, and all we'd hear after the game is everything we did wrong. Because of that, I'd say we didn't play hard for him. We played hard for each other."

Roger settled into his new life as a college sophomore, spending his fall taking classes, hanging out in his dorm room, working out with the baseball team and blowing what seemed to be a bottomless supply of quarters at the local video arcade, where Pac-Man and Gallaga became temporary obsessions. He would call Randy to complain or brag or pick his brain, but he relied equally on the reassurances of his new teammates.

The Longhorns began mandatory conditioning training for the upcoming season on January 21, 1982, only two days after receiving the news that John Machin, the team's top returning left-hander, had signed a contract with the Philadelphia Phillies. His departure left a gaping hole in a pitching staff that had already lost its five best arms from a 1981 squad that had gone 62-11. "We're still going to go to work and try to act as if nothing happened," Gustafson said. "We've got people who I still think we can win with."

Listed as the number two starter behind sophomore Calvin Schiraldi, Clemens quickly established himself as an elite Division I talent. One year removed from beginning the season 8-0 for San Jacinto, Clemens won his first seven decisions as a Longhorn. In sharp contrast to Schiraldi, a quirky, laid-back kid out of Westlake, Texas, Clemens was a bundle of electricity. In the immediate aftermath of a five-hit, 10-strikeout wipeout of Wichita State on March 1 (a 12-0 Longhorn romp), Clemens bragged to the *Daily Texan,* "They call me 'Goose,' and I sure like to see goose eggs up there on the board. I went straight at 'em with hard stuff. It was 85 percent fastballs. I ripped off a couple of good curves for strikeouts."

In truth, Clemens called himself "Goose" and desperately wanted his teammates to follow suit. Through his first eight starts, Clemens led the Longhorns with fifty-five and a third innings pitched, fifty-four strikeouts and seven wins. "Roger would just rear back and throw it at a hitter, and his ball exploded," says Johnny Sutton, a Longhorns outfielder. "We had some great, great pitchers on that team, and Roger was as good as it got."

ACCORDING TO HIS LIFE story, which he now tells by rote, Roger Clemens walked a straight-and-narrow path at Texas that had him either playing baseball, playing video games or hanging out with his girlfriend, Cindy Figg, a pretty UT golfer who would later compete on the LPGA tour. He was the type who would greet strangers with a firm handshake and a kind word and always look people in the eye. "A bunch of us ran wild, and it hurt our games," says Denny. "But not

Roger. It's almost as if he knew his destiny and he didn't want to ruin it by getting in trouble."

Yet, like all undergrads, Clemens had his moments.

On a warm Austin night midway through the 1982 season, Clemens and a couple of teammates headed to an Austin watering hole called "The Keg." While they were hanging out, talking to some coeds, and mingling with their peers, outfielder Rich Thompson, a subpar baseball player who excelled on the Texas football team, was accidentally bumped by a short, stocky kid wearing a fraternity T-shirt. Some beer spilled onto Thompson's ostrich boots. "Oh, I'm really sorry," the culprit said. "I didn't mean for that to happen."

"Don't sweat it," said Thompson. "No big deal."

As Thompson casually walked away, he heard Clemens barking from behind.

"Hey, motherfucker! Hey, motherfucker! What the fuck are you doing?"

"It was an accident," the fraternity member said. "Sorry, man."

"Fuck you!" Clemens screamed. "Do you wanna make a go of it?"

The frat boy and three of his brothers huddled in the middle of the bar. They didn't know who Roger Clemens was. They didn't care who Roger Clemens was. "Yeah," he said. "I'll make a go of it, you son of a bitch." With that, Clemens tapped an incredulous Thompson on the shoulder and said, "Let's go get 'em."

"Truthfully," says Thompson, "I thought Roger was being pretty stupid. It was some spilled beer. Who cares? But I had to stand up alongside a teammate."

Upon exiting the bar, Clemens and his opponent entered a ring of onlookers and began to wrestle. "The next thing I know, the fight is coming my way, and the whole thing turns into a melee," says Thompson. "I get pushed to the ground, I beat the shit out of a frat guy, Roger gets in some punches and takes some punches. But Roger hit one guy in the head, and afterward his pinkie really started to swell."

The following day, Thompson was called into Gustafson's office. "Rich," said Gustafson, "what the hell were you thinking? You were there with Roger. You were standing right next to him. So why the hell didn't you protect him or get him out of there? You're a big guy. What in the world were you thinking?"

By the time he slunk away, the six-foot-one Thompson felt two inches tall. Clemens' hand would recover, but Thompson never forgot the sting of Gustafson's words. "I meant nothing to him," he says. "And Roger was everything."

ALTHOUGH THEY ENTERED 1982 with multiple question marks, the Longhorns emerged as the class of collegiate baseball. With a pitching staff anchored by Clemens and Schiraldi, and the steely leadership of junior shortstop Spike Owen, Texas began the season by winning its first 33 games—one short of the NCAA record set by the '77 Longhorns.

On March 26, 1982, the Longhorns traveled to the University of Houston to face the Cougars. With the record within their grasp, it was a game Texas players *desperately* craved. So, for that matter, did Gustafson, who possessed a profound appreciation of NCAA history. "Coach did something that week that I never understood," says Mike Konderla, a standout relief pitcher. "That I'll never understand." In the days leading up to the game, Clemens had been experiencing discomfort in his right shoulder. He was diagnosed with bursitis and advised to rest for a week or two. Yet with his sights set on the record, Gustafson started Clemens against the Cougars. "He wasn't throwing above 82 mph," Konderla says. "There was no way Roger should have been out there." To no one's surprise, Clemens was pounded for four runs in two-thirds of an inning. The Cougars won, 4-3.

"Coach probably thought Roger at 82 mph was better than most people at 92 mph," says another Longhorn. "But it wasn't right. Roger wasn't one to take it easy or to ask out of a situation. He tried his best, but he really could have done damage to himself. It was bullshit." Teammates never forgot Clemens' effort that day. It was, in many ways, the personification of Randy's lifelong lessons: *Never give in; go harder and harder and harder; to hell with pain.*

The remainder of the season was frustrating for Clemens. He sat out for two weeks after the Houston start, skipping a road trip to Texas Christian University and spending much of his time with the Longhorn trainers. "Roger was the hardest worker we had," says John Turman, the team's student manager. "Coach had this workout plan for the pitchers on the day after their starts, and Roger was the only one who followed it. His reason for living was to kick ass in baseball. When that was taken away, he became very depressed." Clemens returned to pitch against Rice University on April 25, allowing three runs in three and a third innings before being pulled by an agitated Gustafson. Texas won its 13th Southwest Conference title in 15 seasons, but Clemens limped down the stretch. Wrote Steve Campbell in the *Daily Texan:* "Clemens, owner of a 93 mph fastball, got off to a 193 mph start. He won his first seven games, had a 2.08 ERA and looked like Tony Arnold's heir to the All-American throne. When bursitis suddenly brought Clemens' fastball closer to the speed limit, he became of little use."

Clemens rebounded to pitch well in Omaha at the College World Series, dominating Oklahoma State in a 9-1 opening-round rout, then falling 2-1 to Miami. That the Longhorns were eliminated by Wichita State should not have dampened what was an otherwise brilliant season. But, Gustafson being Gustafson, optimism was not allowed. Clemens' 12-2 record? The Longhorns' 59-6 record? A 33-game winning streak? *So what? We lost our final game.*

"We deserved to be proud," says Schiraldi. "But we weren't. We were deflated and hurt. But we were also determined. This wouldn't happen again."

• • •

FOLLOWING HIS SUMMER OFF, Roger Clemens returned to Austin secure in the knowledge that this would be his final year of college. When asked, he would utter the standard lines about valuing an education and possibly completing a degree. But Clemens wasn't seeking a future in business or finance. He was a ballplayer—one who increasingly came to be viewed as a high pick in the June 1983 amateur draft.

Like their star pitcher, great things were expected of the Longhorns in 1983. Though now without Owen, the swift shortstop who had been drafted in the first round by the Seattle Mariners, Texas returned what many still consider to be the greatest pitching staff in the history of college baseball. Along with Clemens, Gustafson boasted a rotation of Schiraldi (13-3, 3.68 ERA in 1982) and Mike Capel (9-0, 3.68 ERA), as well as the game's most ferocious closer, the hard-throwing Kirk Killingsworth (9-0, 0.80 ERA). "Those guys were tough and mean," says Doug Hodo, the Longhorns' designated hitter. "And they fed off each other." All four pitchers were highly skilled and extremely close-knit. "Roger and I had a conversation in our hotel room one night," recalls Killingsworth, who went by the nickname "Killer." "We decided that, for 1983, we would establish the Don Drysdale theory of pitching. Which was 'If you hit one of my hitters, I'll hit two of yours.' We had four guys who could throw 92, 93 mph and command the plate, and we needed to intimidate our opponents."

Did it work? Killingsworth still recalls visiting teams arriving at Disch-Faulk Field and snapping photographs of the Longhorn pitchers as they loosened up during batting practice. "Hell, at that point we knew we'd won," he says. "We were inside their heads."

For the Longhorns, the goal was a College World Series title—period. On the first day of practice, Clemens arrived wearing a white cutoff T-shirt that read THINK OMAHA. He proceeded to unleash a

series of batting practice fastballs—harder and harder and harder—
that set the tone for the season. "The first time up against Roger
that initial day, I hit a line drive off of him that knocked him off the
mound," says Robert Gauntt, a freshman first baseman. "Well, he proceeded to strike me out seven times in a row with sliders. I didn't even
know what a slider was."

Texas, the nation's top-ranked team, opened with an unconvincing
doubleheader sweep of Division II Midwestern State, then split four
games with the University of Texas–Arlington. Against Clemens, the
Mavericks rolled to a 10-6 landslide, turning three singles, four dou-
bles and a UT error into seven runs. "Some of our more experienced
pitchers—Clemens, Schiraldi and Capel—have been way below par,"
Gustafson said afterward. "But I'm not going to get panicky yet."

Gustafson's words were spoken on a Tuesday. The following afternoon, Clemens lost his second straight start, this one a 3-2 heartbreaker
to Texas Lutheran, a school that—like Midwestern State—had never
before defeated the Longhorns. Clemens held the Bulldogs scoreless
for eight innings before allowing a game-winning homer to someone named David Dahse. Afterward, Clemens blew off the assembled
media (well, Ed Combs of the *Daily Texan*), dismissively explaining
away the defeat with "It's just one of those things" as he walked out
the door.

Clemens was at a loss, but, in hindsight, it's easy to understand his
struggles. Here was a young man, not yet 21 years old, pitching for
his life. When he was a sophomore, the major league scouts came to
UT games, but Clemens rightly assumed they were primarily gaug-
ing the juniors. Now, however, the scouts were here to see him. The
frumpy men with the notepads and radar guns symbolized a ticket
to a better life; a chance to assist his mother, Bess; to help Randy and
Kathy settle down and start a family. Clemens wanted to win for the
Longhorns. But mostly, he needed to win for himself. The pressure
was immense.

A couple of days after the Texas Lutheran embarrassment, the Longhorns held a closed-door meeting that turned ugly. The returnees blamed the team's six junior college transfers for not playing well. The junior college transfers blamed the returnees for not making them feel welcome. (Nobody blamed Clemens, and how could they? He had spent the hour leading up to the meeting running pole to pole in the outfield, a lead vest weighing down his body.) "The meeting was uncomfortable," says Turman. "But when it was over, everyone walked out of the room on the same page. We were a team again."

Over the following two months, Clemens improved. On May 1, his record stood at 9-2 with a 2.31 ERA, and the Longhorns were en route to securing yet another Southwest Conference title. A popular debate among college baseball diehards concerned Clemens and Schiraldi, and, specifically, which junior would be more coveted come draft time. While Clemens' stock had dropped from the previous season, Schiraldi was emerging as the nation's transcendent pitcher. He entered May with a sterling 9-1 record and 1.43 ERA and, says Killingsworth, "was even better than the numbers."

Unlike Clemens, who seemed to release every kilowatt of energy into each pitch, Schiraldi looked downright loosey-goosey. He was nicknamed "Nibbler" for his tendency to pick, pick, pick at the plate with a wicked slider, and his Fidrychian mannerisms elicited laughter from the bench. Clemens worked out with a Mr. Universe's intensity, while Schiraldi ate pizza and burgers, drank beer and slept late. "I never put as much into it as Roger did," Schiraldi says. "Not even close." On the other hand, Clemens lacked the perspective to deal with setbacks. Every loss, every bad pitch, was like a deep wound. Schiraldi, meanwhile, shrugged and moved on. "If you'd asked me who would become the bigger star, I would have picked Calvin," says Bryan Burrows, the Texas infielder. "Both were gifted, but Calvin could stomach the ups and downs."

Schiraldi certainly never suffered an emotional meltdown like the one that overwhelmed Clemens on May 3, 1983, when the Longhorns traveled to Tulsa to face Oral Roberts University. In one of his worst outings, Clemens gave up a run in the first, two more in the second and a two-run homer in the sixth in a 6-1 loss to the far-inferior Titans. Though he had experienced his share of ups and downs, this was a new low for Clemens, whose right shoulder continued to hurt. He could grudgingly accept a beating at the hands of, say, Cal State Fullerton or Oklahoma State. But Oral Roberts?

For the first time in his life, baseball was supplying little joy. The 15 to 20 scouts attending each game, their radar guns pointed to the mound like some sort of firing squad, helped turn a confident pitcher into a second-guessing bundle of nerves. Clemens heard the gossip from the scouts—his fastball flattened out as the game went on; his velocity came and went; he was soft. "Never mind that I was pitching nine innings on Friday nights, then coming back and pitching in relief the next day," Clemens wrote in his autobiography. "I got frustrated by it all."

As soon as he was pulled against Oral Roberts, Clemens retreated to the dugout, wrapped a towel over his head and bawled. "I'll always remember that," says David Seitz, a Texas pitcher. "Roger was just devastated." While the game continued, Clemens headed for the Longhorns' clubhouse and began to change into his street clothes—a serious no-no under Gustafson's rules. "Roger, what are you doing?" asked Turman. "What's goi—"

"I'm done!" Clemens screamed. "Done! I'm going back to Austin. I don't wanna play baseball anymore!"

Turman ran into the dugout and fetched Gustafson. The coach rushed back to the clubhouse and sat down beside Clemens. "You don't want to do this," Gustafson said. "You have too much going for you to quit right now. Don't let one bad start put to waste a lifetime of hard work. Don't do this."

Moved by his coach's uncharacteristic empathy, Clemens collected himself and returned to the dugout. "I'm not sure if people realize how close Roger Clemens came to never being Roger Clemens," says Killingsworth. "He was serious about leaving. It wasn't just a passing thought. Roger may well have been done."

TO NOBODY'S GREAT SURPRISE, Roger wasn't done. If anything, the meltdown proved therapeutic. For one and a half years, Clemens had been living his lifelong dream of pitching for the University of Texas—but was he even enjoying the experience? With Randy's grim pursuit of winning and Gustafson's strictness, Clemens had forgotten to embrace the moments. The sunny days. The green grass. A clean baseball. The pop of a ball into the catcher's mitt. The boyish giddiness. The camaraderie. That's why he had first fallen for the game back in Butler Township—and why he was about to fall for it once again.

Although Texas struggled for much of the season, it survived the NCAA Central Regional play-offs (twice beating a Mississippi State squad that featured three future major league All-Stars—Will Clark, Rafael Palmeiro and Bobby Thigpen) to reach the school's 22nd College World Series. With a 61-14 record, the Longhorns were considered the class of the eight-team field. They opened with a 12-0 clubbing of James Madison and on the night of June 6 were due to meet a hated rival, Oklahoma State. Clemens was scheduled to start.

As if the clash with the Cowboys were not a big enough worry for the righty, June 6 was also the day of Major League Baseball's annual draft. The day of reckoning.

Picking first, the Minnesota Twins took pitcher Tim Belcher of Mount Vernon Nazarene College. No surprise there. The Reds, going second, went for shortstop Kurt Stillwell from Thousand Oaks High School, and as the Rangers prepared to pick third, Clemens believed his time had come. Texas, after all, was close to home, and the team had sent multiple scouts to watch him pitch. "Man, I would love to be a Ranger," Clemens told Schiraldi. "That'd be great."

To his chagrin, the Rangers grabbed shortstop Jeff Kunkel of Rider College. The ensuing two hours hit Clemens with one disappointment after another. Some scouts had told him he would be a top 10 pick, but as names such as Stan Hilton (A's) and Robbie Wine (Astros) and Ray Hayward (Padres) came and went, Clemens stewed. "The word was that he lacked the heart to finish games," said one scouting director. "What scouts forgot was that he was starting games on Friday nights and relieving on Saturday afternoons. That's too many innings."

Finally, with the 19th selection, Clemens, who often sported a New York Yankees cap around campus—was drafted by the Boston Red Sox.

The Boston Red Sox?

"As far as I was concerned," Clemens wrote in his autobiography, "Boston was a foreign country."

Eight slots later, the New York Mets grabbed Schiraldi, and teammates Mike Brumley (Red Sox), Killingsworth (Rangers) and Capel (Cubs) were selected as well. "I would have picked Roger ahead of myself, too," says Schiraldi. "He was just a harder worker."

With a weight off his shoulders, Clemens took the mound and pitched well against an Oklahoma State lineup built around Pete Incaviglia, the NCAA's leading home-run hitter. At the conclusion of the first inning, Clemens was walking toward the Texas dugout when he crossed paths with the enormous Incaviglia. "Fuck you guys!" he snarled, sticking a finger in Incaviglia's chest. "You guys aren't worth shit!"

"Roger, what in the world are you doing?" Turman said in the dugout. "That guy will kill you."

"Ah, fuck him," Clemens replied. "I'm just pumped up."

Clemens went eight and a third innings, allowing four runs while striking out 12. With the Oral Roberts disaster behind him, Clemens left the game with his head high, sat down on the bench and cheered his teammates. When the Longhorns won on a Jamie Doughty RBI in the 11th, Clemens engulfed the hero with a fierce bear hug. "That kind of win is Texas baseball," Clemens said afterward. "We didn't play up to par, but we kept plugging. We came back."

Five days later, on a warm summer afternoon in the beef capital of the world, Roger Clemens capped off the dream in the championship game against Alabama. With his mother and siblings in attendance, Clemens pitched a complete-game seven-hitter, winning 4-3. Leading by two runs in the bottom of the ninth, Clemens allowed a double to Dave Magadan, the Crimson Tide star, then an RBI single to Allan Stallings. "Roger was furious," says Burrows. "And when he'd get angry, he'd become unhittable."

Having seen enough, Gustafson approached the mound, content to let his ace watch the remainder of the game. "I'm not leaving," Clemens told his coach. "Not now. No way in hell."

The headmaster of baseball's elite program retreated back to his seat alongside the water cooler. Catcher Jeff Hearron, the team's resident cutup, looked at the snarling, foaming Clemens, waited until Gustafson was out of earshot and cracked, "Man, you look like Secretariat with all that drool. Calm the fuck down." Clemens easily retired the next two hitters, shouting "Oh yeah!" as the final out—an infield pop-up—landed gently in Brumley's glove at shortstop.

He was mobbed by teammates, who tackled him to the ground. As Clemens emerged from the pileup, he raised his arms and screamed toward the heavens, "You tested me, you motherfucker! Don't test me!" Life had often been hard for the pitcher who lost two fathers and was raised in relative poverty, who watched his mother work three jobs and who dreamed of an escape. But now, with the pressure off and the future limitless, the prevailing emotion was relief.

That evening, Texas' conquering heroes returned to the Omaha Holiday Inn and—still wearing their dirt-covered uniforms—tossed one another into the outdoor swimming pool. There were stories to be told and beers to be chugged and glorious achievements to be cherished for one final collegiate moment.

Going Pro

In the summer of 1983, there could be no greater baseball opposites than Roger Clemens and Ronald Davis.

Having signed for $121,000 with Boston shortly after the College World Series, Clemens was a Red Sox bonus baby, the highly touted prospect who—with a mid-90s fastball and Bob Gibson's snarl—was all but guaranteed a major league future.

Having signed for $4,000 with Detroit after going undrafted out of tiny Delta State (location: Cleveland, Mississippi), Davis was a Tigers nobody, a moderately competent first baseman who—boasting a Swiss cheese bat and Steve Balboni's swiftness—would be lucky to attend a major league spring training in his lifetime.

The only thing the two men seemed to share was geography: On a July night in 1983, both ballplayers were standing inside Chain O' Lakes Park in Winter Haven, Florida, for a Florida State League game between the Class A Lakeland Tigers and the Winter Haven Red Sox.

Up until that evening, Roger Clemens was everything the Boston franchise had dreamed of. He had joined Winter Haven in late June while the team was on a road trip to Fort Lauderdale. After spending his first day becoming acquainted with his teammates, he threw a brief bullpen session. The performance was one most of Winter Haven's players still remember.

Cliché be damned, the ball seemed to explode from Clemens' right hand like some sort of nuclear weapon. With each grunt and release, Clemens unleashed a bullet that slammed into catcher Billy Joe Richardson's glove. *Ooof*-pop! *Ooof*-pop! *Ooof*-pop! Standing nearby were a handful of his new Winter Haven teammates, mostly low-grade talents with thin résumés and futures selling medical supplies and teaching third grade. They were there to see the hyped new kid, to hope, in a common jealousy that runs through minor league sports, that he wasn't as good as advertised.

Damn. He was even better.

Fastballs that hit 96 mph on the radar. Pinpoint control. A sadistic slider. "It was beyond belief," says Pete Cappadona, a Winter Haven pitcher. "I remember talking to Tom [manager Tom Kotchman], and we just looked at each other and I said, 'He ain't gonna be here for very long.'"

Clemens pitched just four games and 29 innings for the Class A Sox, compiling a 3-1 record with a 1.24 ERA and—most amazing— 36 strikeouts and *zero* walks. "Class A pitchers walk loads of people," says Daniel Weppner, a Winter Haven reliever for a team that finished 49-84 and in last place in the Northern Division. "It's what they're supposed to do." Following his debut start, a five-inning, nine-strikeout 3-0 cakewalk over St. Petersburg during which he fanned the first five hitters ("Besides having my first child," says Richardson, "my greatest thrill is having caught Roger's first pro start"), teammates began chalking a *K* on the dugout wall every time Clemens set someone down on strikes. "That's something fans do, not players," says Mark Meleski, a Winter Haven infielder. "But he made fans out of us all."

Clemens stayed in a room with a kitchenette at the rickety Winter Haven Holiday Inn and was perpetually accompanied by a brown briefcase that contained scouting reports of opposing teams' hitters. He would eat a couple of meals with teammates at Sally's Shrimp Boat, where alligators would swim to the deck in search of food, and have an ice cream or two at Andy's Igloo. Otherwise—*yawn*. "He kept to himself and was always respectful," says John Michael Roth, a Winter Haven outfielder. "You could tell he was focused on one thing, and that was moving up the ladder as quickly as possible."

Yet here Clemens now stood, in the center of Chain O' Lakes Park, making his fourth start and focused on something beyond personal glory. Two days earlier, in a game against the Tigers on the road, Mike Brumley, Clemens' friend and former Texas teammate, was playing shortstop for the Sox when Lakeland rallied. With Davis on first and one out, a Tiger named Reggie Thomas hit a hard shot to Winter Haven second baseman Chris Cannizzaro, who fielded the ball cleanly and threw to Brumley. Initially thinking the ball had reached the outfield, Davis found himself hung up between sliding and not sliding. "So I made my body roll into second, and I took Brumley out really hard and flipped him over," he says. "I certainly wasn't trying to hurt the kid."

As he jogged off the field, Davis heard the jawing from the Winter Haven dugout. "You'll get yours, you son of a bitch!" Clemens screamed. "I'll see you in two fucking days!"

Now Clemens was pitching against the Tigers, anticipating his chance for revenge. In the first inning, he struck out the leadoff hitter, Chris Pittaro. He struck out the second hitter, Lorenzo Arce. He struck out the third hitter, Virgilio Silverio. In the second inning, he struck out the cleanup hitter, Thomas, and the fifth hitter, Rondal Rollin. "Roger was just throwing BBs," says Cannizzaro. "They couldn't touch him." As he squatted in the on-deck circle, preparing to hit, Davis thought about the warning his manager, Ted Brazell, had issued before the game: "Watch out tonight. Clemens will be coming after you."

When Rollin was retired, Davis, a left-handed hitter, walked up to the plate, took a couple of practice cuts and dug in. Born and raised in tiny Laurel, Mississippi, Davis had long dreamed of escaping his small town to play professional baseball. "I loved the chance to meet the people from different countries—the Dominicans, the Mexicans," he says. "People heard I was from Mississippi and they'd ask if we had paved roads." Though he was a good enough collegiate ballplayer to be named a Division II All-American, Davis was more space filler than prospect. "I knew what I was," he says. "I had my limits."

As Davis looked out at Clemens, he was no longer thinking about getting beaned or having to duck or Wayne Dyer's 10 keys to self-preservation. "I just wanted a hit," he says. "The same as always."

Clemens wound up, unfolded his six-foot-four frame and let loose a fastball that traveled directly from his hand to the back of Davis' head. *PUH!* The sound was dull, like a fist pounding dough. The ball was thrown so hard that it ricocheted off Davis' helmet and into the stands. Davis took a couple of steps forward, wobbled, then fell to the ground like a drunkard following one last shot of Jägermeister. When he finally rose, Davis tried charging the mound but was overcome with dizziness and dropped again. "I understood him throwing at me," says Davis. "I can respect standing up for a teammate. But he threw at my head. At my head! You don't mess with somebody's career like that." Davis was taken to the nearby hospital. Clemens remained in the game and struck out 15 Tigers. Ed Kenney, Boston's farm director, was watching from behind home plate. He was dazzled. The kid had guts. It would be Clemens' final Class A start.

Following the game, one Winter Haven player after another approached Clemens' locker to shake his hand. He had defended a teammate—the ultimate act of baseball decorum. "That's what you're supposed to do," says Steve Ellsworth, a Winter Haven teammate. "It speaks to what type of competitor Roger was."

Yet for a man who would go on to make a reputation off of brushing back opposing hitters, Clemens was surprisingly shaken. A couple of days after the game, Davis received a handwritten letter of apology, with Clemens (laughably) insisting he had been aiming for the leg, not the skull.

"I never really forgave him, because I know it was 100 percent intentional," says Davis, who retired after the '84 season and now works as an electrical technician. "But, heck, I can always say I was the first professional baseball player Roger Clemens beaned."

ALTHOUGH CLEMENS WOULD SPEND the first 16 years of his major league career burdened by the dreaded "He's never won the big one" label, such was—technically—not the case.

In 1983, Clemens won the big one.

Granted, it was an Eastern League championship with Double A New Britain.

Upon his arrival in Connecticut, Clemens entered the clubhouse of Beehive Field and was warmly greeted by Rac Slider, the New Britain manager and a man whose mannerisms must have felt familiar to the young pitcher. A 49-year-old baseball lifer, Slider had been raised in Simms, Texas, a middle-of-nowhere ranching town that taught the rugged, take-no-crap mind-set Clemens had adopted as his own. "I believed in being tough," says Slider. "You don't do your job, you have to answer to me."

Before Clemens' arrival, Slider had been briefed on what was at stake here: namely, the future of the Red Sox. Slider was not to overwork Clemens. The pitcher was never to throw more than 100 pitches or enter a game in relief. Slider's job title was officially "manager," but in this case, he was primarily a caretaker. Nurture the kid, teach him a few things—and, by the grace of God, don't screw anything up.

Knowing that Clemens was being babied, it would have been easy—expected, even—for New Britain's other players to loathe the kid. To some extent, they did. "Roger was nice enough," says Gary Miller-Jones, New Britain's second baseman. "He had a very high opinion of himself, which a lot of us didn't like. But it's hard to criticize that, because his attitude was part of the package. He believed he was a major league pitcher, even when he wasn't. Were some of us jealous? Of course we were. Some of us had been in Double A for three or four years, and this young guy's shooting through the organization. How would you feel?"

Any resentment, however, was dulled by the unassailable truth that Clemens was brilliant. For the other New Britain pitchers—a highly regarded group that included future big leaguers Ellsworth (who had also been promoted) and Jeff Sellers—it was surely similar to what Antonio Salieri had endured when watching the young Mozart at work. "He was a phenomenon," says Clinton Johnson, a New Britain right-hander. "His fastball was insane. His slider was sharp. He had complete command of the strike zone. I saw him throw, and I thought, 'This boy is ready for the big leagues right now.'"

"Catching Roger was as easy as drinking a glass of water," says Jeff Hall, a New Britain catcher. "You start on the black and keep going until the ump calls a ball. That was all it took. He did the rest."

As was the case in Winter Haven, Clemens largely kept to himself in New Britain, preferring a bucket filled with quarters at the local video arcade to nights out with teammates. At the tail end of an era when ballplayers lived hard and played harder, Clemens merely played hard. "He didn't drink, didn't smoke, didn't swear," says Hall. "He wasn't a loner, but he didn't buddy up to people. He was there to pitch."

In seven starts, Clemens went 4-1 with a 1.38 ERA. He struck out 59 over 52 innings, walking just 12. With a 72-67 record, New Britain charged into the Eastern League play-offs intent on winning a title. "He was going to be brought to me for the final month," says Tony Torchia, manager of Triple A Pawtucket. "But we were pretty bad, and I urged the franchise to get him some Double A play-off experience. I felt there was more value in that environment, and they agreed."

The Sox faced the Reading Phillies in the best-of-three first-round series, and Slider named Clemens his opening-game starter. As opposed to the riffraff he had faced at Winter Haven, Reading's lineup was stocked with future big leaguers like Juan Samuel, Darren Daulton and Jeff Stone. The Phillies were 96-44 and, had anyone cared to bet on a Double A play-off series, would have been prohibitive favorites. In a team meeting before the opener, Slider gathered his men around him. "Most of you guys will never reach the major leagues," he said. "To you, these play-offs represent your best shot at getting a ring. So don't hold back. Don't keep anything inside. Let it all out."

As Clemens warmed up to start the game, he was approached by the home plate umpire and told that his glove was illegal. Reading manager Bill Dancy had issued the complaint—a not-especially-subtle attempt to rattle the kid. "All that writing," the ump said. "It's distracting." Sure enough, while still at Texas, several female friends had sneaked into his locker and, believing the Rawlings mitt was an extra, scribbled GOOD LUCK, GOOSE and WE LOVE YOU in black shoe polish. The marks wouldn't wash off.

Clemens agreed to switch gloves but wanted first to complete his warm-ups. With Slider and the New Britain bench ripping into him, the umpire lost his cool. "You change that glove when I tell you, you little fuck!" he screamed. Slider charged the umpire. Clemens charged the umpire. Dancy, grinning ear to ear, was euphoric. His plan had worked—another top prospect was about to unfold under the stress of the postseason.

Clemens, however, was no ordinary phenom. He cooled down, borrowed teammate Charlie Mitchell's glove and dominated the Phillies, holding them to one hit, one walk and no runs while striking out 13 over 10 innings in a 1-0 victory. "We couldn't hit him," says Stone. "He was throwing 97 mph with a nasty curve. He was out of our league." Afterward, Dancy sought out Clemens to shake his hand. "You," he said, "don't belong here."

New Britain defeated the Phillies in three games, and Clemens' final Double A start came eight days later, when he faced the Lynn

Pirates for the Eastern League title. The Sox led the best-of-five series two games to one, and Slider was happy to give Clemens the chance to finish things off. In a game that was never close, Clemens threw a three-hitter, striking out 10 Pirates in a 6-0 rout.

Within a span of three months, Clemens had won two titles. Though he had been with New Britain for less than five weeks, Clemens soaked in the postgame champagne, giddy over the completion of a memorable first season.

AS IF CLEMENS' LIFE weren't enough of a fairy tale, in the aftermath of New Britain's championship he was pulled aside by Slider and told that the organization would like him to spend some time in Boston.

Cocksure on the mound, Clemens could be equally reticent off of it. As he tiptoed into Fenway Park on a late-summer day, his eyes the size of Oreos, the kid from Butler Township, Ohio, had made it. He took in the thick grass, the rows upon rows of seats, the Green Monster. Clemens had been to the Astrodome numerous times as a teen, but this—Fenway—was baseball.

Entering the small, no-frills Red Sox clubhouse, Clemens was flabbergasted to see he had been issued a locker (well, he shared a stall with a batboy named Walter McDougal), with uniform number 21 dangling from a hanger. Though he was there strictly as an observer, the gesture from clubhouse man Vinnie Orlando rendered the prospect speechless. The numeral was more than mere digits to Clemens. Randy had worn number 21 throughout high school and college, and he and Kathy had been married on December 21, 1975. When Clemens had signed with the Red Sox, he had bought his mother a ring encrusted with 21 diamonds.

In his weeklong visit to Boston, Clemens the baseball phenomenon was treated like a clubhouse boy. Few players spoke with him, acknowledged him, engaged him in so much as prolonged eye contact. During games he sat in the press box. "Back then the Red Sox veterans treated young guys like we weren't even there," says Lee Graham, an outfielder who played five games with Boston in 1983. "It was like you were a fly on the wall, and you'd better not open your mouth."

In the major leagues, it was nothing special to see a guy throwing 94 mph with pinpoint control. This was the terrain of Tom Seaver and Nolan Ryan and Ron Guidry and dozens of other similarly skilled professionals. Clemens' bullpen sessions hardly raised eyebrows, but his work ethic did. With his season completed, Clemens had earned the right to kick back. Instead, he was running pole to pole in the Fenway outfield; doing sit-ups and push-ups beneath the stadium; lifting weights as the other players spent the pregame hours smoking cigarettes, playing cards and eating hoagies. "My first impression was 'This is the hardest worker I've ever seen,'" says Dave Stapleton, Boston's first baseman. "Young players come and go, and they usually don't resonate. Roger resonated."

IN JANUARY 1984, WHILE home in Houston, Roger ran into an old Spring Woods High classmate named Debbie Godfrey. Perky yet tough, with wavy light brown hair and an athletic physique, Debbie was a ballet, jazz and tap dance instructor who—like Roger—had been raised in the lower-middle-class environs of suburban Houston. Her family lived in the rundown Victorian Village apartment complex across the street from the high school, though Debbie's optimistic confidence concealed any despondency. "We have a lot in common," Debbie once said. "We both grew up knowing hard times. My mother was divorced. We didn't have much."

Although Roger and Debbie were friendly in high school, it had been primarily a "Hi!"-and-"Bye!" relationship as they passed each other in the hallway. Debbie had dated one of Roger's baseball teammates, a kid he didn't particularly care for. Now, in the early winter of 1984, Roger and Debbie were brought back together. A mutual friend had arranged an encounter, telling Roger it was a blind date and Debbie that it was merely a gathering of long-lost chums. "My first impression of Roger was 'What a tall, handsome man!'" she said. "More than that, he seemed responsible. He always did everything he said he was going to do. And he was sweet. He wanted only to talk about what I was doing. We met on the 10th. Our first kiss was on the 19th."

In Debbie, Roger found not merely a lover but a sports fanatic and workout partner. In the midst of auditioning for the Dallas Cowboys' cheerleading squad for a second straight year (she failed to survive the final cut), Debbie was obsessed with fitness and righteous eating. In Roger, Debbie found a man who held doors open and answered everyone with "Yes, sir" and "Yes, ma'am." He was a kid in a giant's body, a surprisingly affectionate lug who treated his mother like a queen and placed family above all else. If there was an arrogant side to Roger, Debbie sure didn't see it. Plus, unlike the vast majority of Texas baseball players, Roger chewed tobacco but once a year, when he went on his annual hunting trip. His teeth were as white as whole milk.

At age 21, Debbie considered her defining life moment to be November 22, 1963, when—as a young child—she had been with her mother near the Texas School Book Depository in Dallas when John F. Kennedy was assassinated.

Soon, there would be two new ones.

In May, after asking the permission of her mother and stepfather, Roger proposed to Debbie. By year's end, they were married.

IN FEBRUARY 1984, CLEMENS reported to spring training in Winter Haven, convinced that he would make the Red Sox starting rotation. If anyone doubted his intentions, they only needed to view the rear of his black GMC truck, which featured a customized sox–21 license plate.

Like anyone coming off of two championships, a 9-2 professional record and a buffet of experts proclaiming him "The next . . ." [fill in the blank with Nolan Ryan, Bob Gibson or Tom Seaver], Clemens looked at Boston's so-so collection of returning pitchers and knew he belonged. In 1983, Boston had endured a forgettable 78-84 season. Surely, manager Ralph Houk would be sold after one glimpse of Clemens' blistering stuff.

If Clemens was struck by one thing during that initial spring, it wasn't Jim Rice's power, Dwight Evans' throwing arm or Wade Boggs' bat control. No, it was the lack of a team fitness regimen. Having spent much of his life outrunning, outlifting and outhustling the competition, Clemens was dismayed by Houk's glaring indifference to physicality. "Our workouts consisted of something like six 60-yard dashes across the outfield," he wrote in his autobiography, "and by the third week I was in worse shape than when I reported. I kept figuring there must be something else coming, so I only did a few extra sprints. Finally I realized that's all there was."

An exasperated Clemens developed his own program, drawing scorn from a handful of Red Sox veterans. With each extra sprint, each additional push-up, Clemens was putting the other players to shame. "If anyone felt threatened, they probably needed to look in the mirror," says McDougal. "Roger did what he knew—busted his rear."

Though his numbers were only so-so (1-2 with a 6.60 ERA), Clemens showed enough to make the big-league roster. "He's got good poise—there's no question about that," Houk said in late March. "It's not like he's 18 years old. He's been pitching against good competition for a long time." Despite the praise, the ace-in-training had no chance of sticking. Had the Red Sox begun the season with Clemens on the roster, he would have been eligible for arbitration after two years. What was the rush? "I knew he had a good spring, but we had some good young pitchers that year," Houk said. "I felt going down for a month wouldn't hurt him."

On March 26, one day after Clemens was charged with six runs on eight hits in three innings against Pittsburgh, Houk called the 21-year-old into his office and told him he would begin the season at Triple A Pawtucket. "But don't get too comfortable," Houk told his despondent pitcher. "I have a feeling you won't be there for long."

Clemens was upset, but he refused to show others his true emotions. After retreating to the corner of the locker room for a brief cry, he reported to Torchia, the Pawtucket manager. His new skipper was immediately impressed. "I've always had this small method to learn about a guy," says Torchia. "It was Roger's second day in minor league camp, and we were getting ready to play a spring training game in which he wasn't pitching. So I said, 'Roger, would you mind being a batboy?'"

"Sure, Skip," Clemens said. "I'd be happy to!"

"So that was his role for the afternoon," says Torchia. "And he did a helluva job. I'll never forgot that."

Any remorse over the demotion dissipated when Clemens relocated to Pawtucket, Rhode Island, and found, to his surprise, bliss. This wasn't Winter Haven. This wasn't New Britain. This was a vibrant small city with a die-hard Red Sox fan base and a nice ballpark, McCoy Stadium. Most of the team lived within walking distance of the park and after games would usually retreat to the local bar, My Brother's Pub, for beers, wings and conversation.

As he had in the two previous minor league stops, Clemens quickly adjusted to a new league. In seven games and 46⅔ innings with Pawtucket, he went 2-3 with a 1.93 ERA and 50 strikeouts. He struck out 11 and allowed just three hits in a 16-0 win against Syracuse. He tossed a four-hitter, fanning nine, versus Columbus. "The games Roger lost were all close," says Torchia. "With him, there was no such thing as a terrible performance."

One month into their season, the Boston Red Sox had an off day, which gave pitching coach Lee Stange the chance to drive to Pawtucket and watch Clemens start against Tidewater. At the time, Boston was 13-17, and its pitching staff was in shambles.

That night, fighting sporadic rain and temperatures in the low 50s, Clemens struck out nine batters in a 3-0 loss to the Tides. It wasn't Clemens' best start for Pawtucket. "But," says Torchia, "a picture is worth a thousand words. Roger's picture was worth even more."

Following the game, Stange pulled Clemens aside. "I don't have the final say, so this isn't official," he said. "But I believe you just made your last minor league start."

The next morning, May 11, 1984, the news was official.

Roger Clemens was coming to Boston.

7

Rah-jah in Beantown

In the hours leading up to his first major league start, Roger Clemens did not spend most of his time with Gary Allenson, the sixth-year catcher who would be calling the game. He didn't spend the time with Ralph Houk, the veteran manager; Lee Stange, the wise pitching coach; Bruce Hurst; Bobby Ojeda; John Henry Johnson or any of the other experienced pitchers who might have been able to provide insight.

No, as the Red Sox prepared for the debut of baseball's most highly anticipated mound prospect since David Clyde's arrival in Texas 11 years earlier, Roger Clemens met with his brother Randy.

With the rookie's heart pounding, his hands sweaty and his thoughts darting, the two siblings sat in the bowels of Cleveland's antiquated Municipal Stadium and talked.

For Roger, here, at last, was the realization of a lifelong dream. The poor, chunky kid from Ohio had come back to do exactly what he had promised friends and family members all those years ago. Bess had flown in from Houston with Debbie, now Roger's fiancé. Kathy had come along with Randy from their home in Troy, Ohio. Roger's grandmother and aunt arrived from Detroit. All told, Roger needed 15 tickets for his debut—a Clemens family reunion held in the stands of one of Major League Baseball's worst stadiums.

Lost in the euphoria was a simple question: How did Randy feel about all this? *He* was, after all, the Clemens brother who was supposed to have made it big in sports, who had seemed destined to be dribbling the ball down the parquet floor of the Boston Garden or beneath the rafters of Madison Square Garden. *He* had been the small-town star destined to put tiny Butler Township on the map. "If there were a Clemens who was going to go on to be a major national sports star, it was Randy," says Bob Costello, a former Butler Township coach. "He was the one."

Instead, Randy Clemens was a nobody basketball coach, still at Troy High School, still fantasizing of a college scout knocking on his door and wisking him away to assist at UCLA or Indiana or North Carolina, still allegedly battling substance abuse problems. About to begin his fourth and final season at Troy, Randy's reputation in the Dayton area was in tatters. His Bobby Knight wanna-be shtick had grown tired—the taunting and yelling and snarling along the sideline, the audibly cursing-out of referees for the tiniest of mistakes. "He was a great coach, except for his behavior on the bench," says Larry South, his lifelong friend and a Troy assistant coach. "The kids loved him because he was one of them. But he used a lot of profanity, and he didn't think about how that came across."

Those who knew Randy well say he was simultaneously pleased and haunted by his little brother's success, and that any triumphs Roger enjoyed were often claimed by Randy as his own. *I helped Roger with this. I taught Roger that.* Perhaps that's why, when Roger was wrapping up his collegiate days, Randy insisted that he not hire an agent to negotiate with the Red Sox. "I'll represent you," he said. "At least you'll know I have your best interests at heart." So Randy, not Scott Boras or Leigh Steinberg or Jerry Maguire, hammered out the $121,000 deal— one that, in his defense, was deemed fair by all sides.

"Randy saw Roger as his ticket," says South. "I don't know that Roger knew his brother viewed him that way. He probably didn't, because Roger idolized Randy. But Randy always thought—after all the times he'd helped Roger—that eventually Roger would lead him to a big-time job in college or professional sports. I'm sure he wanted to be living Roger's life, but he would have been happy with whatever the next best thing was."

So how did Randy feel about Roger Clemens making his big-league debut? Proud, surely. But, as he watched his brother warm up in the bullpen, also remorseful.

The family's star was on the field.

The older brother was in the stands.

THE DEBUT DID NOT go well. It wasn't the worst game a rookie Red Sox pitcher has ever thrown, but when contrasted with the 1984 premieres of peers like the Mets' Dwight Gooden (five innings, one earned run) and Seattle's Mark Langston (seven innings, two earned runs), Clemens' five and two-thirds innings, 11-hit, four-earned-runs, four-strikeouts showing in a 7-5 loss hardly goes down as a Hall of Fame–worthy beginning.

In one regard, perhaps, Clemens was doomed from the outset. Unlike Gooden, who made his first major league start before 18,925 spectators inside the clean, crisp Astrodome, Clemens found himself submerged in baseball hell. With blustery Lake Erie cutting through Municipal Stadium and a fierce cold spell keeping temperatures in the low 40s, Clemens took the mound for the bottom of the first, looked up into the stands and saw . . . wood. Lots and lots and lots of wood. In a stadium that held 70,000, there were exactly 4,004 paid customers and

65,996 empty seats. "I remember it being real cold," Clemens would say years later. "I remember my wife telling me that while we were hitting, she'd go stand in the ladies' restroom just to stay warm."

After Boston went down without scoring in the top of the first, the Indians came to the plate and, following manager Pat Corrales' blueprint, attacked. Brett Butler grounded out and Tony Bernazard flew out, but left fielder Pat Tabler singled, then stole second. Designated hitter Andre Thornton followed with an RBI single, then swiped second as well. At that point in their careers, Tabler and Thornton had stolen 32 bases in 1,314 combined games. They possessed the speed of Rickey Henderson—had Henderson played with refrigerators tied to both of his feet. "But Roger was a 1.9 [seconds] to the plate, as slow as hell," says Allenson, his catcher. "At that point, he had no real concept of keeping opposing runners in check."

While Clemens ended the first having surrendered but a single run, it would be a trying night. The Indians stole a franchise-record seven bases off of the rookie, including two by the lumbering Thornton. (After the game it was brought to Clemens' attention by teammate Marty Barrett that he was tipping his pitches—whenever he threw a curveball, he raised the pointer finger on his left hand.)

By the time Houk strolled to the mound to remove his starter midway through the sixth, Cleveland's small army of loyalists was mercilessly heckling Clemens. He ended the night with a no decision in the 7-5 Boston loss, but with his ego bruised. This wasn't quite how he'd imagined it. Afterward, Houk called the rookie into his office and assured him that, before long, he would be dominating the likes of Cleveland. "Teams will try and jump on you for a while, and sometimes they will," Houk said. "But they'll learn what you're made of. Just keep bringing it."

"What really impresses me about [Roger] is his poise," Houk told the media. "Sure, he was nervous, it being his first major league start and having all his family there. But we screwed up all kinds of plays, they got all the cheap hits and he never got rattled. There's no question about it. He's going to be a good one."

CLEMENS DIDN'T HAVE TO wait long for his first major league win. Five days after the Indians debacle, the Red Sox traveled to Minneapolis' Metrodome to meet the adequate Twins. As in Cleveland, Clemens fell behind 1-0 after the first inning and ended the third trailing 3-2.

Then, for the first time as a big leaguer, Roger Clemens looked spectacular. Over the next two innings, he struck out four of seven batters faced, including Tom Brunansky and Kent Hrbek, the Twins' most dangerous sluggers. With his mid-90s fastball cutting in and out, up and down, Minnesota's hitters appeared baffled. Although Brunansky homered in the sixth, Clemens whiffed Gary Gaetti, another All-Star-caliber hitter, to kill any rally hopes. The beauty of the moment wasn't Gaetti going down on a high fastball, but the pitch that preceeded it—a changeup that turned the hitter's knees into Jell-O. Clemens got through the seventh, ending the inning with a Tim Teufel fly-out to second. When Clemens reached the dugout, Houk wrapped his arm around the kid's sweaty neck and told him that Bob Stanley, one of the league's better closers, would handle things from there. Clemens received high fives and backslaps from his veteran teammates, all of whom grasped the importance of the moment. Many achievements are celebrated in the course of a 162-game baseball season, but few with the Bar Mitzvah–like euphoria of a pitcher's first victory. When Hatcher ended the game by grounding out to first, Stanley pumped his fist and presented Clemens with the game ball. The Red Sox won, 5-4.

It was May 20, 1984, and Roger Clemens was 1-0.

Although Boston's players would have relished the occasion for any of their young pitchers, there was something about Clemens that appealed to their inner hard-asses. Yeah, he was cocky, with the strut and the scowl and the vanity license plate to prove it. But he was also respectful. Back in the early 1980s, before rookies were gifted with million-dollar payouts and endorsement deals for Gatorade and Kentucky Fried Chicken, they were expected to show up, work hard, listen intently and shut the hell up. No team embraced this ethos more than Boston, where over the course of decades the superstars—from Ted Williams to Carl Yastrzemski to the present duo of Jim Rice and Dwight Evans—projected a regal aura. "You knew your place with the Red Sox," says Reid Nichols, a utility infielder from 1980 to 1985. "And your place was usually pretty silent and isolated."

Naturally quiet to begin with, Clemens didn't have to work hard at keeping his head down and his thoughts to himself. When the media surrounded his locker after games, his replies contained all the pizzazz of an onion ring. "I gave my all for the team" and "This was a hard-fought win" were some of his standard platitudes. Most important, Clemens busted his tail. "Usually young guys rely only on their talent early on, then realize they need to work harder as they get older," says Rick Miller, a Boston outfielder. "But Roger seemed to realize he had to work hard right away. When I came up, we were told not to lift too many weights. Well, Roger lifted all the time. In baseball, most players don't love running. Well, Roger was always running. If you were one of the veterans, you looked at this kid and, after getting over any feelings of being threatened, immediately approved."

What especially aided Clemens' cause was the respect he earned from Rice, the 31-year-old All-Star slugger who was known by media and some teammates to be moody and abrasive. Fair or not, many African American ballplayers still looked at their southern white teammates (despite his Ohio roots, Clemens was known as a Texan) with a skeptical glare, wondering where their loyalties fell in the Mason-Dixon divide. The Red Sox, after all, were the last major league franchise to play an African American, and, as Howard Bryant detailed in *Shut Out,* his brilliant book on race and baseball in Boston, racial tensions poisoned the clubhouse for decades. "Clemens and Rice were pretty close, and a lot of that had to do with Roger giving Jim his due as a leader," says Bryant, a former writer for the *Boston Herald*. "Whether he was brought up with blacks or not, Roger seemed to identify with the black guys on the Red Sox, because a lot of them—starting with Rice—were dogged like he was."

Rice and Evans would take Clemens out for dinner, talk strategy with him, engage him on team flights and offer tips on how to handle the press. (Asked by a reporter what sort of music the team listened to, Clemens wisely replied, "Whatever Jim Rice wants.") Clemens was tagged "Super Rook," "Big Tex" and "Top Gun," but not in the mean way monikers are sometimes affixed to irritating newcomers. It was flattery. Soon his nickname was, simply, "Rocket." The tag stuck.

"There was nothing not to like about Roger," says Dennis "Oil Can" Boyd, a fellow starting pitcher. "When you behave like he did, you earn the trust and respect of your teammates."

Boyd, an eccentric 24-year-old right-hander with a funky delivery and funkier mannerisms, learned to love Clemens during a road trip to Baltimore. On the night of June 25, 1984, shortly after he helped pitch the Sox to a 7-4 victory over the Orioles, Boyd visited a nightclub in one of Baltimore's rougher sections. While trying to hail a taxi, he was robbed at gunpoint and stripped of his wallet, watch and much of his clothing. "Hell, I returned to the hotel damn near naked," he says with a laugh. "Well, the next day a guy from a pawnshop calls and says he has my watch, which had my name engraved on the back." Clemens, whose road locker was three down from Boyd's, overheard the conversation.

"Can, you got mugged?" he asked.

"Yup," said Boyd. "I sure did."

"Where the hell was it?" Clemens asked.

Boyd named the street where the incident occurred.

Clemens stood up. "We're going there tonight!" he screamed. "I wanna get names, I wanna get numbers! You don't do that to Oil Can Boyd!"

Boyd initially thought his teammate was joking. He wasn't. "He wanted to head down there after the game and beat some guys up," Boyd says. "I might be crazy, but I'm not *that* crazy. I told Roger to forget it. But I've always remembered that loyalty."

Though Houk and his staff believed Clemens' first victory was a gateway to greater things, the following few weeks proved difficult. Clemens allowed five or more runs in three of his next four starts, and, following a June 12 beating against the Yankees, his ERA ballooned to 7.38. The stuff that he had relied on in college and the minor leagues was no longer cutting it, and a dejected Clemens began to question aloud whether—as the local media was suggesting—he should still be toiling in Triple A. A kid who had never pitched timidly was now pitching timidly. He looked out at the Don Mattinglys and Eddie Murrays and Jack Percontes of the league and wondered if he truly belonged. Less than three years ago he was a nobody junior college charity case. Had it all come too fast? Too easily? Was he simply not good enough?

That's when Boyd and Bobby Ojeda, two of the team's better starters, sat down with Clemens for a much-needed talk. "You're being stupid, and you're not a stupid person," said Boyd. "This is the major fucking leagues, and you need to learn to pitch here."

"But I know I can throw my fastball past these guys," Clemens said.

"No," said Ojeda, a cagey left-hander with a mop of curly brown hair atop his head. "Not here."

"Heat ain't everything," Boyd said. "Guys at this level will swing and miss, but you're not throwing it *by* them. They're just missing. Give 'em a straight fastball at 100 mph and they'd fucking kill it. You've got a curveball, you've got a slider. Fucking use 'em."

Clemens nodded. On the night of June 22, he made his fourth start at Fenway, still a confounding place to pitch for the young Texan.

Clemens wasn't quite sure what to make of the Green Monster, the glowing CITGO sign or the abrasive diehards with their seallike barks of *"Rah-jah!"* Having been denied a World Series title since 1918, Boston fans were desperate. In Clemens, they believed they had found their redeemer. So as he walked to the mound on that breezy Friday night, the fans stood up and applauded.

In what would go down as one of the best performances of his rookie year, Clemens overwhelmed the Toronto Blue Jays, scattering six hits while striking out nine in an 8-1 victory. He threw only 118 pitches, walked none and snapped his team's eight-game losing streak. "They told me to let it go," he said afterward, "and that's what I did."

Clemens didn't perform terribly over the remainder of the season, but he didn't perform brilliantly, either. He went 34 days without another victory, usually pitching just poorly enough to win or lose, depending on the opponent. Were there one thing going for the frustrated righty, it was that Boston, a rebuilding club that would win 86 games and place fourth in the American League East, had been out of the pennant race since May. The postseason hopes of a city did not rest with a rookie.

ON THE AFTERNOON OF August 21, Clemens reported to Fenway Park for his evening start against the Kansas City Royals. As his teammates went about their routines, taking BP, loading up on pine tar and wrapping their wrists in tape, Clemens sat at his locker and fretted.

He twirled his right arm a handful of times. He pressed on his elbow and shoulder. Picked up a sneaker, lifted it into the air, put it down.

"Can," he said to Boyd, "I'm not feeling good."

Boyd ignored Clemens—he'd heard this one before.

"Can, really," he said. "Something's wrong with the arm."

"Dammit, Roger," Boyd replied. "Just don't worry about it. You're young—go pitch."

That night Clemens' stuff, to cite Boyd, was "filthy." Fastballs that painted the outer tip of the black. Curveballs that broke from elbows to knees. Clemens struck out 15 Royals in an 11-1 Boston rout.

After the game, Clemens told the media, "I probably had my best fastball since I've been here." When the press, left, however, he sat down beside Boyd, dejected. "Can," he said, "that wasn't my fastball."

"Hell," Boyd replied, recalling the 95-mph velocity, "then give it to me. I'll take it."

"No, I'm serious," Clemens said. "My arm ain't feeling good. I wasn't myself out there."

"Roger," Boyd said, "you struck out 15."

"I'm telling you," Clemens said. "I'm telling you . . ."

He made two more starts in the 1984 season, both against the Indians. The first was brilliant, the second painful. Clemens left in the fourth inning, his forearm throbbing. Of Cleveland's 11 outs, seven had come by strikeout. But Clemens felt as if a hot brand was being stabbed against his body.

The injury, a strained tendon, was minor. The fear, a savior doomed by arm trouble, was major. With the play-offs a mathematical impossibility, the Red Sox shut Clemens down for the remainder of the season.

His final numbers, 9-4 with a 4.32 ERA, were solid but unspectacular. Clemens placed sixth in AL Rookie of the Year voting, but those who watched closely knew something much of the country had yet to learn. "You may well have looked at the numbers and thought, 'Good pitcher,'" says Hurst. "But if you were there every day, it was easy to know Roger Clemens was about to become a superstar. A major, major superstar."

CHAPTER

8

The Can

In the history of Major League Baseball, where men from disparate backgrounds are tossed together like ingredients in a salad, oddball alliances are inevitable. Within the confines of the clubhouse, blacks and whites play cards, Dominicans and Japanese share chewing tobacco, old and young guzzle beers, liberals and conservatives share *Playboy*s—and Roger Clemens and Dennis "Oil Can" Boyd became close friends.

Throughout his relatively sheltered life, surrounded by blue-collar, lower- and middle-class peers, Clemens knew what to expect of people. They liked a good ball game and a cold beer. They kept their opinions to themselves and their emotions largely in check. They tried not to brag excessively and conformed to a certain 1950s-style respectfulness. *Yes, sir. No, sir. Please. Thank you.* They were, 98 percent of the time, white.

Then, in late 1983, the Rocket met the Can. They first stood side by side during batting practice before a game at Fenway, when Boyd was a young pitcher trying to establish himself and Clemens was the hot-shot minor leaguer making a brief visit with the big club. Clemens was white. Boyd was African American. Clemens was big and burly. Boyd, standing at six-foot-one and 155 pounds, looked like a twisted pipe cleaner. Clemens threw heat, heat and heat. Boyd was all junk. Clemens spoke quietly, in three- and four-word sentences. Boyd rambled for hours.

"We hit it off right away," says Boyd. "There was something about Roger that I immediately loved. The authenticity."

Born and raised in the poorest part of Meridian, Mississippi, Boyd had learned the game of baseball at the Lake Erie Ballpark on 10th Avenue, a couple of streets over from his family's ramshackle house. It was where four generations of family members had played, including his father, Willie Boyd, who had pitched against Hank Aaron and Willie Mays at the field. "People ask me where I come from," Boyd once said, "and I tell them, 'I come from baseball.'"

Gifted on the mound since early boyhood, Boyd's dazzling assortment of pitches was rivaled only by his even more dizzying assortment of moods. At age 12 he was sent to the school psychiatrist because of his tantrums, and at age 17, while playing in a semipro game in Meridian, he nearly tossed his career away. "[An umpire] threw me out of the game because you can't swear on the ball field," Boyd said. "I went wild. I took my uniform off and left the park in my underwear. I sat in my daddy's car, crying, kicking, cussing, fussing. The next day my daddy said there were a lot of scouts in the ballpark, and they all left."

Two years later, while pitching for Jackson State, Boyd became so enraged by the chants of "Nigger!" from an opposing team that he chased a player to first base and punched him in the mouth. "I just lost it," Boyd said. "I just absolutely lost it."

But that was Oil Can Boyd—emotionally immature, unable to handle success or failure, cocksure and crazy. "First time I met Dennis, he said, 'Hi, I'm Dennis "Oil Can" Boyd, and I throw 100 mph,'" says

Pat Dodson, a Boston first baseman. "I started calling him 'Trash Can,' because he talked so much garbage." Teammates tended to tiptoe past the Can's locker, fearful of being trapped in a 50-minute monologue to nowhere. "Dennis once screamed at my roommate, 'I've got a .45, and I'm gonna shoot you!'" says Tom Bolton, a Red Sox pitcher. "He was *way* out there." Coaches offered him as little advice as humanly possible. Opponents viewed him as some sort of Looney Tunes character.

Clemens *loved* him.

To Clemens, Boyd was real. He said what he thought and held nothing back. His skin was as thick as a tire; his laugh filled up an auditorium; his insults stung like a poisoned dart. You could have a screaming argument with the Can, and 20 minutes later he'd be slapping you on the back, chuckling.

That's why, after the 1984 season, Clemens not only invited Boyd to his November wedding in Houston but asked him to serve as one of the groomsmen. Boyd and his wife, Karen, drove the 520 miles from Meridian to Houston for the event. "Debbie threw the bouquet right into my hands," Boyd says. "She was just the sweetest thing, that girl."

In Boyd, Clemens saw someone in need of a friend. He didn't care that he was black or profane or, quite often, three tomatoes short of a salad. Clemens stepped up and served, in a sense, as Boyd's translator, explaining to teammates that the speak-first, think-second pitcher was a genuinely good man who meant, oh, 60 percent of what he said. He took Boyd out to dinner on the road, went with him to movies and, on occasion, theme parks. If other Sox players didn't want Boyd around for a team gathering, well, Clemens usually didn't attend, either. "Roger thought he could mentor Oil Can and sort of calm him down," says John Leister, a Boston pitcher. "Oil Can was the rebel of the Red Sox, and Roger saw someone who he could help mature and develop."

All of this explains why Clemens was shocked when he arrived in Winter Haven for spring training in February 1985 and found that Boyd was bad-mouthing him. Because they lacked significant major league experience, Clemens, Boyd and Al Nipper—all free agents, all close friends, all part of Boston's vaunted young rotation—could have had their contracts automatically renewed for the upcoming season. Yet Lou Gorman, the team's GM, said, "we want to be fair to them," noting that the trio represented the future of the organization. "We'll keep talking," he said in February at the beginning of spring training, "and they'll be permitted to start working out on schedule Friday even if they're not signed."

For Boyd, this wasn't enough. The Can told *The Boston Globe* that, without question, he deserved more money than either Clemens or Nipper. It was, from his vantage point, an issue of respect—the Boston Red Sox needed to respect Oil Can.

Not long after the words escaped Boyd's lips, Boston's army of reporters marched over to Clemens' locker. A potentially roster-dividing war of words was eagerly anticipated. Yet instead of taking the bait, Clemens did something that not only impressed teammates but set a new tone for what had traditionally been a team with poor clubhouse chemistry: He gave Boyd the benefit of the doubt.

"Can is Can," he said, laughing. "Can is excitable, and he gets upset. I understand it's not personal. He's my friend. I don't hold a grudge."

Shortly after learning of Clemens' reaction, Boyd approached the blooming ace, extended his hand and apologized. "You've been good to me, Rocket," he said. "I shouldn't have dragged you into this." Clemens gave Boyd a slap on the back. "No big deal," he said. "We're deeper than that."

The two pitchers both eventually signed for roughly $140,000 ("I'm all right," Boyd said of the deal. "I'm not satisfied, but I'm all right"), and the bond endured. They spent hours in the clubhouse talking about everything from pitching strategy to the World Series championship they planned on one day bringing to Boston.

"Roger is a friend for life," says Boyd. "Whenever I've needed him, he's been there for me. And whenever he needs me—and I mean whenever—I will drop everything to be by his side. You don't love that many people in your life. But I love Roger Clemens."

ARMED WITH THE HIGH expectations that usually accompany a stellar young rotation (no starter was older than 29), baseball's best hitter (third baseman Wade Boggs, who would bat .368) and a new manager, John McNamara, the Red Sox expected to contend for the 1985 American League pennant. "Boston," wrote John Franks of UPI, "has the hitting and fielding to win it all."

Instead, they stunk.

The biggest disappointment was Clemens, who throughout the 81-81 season battled one health woe after another. On July 8, with his record 6-4 and the Sox eight and a half games behind Toronto in the AL East, Clemens was placed on the 15-day disabled list with inflammation in his throwing shoulder. He had been scheduled to start the day before against the Angels at Anaheim, but while warming up felt a pain that he described "as if someone stuck a knife in the back of my shoulder." Clemens begged Bill Fischer, the first-year pitching coach, to let him play. "Forget it," Fischer barked. "You're going back to Boston." After Clemens walked from the field into the clubhouse, he lost it. He tore off his jersey, buttons flying left and right, whipped his glove into a nearby trash can and his pants and socks into another trash can. Finally he leaned against a wall and began to wail. "Why me?" he screamed. "Why me? Why me? Why me?" Tears streaming down his cheeks, Clemens left the stadium in T-shirt and shorts and took a jog around Anaheim.

Major league clubhouse tantrums are generally addressed in one of two ways: Either the guilty party is shipped off to Triple A Bumble-hell and never heard from again, or the incident is dismissed. Clemens' flip-out, however, resulted in a curious reaction. Boston's players applauded his anger. This wasn't Boyd whining about money or respect. Randy had always taught Roger that a winner never lets down his teammates. Never. It doesn't matter if you're hurting, grieving, drained, confused—you damn well better pitch. "You had to admire that about Roger," says Boyd. "Nobody wanted the ball more than he did."

But now, his health in peril, Clemens was lost. As he ran through Anaheim's Mickey Mouse–pocked streets, his mind raced. He considered developing a gimmick pitch—a knuckler, perhaps. Or a big loopy curve. Maybe he could reestablish himself as a position player. "I couldn't stand the idea of being one of those could-have-beens," Clemens said. "I was really hurting, and I didn't know why. Or why me." He had been conditioned to handle many scenarios—late-game rallies, blowouts, no-hitters. But not this.

Clemens returned from the DL on August 3, put on his most optimistic game face, but never felt right. He pitched two more times, then was a last-minute scratch before his August 18 start against the Yankees. "Things got so bad that while I was warming up I got into an argument with a Yankee fan," he said. "It was on purpose, just to get up, to get my adrenaline going. But I was fooling myself. I had nothing."

"I saw Roger cry like a baby that day," says Fischer. "He thought he was done."

Through his first 22 years, Clemens had faced nothing like this. "I just want to know what is wrong," he told the *Sporting News*. "Tell me what it is. Tell me what's causing this pain."

On August 23, Arthur Pappas, the Red Sox team physician, recommended that Clemens undergo surgery to repair what he called a "small flap tear" in the cartilage disk surrounding his right shoulder. The minimum recovery time would be four months.

The operation, conducted by Dr. James Andrews on August 30, took only 20 minutes and was deemed a success. Clemens was throwing by early November, and by spring training he declared himself fit and ready for the 1986 season. "I'm good to go!" he told the media—a confident bellow intended to conceal a bevy of doubts. For the first time since he had been drafted by the Red Sox, Clemens was no longer the can't-miss kid. Through the decades, hundreds of prospects had come in looking like the next Nolan Ryan, only to have injuries derail their dreams.

"We knew Roger was a battler," says Hurst. "But we didn't know what to expect."

ON FEBRUARY 23, 1986, newspapers across the country ran an Associated Press article titled "Clemens Faces Lower Expectations."
Wrote Dave O'Hara:

> Hard-throwing Roger Clemens of the Boston Red Sox is headed into spring training with two primary goals: to start and finish the 1986 season.
>
> "I want to be ready to go all out when the season starts and I want to finish strong," Clemens said Sunday as he checked into the Boston training camp.
>
> Clemens has been considered a "franchise type" pitcher since he was signed as a number 1 draft pick after helping Texas to the NCAA championship in 1983.
>
> However, after a brilliant first year in the minors, the fire-balling right-hander has had arm woes, sitting out the final weeks of both the 1984 and '85 seasons.

Was this what it had come to? Was the goal of the American League's top young pitcher merely to last an entire year?
Sadly, yes.
Clemens reported to spring training and told anyone who asked that his arm was healthy. "I haven't had any setbacks yet," he said on February 26. "So hopefully I won't have one."
Yet armed with a new $220,000 contract, Clemens reared back,

threw his best stuff—and got rocked. In his exhibition season debut against Detroit, the Rocket needed 34 pitches to get through the first inning, permitting four runs, four hits and a walk in an 11-2 loss. "I wanted my arm to get a good test," he said afterward. "And I think it did." His next start was little better—surrendering five hits and three runs in three innings to the Astros. "He's going out there, throwing easily and not hurting," said McNamara. "We consider that encouraging." Then there was the third start, when Clemens was humiliated by the light-hitting Twins. His line: 3 IP, 4 hits, 7 runs, 5 walks, 1 strikeout. "I think he's back," raved McNamara. "I'm not discouraged by the figures, I'm encouraged by the way he's throwing the ball."

That, of course, was pure spin. When players struggle, managers do everything in their verbal power to turn their struggles around. You hope your guy can fix himself, but you're never quite sure.

After Clemens was clubbed for a fourth straight game, this time a five-inning, nine-hit, three-run debacle against the White Sox, the dread was too profound to hide. Instead of speaking highly of, say, his velocity or his stamina, Clemens looked over the throng of reporters and dejectedly said, "I have no comment to make on my pitching."

Finally, Fischer sat Clemens down.

"You're throwing all breaking stuff," Fischer barked. "How hard do you think you're throwing your fastball?"

"Eighty-four?" Clemens guessed.

Fischer handed him the radar gun readings. "Ninety-three."

"What?" said Clemens. "I'm throwing 93?"

"Yeah," said Fischer. "So how about you stop pitching like a girl and just let it rip?"

When the Rocket made his 1986 debut on April 11 at Chicago's Comiskey Park, a nation of baseball enthusiasts watched with rapt anticipation. Would this be Roger Clemens, potential Cy Young Award winner, or Roger Clemens, 23-year-old has-been? Would his fastball still crackle and pop at 95 mph, or float toward the plate in the mid-80s? Would he breathe fire, or cautiously hope for the best?

The answer left Boston fans giddy. Through eight and two-thirds innings, Clemens allowed six hits and only one earned run in an easy 7-2 triumph. The Clemens who had labored throughout the spring was gone, replaced by a man whose fastball traveled 97 mph, whose slider left opposing hitters shuddering and whose arm seemed as strong in the sixth and seventh innings as it did before the first pitch. "I felt great," Clemens said afterward. "No trouble with the shoulder at all."

His next two starts were equally encouraging, and on the morning of April 29, 1986, Roger Clemens woke up a 3-0 pitcher who once again *knew* he was destined for big things.

He just didn't know a big thing would come that night.

CHAPTER

9

Dominance

On the path to greatness, there is always "*The* Moment."

For Dwight Eisenhower, it came in 1926, when he was named a battalion commander at Fort Benning, Georgia. For Jimi Hendrix, it came while performing "Killing Floor" at the 1967 Monterey Pop Festival. For Joe Montana, it occurred in the waning moments of the NFC Championship Game following the 1981 season, when he rolled to his right and spotted Dwight Clark in the rear of the end zone.

For Roger Clemens, it took place on April 29, 1986, when he and the Red Sox began the day as afterthoughts in Boston's newspapers.

The top billing belonged to the New England Patriots, the defending AFC champions, which, that afternoon, would use their first pick in the NFL draft to select Reggie Dupard, a running back out of Southern Methodist. (The story turned out to be a nonstory: In five pro seasons, Dupard rushed for 704 forgettable yards.) A close second belonged to the Boston Celtics of Larry Bird, Kevin McHale and Robert

Parish, who that night would face Dominique Wilkins and the Atlanta Hawks in game two of the Eastern Conference semifinals.

Roger Clemens starting against the lowly Seattle Mariners? *Yawn.*

Granted, he remained Boston's top pitching hope. But it had been nearly three years since the Red Sox had drafted Clemens out of Texas, and all the "He's the next Nolan Ryan!" talk had grown a bit stale. "It was obvious Roger had a bright future," says Dan Shaughnessy, the noted *Boston Globe* writer. "But a lot of heavily hyped players have come through this town without living up to the talk."

So it was that—despite Clemens' presence on the mound—just 13,414 fans showed up at Fenway on a brisk 57-degree evening to watch the Red Sox face the mediocre Seattle Mariners in the first of a three-game series. The stadium photographer's well, usually packed with representatives of the local newspapers and wire services, was barren save for Jerry Buckley, the team's photographer. The press box, usually filled to the brim, felt like a department store three minutes after closing. In the stands, good seats could be had anywhere. From the broadcast booth, Ned Martin and Bob Montgomery welcomed the audience to yet another New England Sports Network telecast with all the energy of a supermarket pudding sale. "The theme of this series," said Martin, "is hitting!"

Clemens, of course, didn't give a damn. Dating back to boyhood, he rarely noticed the attendance or heard the shouts or cared that so-and-so celebrity in so-and-so row was in the building. No, he was all about the moment, about building up animosity toward the opposing hitter.

With his scheduled start in Kansas City two days earlier having been rained out, Clemens was working on six days of rest. He had woken up that morning with a severe headache, and nothing felt quite right all day. On his drive to the ballpark, he had been stuck in a traffic jam on Storrow Drive, still two and a half miles from Fenway just 45 minutes before the game was supposed to begin. With little time to spare, a motorcycle police officer spotted the pitcher and did a double-take. "Aren't you supposed to be on the mound?" he asked.

"Yeah," said Clemens.

"OK," the officer replied. "Follow me."

With lights flashing and siren blaring, he guided Clemens to the ballpark.

And now Clemens was about to face the one team that had always given him trouble (Clemens was 0-2 with a 9.58 ERA versus the Mariners).

"I came in, did my Superman impression of getting dressed in a phone booth, did some quick sprints, a couple of stretches and started firing away in the bullpen," Clemens recalled. "I remember I didn't throw one strike in the bullpen. Fish [pitching coach Bill Fischer] had his head buried in his hands. He didn't think I'd get out of the first inning. And every time I bent over or did toe stretches, I had a really bad headache. My temples were pounding."

"Then the first guy stepped in, I took a couple of deep breaths and it just started happening."

The game began at 7:18 P.M., with Seattle shortstop Spike Owen, Clemens' former teammate at the University of Texas, entering the batter's box. Upon arriving in Austin as a sophomore, Clemens had immediately looked to Owen as a baseball role model. He was the heart of the Longhorns—their best player and most vocal leader. Now, as Owen dug in, Clemens smirked devilishly. One day earlier, Clemens had played 36 holes of golf with Mike Capel, another former Texas player. "The first time you face Spike, I dare you to bust him off the plate," Capel said. "Throw him a bow tie."

"Really?" said Clemens. "You want me to give him some chin music?"

"Yeah," said Capel. "I'll bet a hundred dollars you don't do it."

The first pitch to Owen was over the plate for a strike. The second pitch was a high, inside fastball that sent Owen sprawling to the dirt. The third pitch, also high and inside, put Owen on his back yet again.

"What the hell are you doing?" Owen screamed.

"Roger sent messages that weren't hard to interpret," says Bruce Hurst. "He liked to establish himself early." Six pitches later, Owen was punched out on a fastball at the knees.

Although he had faced just one batter, Clemens was already working up a sweat. His forehead was dotted with perspiration, as were his cheeks and nose. Beneath his uniform Clemens wore a blue long-sleeved shirt. Despite the cold weather, he was hot.

The next batter, an All-Star outfielder named Phil Bradley, struck out looking, and the third hitter, Ken Phelps, swung through a fastball for strike three. As he walked off the mound, a small silver cross peeking out from beneath his jersey, Clemens received a standing ovation. Bellowed Martin from the broadcast booth, "A rather startling and awesome first inning!"

Clemens struck out two in the second and one in the third. Despite his reputation as an old-fashioned power pitcher, he was masterfully mixing things up. His curveball mimicked Dwight Gooden's, buckling the knees of established hitters such as Gorman Thomas and Ivan Calderon. His slider seemed to zig and zag from plate to black. When Calderon whiffed on three pitches to end the third, his exaggerated swings looked to be something out of the Flintstones—Bam-Bam Rubble wailing away with his club at a passing dodo bird.

"Seattle had some very good fastball hitters," says Dave Stapleton, Boston's backup first baseman, "and they couldn't touch Roger. I mean, people couldn't even pull the trigger. They couldn't even swing their bats."

Between innings, Clemens retreated to the trainer's room beneath the stadium and focused on the upcoming hitters. Having entered the night with a league-leading 166 strikeouts in 19 games, the Mariners swung at everything.

In the top of the fourth inning, with no score, Owen broke up Clemens' no-hitter by singling to right on a hanging curveball. In what was the most impressive sequence of the night, Clemens proceeded to strike out the Mariners' three most dangerous hitters. First Bradley went down on an inside fastball. Then Phelps looked foolish on a wicked slider. Clemens' biggest ally of the night proved to be Don Baylor, the bulky designated hitter who was filling in at first base for the injured Bill Buckner. With two outs, Thomas hit a high pop fly just foul of the first-base line. Baylor, blessed with the agility of a brick, backed up, backed up, backed up, backed up and—*clunk!*—had the ball hit his glove and fall to the ground. "My wife could have made the play!" a fan screamed from the stands. "How much are they paying you, Baylor?" Given another chance, Thomas whiffed on a fastball over the heart of the plate.

"Don was a terrible defensive player," says Stapleton. "Great guy, great hitter, no glove." Stapleton laughs. "Roger was lucky to have him in there."

By the time Thomas struck out, Fenway Park was abuzz. After four innings, Clemens had nine strikeouts. The 13,414 sounded like 100,000. Clemens left the field at the end of each inning greeted by a thunderous standing ovation. Charting the game from the bench, Hurst would turn toward Dennis Boyd and Al Nipper and say, "Man, Roger's got nine strikeouts . . . 10 strikeouts . . . 11 strikeouts . . . 12 strikeouts . . . 13 strikeouts . . . 14 strikeouts. What's the record?" It was 19, set by Charlie Sweeney, Tom Seaver, Steve Carlton and Nolan Ryan. Hurst said nothing to Clemens. "Why," says Hurst, "mess with a man's rhythm?"

Clemens entered the top of the seventh with 14 strikeouts, one shy of his career high. He had already tied an American League record with eight straight K's. "The amazing thing," said Rich Gedman, Boston's catcher, "is there were hardly any foul balls at all." Bradley led off and on the fourth pitch swung through a waist-high fastball. The look that crossed his face was not one of anger or resentment or indifference but of helpless acceptance. On this night, he was not good enough to touch Clemens. Not even close.

After Clemens struck out Phelps for the third time, Thomas walked to the plate, fell behind one ball, two strikes, then launched a solo home run to dead center field. With his bushy handlebar mustache and a 12-pack gut, Thomas looked to be more beer-softball-league masher than major league player. Yet now, in the midst of jogging the bases after his 257th career homer, Thomas smiled as Fenway fell quiet. A place that had endured so many heartbreaks seemed prepared to accept another one. Trailing 1-0, Clemens might strike out 18 or 19 or 20 . . . and lose.

The Red Sox fought back in the bottom of the inning, and Dwight Evans' three-run homer put his team up, 3-1. By this point, the local radio and TV stations, as well as the *Herald* and *Globe,* had caught wind of what was transpiring and sent over every available hand. Larry Whiteside, the *Globe*'s columnist, had started the evening at Fenway, watched a couple of innings, then left to cover the Celtics-Hawks play-off game. In the middle of the basketball game, the Boston Garden scoreboard flashed: "Roger Clemens has 12 strikeouts after five innings." A loud cheer filled the building. Whiteside gulped and looked at Vince Doria, a *Globe* sports editor. "Weren't you over at Fenway earlier?" Doria asked.

"Yeah," said Whiteside. "But Clemens only had five strikeouts when I left."

That was after two innings.

By now, Fenway was in a tizzy. Along the centerfield wall, a handful of college kids from nearby Newton had begun posting a red cardboard *K* for every strikeout. "I was sitting in the bullpen, trying to count all those K's," says Matt Young, a Seattle reliever. "You're always rooting for your own team, but I'm also a fan of history. We were a terrible team, he was a great pitcher. I could see where this one was heading." Clemens charged out onto the field to start the eighth, blew away the overmatched Calderon on three pitches, gave up a single to Danny Tartabull, then struck out Dave Henderson on a pitch so fast that Montgomery, the announcer, cracked, "That ball *sounded* high."

"Roger's fastball was coming in at about 120 miles an hour, his slider about 110," Henderson later said. "We all broke out our pepper swings after a while, just trying to make contact."

When pinch hitter Al Cowens flew out to center to end the inning, Fenway's denizens exploded. Clemens was two strikeouts away from breaking the record.

"I knew he was doing something special, but I didn't know how special until they started flashing his strikeout totals on the scoreboard," says Vic Voltaggio, the home-plate umpire. "Nothing, and I mean absolutely nothing, was ever more amazing than Roger's performance that night. He had complete control of that game from the first pitch until the end." This from a man who would work three no-hitters over the course of his 20-year career.

The Red Sox failed to score in the bottom of the eighth, and few in attendance complained. Nobody at Fenway was interested in watching Baylor or Evans face Mike Moore (who, for the record, pitched a solid game, allowing eight hits and three runs in seven and a third innings). This night was all about Roger Clemens. Sitting in the clubhouse while his teammates batted, the pitcher was nudged by Nipper, who said, "Rocket, do you realize that you're one away from tying the strikeout record?" Clemens barely acknowledged the news. He was locked in.

As Clemens walked onto the field to begin the ninth, Nipper looked at Charlie Moss, the Boston trainer, and said, "He's not the type to be affected by knowing. Watch."

Owen, the Mariner who had looked most comfortable hitting against his former teammate, led off and refused to merely lay down his bat. He took a fastball for strike one, then a ball, then made contact with a high fastball that rolled along the third base line before angling foul. "Somehow you get the feeling," Martin said, "these fans are glad that went foul." Clemens' follow-up offering was a letters-high fastball that Owen futilely chased for strikeout number 19. The ball was clocked at 96 mph—in the *ninth* inning.

The record was now one K away. Bradley walked up to the plate like a man who, according to *Sports Illustrated*'s Peter Gammons, "was approaching his execution." A 27-year-old speedster from Macomb, Illinois, Bradley was a quiet man who dreamed of owning a farm and whose greatest boyhood joy, he once told *Sports Illustrated,* came from, "castrating hogs."

Unlike, say, Thomas, a 13-year veteran who handled setbacks with the same casual demeanor as he did triumphs, Bradley was intense. A three-time All–Big Eight quarterback at Missouri, he had never forgotten the sting of being ignored in the 1981 NFL draft. Despite playing for the lowly Mariners, Bradley considered himself a winner. He most certainly had no interest in becoming a footnote of history.

The first two pitches were out of the strike zone. Bradley took both. The next two offerings were fastballs over the plate, both mid-90s in velocity, both ignored by Bradley. Finally, with the count 2-2, Clemens wound up, uncoiled and released another fastball. The pitch sailed past Bradley's stiff body and into Gedman's glove.

Strike three.

"A new record!" Martin screamed. "Clemens has set a major league record for strikeouts in a game!" Wade Boggs, Boston's third baseman, ran over to shake his teammate's hand. Having run out of room, the kids from Newton posted their 20th red *K* above the line of 19 others. The fans stood for a deafening ovation. In the dugout, Moss told Hurst, "We should get that ball to save it."

Hurst laughed. "Charlie," he said, "that ball ain't going anywhere."

That Phelps, the final batter, grounded out to shortstop took nothing away from the occasion. As Stapleton, now playing first, gripped the final out, Boston's players burst from the dugout and engulfed their teammate in hugs and high fives. Shortly thereafter Bill Fischer, the pitching coach, presented Clemens with the official game lineup card. He signed it "Best Game I Ever Saw Pitched." For several minutes inside the clubhouse, Clemens and Gedman—battery mates and close pals—were nearly speechless.

"Man," said Clemens.

"Man," said Gedman.

"Man," said Clemens.

"Man," said Gedman.

Nolan Ryan sent a congratulatory telegram. Ted Kennedy and Michael Dukakis phoned, as did Peter Ueberroth, baseball's commissioner. Hurst pulled Clemens aside and said, "Roger, your life has officially changed."

"It's great," Clemens said afterward. "It's unbelievable, spectacular and everything else that goes with it. It's hard to explain. It hasn't sunk in yet. I'm just happy there's someone up there looking over me. I thank the man in the sky for what I did tonight."

Of Clemens' 138 pitches, a remarkable 97 were thrown for strikes—and only 29 of those were even touched. He walked no one and didn't have a three-ball count from the fourth inning on. "Two things make Clemens unusual among power pitchers," said Mariners manager Chuck Cottier. "First, his fastball explodes down in the strike zone, and, second, the only others with his control were Koufax—at the end—and Bob Gibson."

If Clemens was the evening's most fortunate man, the runner-up was Joe Hickey, a Center Barnstead, New Hampshire, resident who had made the two-hour drive to Fenway. "Actually, I wanted to go to the Celtics game," he said. "But there was no way for me to get any tickets. So I said, 'What the heck . . . go to Fenway?'" Sitting in a seat just to the left of home plate, Hickey, a 45-year-old amateur photographer, had an early feeling this would be a big night for

Clemens. So he shot pictures of every Seattle strikeout. When Bradley approached the plate in the ninth inning, Hickey was ready. "I got Voltaggio just as I wanted him," he said, "with his arm, leg and foot stuck out there and making the call." Because nearly all of Boston's professional sports photographers were elsewhere, Hickey was the only person to capture the final moment. He sold copies to several outlets, including *Sports Illustrated* and the Baseball Hall of Fame, and was profiled in the *Globe* by columnist Michael Madden. Best of all, he had a copy autographed by Clemens, Voltaggio, Gedman and center fielder Steve Lyons—all of whom appear in the image. (Bradley refused to sign.)

Late that night, Clemens tossed and turned, unable to file away the 20 strikeouts in his head. The next afternoon, back on the Fenway infield for batting practice, Clemens was approached by Thomas. With a smile peeking out from beneath his mustache, the burly Seattle slugger extended his hand. He was holding a clean baseball and wanted Clemens' signature.

"Kid," he said, "they told me you throw the ball hard but that you also throw it straight. Kid, you throw the ball really hard, but it ain't so straight."

Roger Clemens had arrived.

He was no longer the kid with the potential but the man with the talent. *Sports Illustrated* placed him on its May 12, 1986, cover, alongside the headline LORD OF THE K's. *People* magazine, ordinarily the terrain of Burt Reynolds and "Ten Easy Steps to Weight Loss Success," ran a profile, complete with a photograph of Clemens sitting in the Fenway stands, dressed nattily in an Izod shirt, blue jeans and python boots. Clemens made the rounds of national television and radio, offering very little of substance but charming all with his Texas drawl and crooked smile. "My jaw," he said in the midst of it all, "has become very sore." During a visit to Massachusetts, Corazon Aquino, the president of the Philippines, told an audience, "I'm happy to be back in

Boston, especially happy now that Roger Clemens and the Boston Red Sox are going to win the World Series."

Clemens followed up the 20-strikeout masterpiece with a 10-strikeout stifling of Oakland. He improved to 8-0 on May 25 by beating the Texas Rangers on a two-hitter and returned seven days later to strike out nine Twins in another Boston victory. His emergence was hardly damaged by the fact that the Red Sox, often the laughingstocks of baseball, featured one of the game's best young rotations (Clemens, Boyd and Hurst combined to go 53-22), its top batsman (the .357-hitting Wade Boggs), a trio of crusty hitters who could still crush the ball (Jim Rice, Dwight Evans and Bill Buckner) and a manager, John McNamara, who specialized in pressing the right buttons while leaving well enough alone. "When you have someone like Roger, you're automatically a contender," says Fischer. "No matter what else happens, you know you're going to win every time Roger pitches."

When he had been just another young starter, Clemens seemed either shy or mysterious and sometimes both. But now, with three, four, five, six, seven, eight reporters waiting by his locker to write this profile for *The Washington Post* or that feature for the *Los Angeles Times,* Clemens was exposed as something of an unsophisticated bumpkin. When, in the months following the 20-strikeout game, he was asked about having shipped his hat, glove and spikes to the Hall of Fame, Clemens told a reporter that he had enclosed a note reading, "Rest of me to follow later." The comment, which surely entered and departed Clemens' brain without a second's consideration, came off as excessively arrogant—as did his propensity for screaming "Swing a little harder!" at opposing hitters who took big cuts. That was nothing compared to his confession to a *People* stringer named Cable Neuhaus that, having to spend so much time in Boston, he had recently purchased a .38 caliber handgun so that Debbie, his wife, could protect herself. "I'd rather be tried by twelve," he said, "than buried by six." He added that while he enjoyed being a member of the Sox, "the people in Boston never smile." That *People* never ran the quotes was both an indictment of the magazine's news judgment and a huge favor to the pitcher. In the most hypersensitive of American cities, the words would not have gone over well.

When Clemens spoke to the press after games, his replies often came off as either rambling, incoherent, or rambling *and* incoherent. "He was special; he knew he was special and he was often difficult to cover," says Dan Shaughnessy, the *Boston Globe* writer. "Roger probably felt we had it out for him, and some writers probably felt Roger wanted to make their lives more difficult than necessary."

Despite the mounting mutual hostilities, even the Boston press could not deny the magnificence of Clemens' season. On June 6 he improved to 10-0 with a complete-game four-hit shutout against the Brewers, and five days later he picked up victory number 11 by limiting the Blue Jays to one run over eight innings. Through the end of June, the Red Sox were 49-25 and eight games ahead of New York in the division. Raved Thomas Boswell of *The Washington Post:* "[Clemens] could be the Fenway Messiah—often sighted but never confirmed."

On June 27, Clemens became the fifth major league pitcher ever to begin a season 14-0 by dominating the Orioles 5-3 before 52,159 fans at Baltimore's Memorial Stadium—the second-largest crowd in the building's history. Much like Babe Ruth, Mickey Mantle and Reggie Jackson before him, Clemens was becoming an event in and of himself. *See the amazing Rocket and his 100-mph fastball!* He was The Story of Baseball: 1986, and even after he finally lost—a 4-2 setback to the Blue Jays on July 2 that dropped his record to 14-1—the buzz never died.

Thanks largely to Clemens, the Red Sox were running away with the American League East. They entered the All-Star break with a league-best 56-31 record and led the second-place Yankees by seven games. "It was a dream season," says Hurst. "For Roger, definitely. But for the Red Sox, too. It felt like we could do no wrong."

•   •   •

ALTHOUGH ROGER CLEMENS WAS now officially a superstar, the 57th annual All-Star Game, to be held in his backyard at the Houston Astrodome, would lift him to an even higher national level. As July 15 approached, giddy baseball enthusiasts openly pined for a battle of the sport's two top young guns—Clemens and Dwight Gooden of the New York Mets.

Ever since Clemens' first day in the big leagues two years earlier, he had heard the comparisons to New York's already legendary "Dr. K"—and Clemens dug it. During a 1985 season that rivaled the best of Sandy Koufax or Juan Marichal, Gooden went 24-4 with a 1.53 ERA and 268 strikeouts. He was the standard-bearer of modern pitching greatness, and eight days before the game, Dave Anderson of *The New York Times* wrote a piece all but demanding the match-up:

> For fastball aficionados, it's almost too good to be true. If baseball fans could vote for the starting pitchers of the All-Star Game, they would surely choose Dwight Gooden of the Mets and Roger Clemens of the Red Sox. And barring a muscle twinge, baseball's two most compelling pitchers will be firing dueling fastballs, if not dueling Ks, through the first three innings at the Houston Astrodome next Tuesday night.

Yet while most fans and journalists saw Clemens and Gooden as twin pillars of youthful heat, control and domination, those familiar with the two men viewed the meeting as shooting stars headed in opposite directions.

In the aftermath of his historic 1985 season, Gooden—polite, humble, soft-spoken, fearful of trouble—had started to change. Just 21 years old and highly impressionable, he saw the wild partying of his New York teammates and chose to follow along. He started to drink and smoke cigarettes and marijuana and, finally, snort cocaine.

Although he entered the All-Star break with a 10-4 record and 2.77

ERA, Gooden was now merely a very good right-handed pitcher. He was the classic example of what happens when a kid is thrown into the spotlight too swiftly, the classic example of what Boston hoped to avoid with Clemens.

Though as partiers the Red Sox paled in comparison to the high-flying Mets, the team had its fair share of deviants. Guys hit the clubs and slept around and drank to excess. It was the 1980s; surely some experimented with drugs. But not Clemens. "I only need to be a hero to my wife and family," he told *People*. "And I've always been a hero to them." Though time, fame and money would alter his behavior, in the mid-1980s the Boston ace walked the straight and narrow. He saw what drugs were doing to his older brother Randy, and it surely petrified him. On the road Clemens would go out with teammates, have dinner, maybe a beer, then return to his hotel room. "He was just a big kid," says one teammate. "When we went to Texas to play the Rangers, all he wanted to do was go on the water slides at Six Flags. He was an innocent, fun guy." In Boston, Roger was usually at home with Debbie, who was pregnant with the couple's first child. They would play Scrabble or watch television in their sparsely furnished Malden apartment.

"Wild stuff wasn't Roger's way," says Ed Jurak, a Red Sox utility infielder. "He wasn't into drugs, he wasn't into cheating on his wife. He was about one thing, and that was running, lifting weights, throwing and becoming the best pitcher the world had ever seen."

Clemens and Gooden did, indeed, start the All-Star Game, and while the Mets ace was battered around for three hits and two runs in three innings, the Rocket pitched three scoreless frames to win the MVP trophy.

"Roger Clemens," Mets outfielder Darryl Strawberry said afterward, "is going to be one of the greats of the game."

And Dwight Gooden, tragically, would never again live up to the hype.

•　　•　　•

DESPITE ROGER CLEMENS BEGINNING the second part of the season with a 15-2 record, history suggested that the immediate future might not be so kind. Four pitchers had won more consecutive starts to begin a year, and from the time their streaks had been snapped, all four (Rube Marquard, Elroy Face, Johnny Allen and Dave McNally) posted either .500 or sub-.500 records through season's end.

Not one to follow the pack, Clemens won his first three games after the break, prompting Tom Seaver, the legendary right-hander acquired by Boston in late June, to respond to the question "How can you help Roger?" with a memorable line: "Two things. At home, tell him what time the game starts. On the road, tell him what time the bus leaves."

On July 30, Clemens stepped onto the mound at Chicago's Comiskey Park sporting a 17-2 record and 2.50 ERA. With White Sox runners on the corners and the score tied at 2 in the bottom of the fifth, Harold Baines hit a roller toward first baseman Bill Buckner, who fielded the ball cleanly and tossed it to Clemens. Though not especially swift, Baines nearly outpaced Clemens to the bag. *Nearly.*

The video replay showed Clemens' foot beating Baines. The reaction of Boston players showed Clemens' foot beating Baines. But Greg Kosc, the first-base umpire, ruled that Clemens had missed the bag. Instead of the Red Sox recording the third out, Chicago's John Cangelosi scored the go-ahead run.

Over the next six minutes, Clemens morphed from cool gunslinger into the Incredible Hulk. Teammate Don Baylor held him back as he charged toward Kosc, spewing profanities. His eyes wide, spittle flying, Clemens' momentum carried his body into Kosc's arm—a baseball no-no. When Clemens saw on the Comiskey scoreboard that Kosc had missed the call, his anger only intensified. He was carried away, horizontally, by Baylor and Rice, screaming vulgarities the entire trip.

"Man, that did become a little shit storm," says Kosc. "In hindsight maybe I should have called [Baines] out because it was so close, but I remain convinced Roger did not make contact with the base."

That the White Sox won, 7-2, wasn't as significant as Clemens' ejection and resulting two-game suspension. Clemens may well have been blessed with an arm from Zeus, but he needed to manage his anger better. Coaches knew it, players knew it. Even Clemens begrudgingly admitted it. If he couldn't control himself in a relatively meaningless game against the lowly White Sox, how would he do come play-off time? "That was probably Roger's one weakness," says Mike Greenwell, a Boston outfielder. "Sometimes he'd get so fired up that he'd lose control."

It mattered not. The Red Sox ran away with the American League East, and Clemens was historically good. During a rocky stretch in mid- to late July, when Boston lost 10 of 13 games, the three wins were all courtesy of Clemens. "When he's pitching and we get three or four runs," Buckner said, "the other team is going to give up. The game is over."

Clemens wrapped up the regular season by winning seven straight decisions and hitting 100 mph on the radar against Detroit. On September 28 at Fenway Park, Boston beat second-place Toronto 12-3 to capture the franchise's first division crown in 11 years. Clemens, who wound up with a 24-4 record that would result in him being named the AL's Cy Young Award winner and Most Valuable Player, mounted a horse and took a victory ride seated behind a policeman. As the colt bucked, Clemens, wrote Leigh Montville of the *Globe*, "waved as if he were Clint Eastwood in the Rose Parade." Though his stated career goal was to one day reach the Hall of Fame, a World Series title placed a close second.

"This," said Clemens, "is what it's all about. This is what I pitch for."

FOR FOLLOWERS OF THE Red Sox, the thought of the postseason—though exciting and even a bit titillating—was usually accompanied by little optimism.

Boston had last won a World Series in 1918, and the decades that followed brought one embarrassment after another.

But maybe, just maybe, this year would be different.

The 1986 Red Sox won the AL East with a convincing 95-66 record, beating the Yankees by five and a half games in a race that never felt especially tight. Yet though the team was very good, what gave the city a true reason to believe was that, for the first time since Luis Tiant's mid-1970s heyday, a legitimate ace led the way.

Never was Clemens' fortitude more evident (or essential) than in the days before game one of the ALCS against the California Angels, when he stared down a pack of frenzied reporters inside Fenway's cramped home clubhouse and said, unequivocally, "I will be 100 percent for game one. No one is going to take it away from me."

In his final regular-season start, Clemens had been hit in the elbow by a line drive off the bat of Baltimore's John Stefero. He had been rushed to the hospital, and the elbow had swelled to the size of a small pumpkin.

In Boston, the city where sports optimism came to die, the widespread belief was that Clemens would miss his first start and maybe the entire postseason. Oddly (and comically), the immediate consensus of Angels fans was the exact opposite: *Of course Roger Clemens will return. He'll probably throw a no-hitter.* A team that had failed to reach the World Series in 25 years of existence, California diehards mimicked their Boston peers in expecting the worst. In the franchise's latest postseason implosion, the Angels had won the first two games of the 1982 ALCS against Milwaukee, only to lose the next three.

Clemens did start the first game, walking out to the Fenway Park mound to a boisterous ovation. The bunting was perfectly hung, the scent of popcorn and hot dogs filled the aisles, and blue and red baseball caps turned the stands into an ocean of color. Play-off fever had returned, and so had Clemens—the man to carry the Red Sox to new heights; the man who hadn't lost a game in more than two months; the man who would finally make people forget the trading of Babe Ruth and the repeated failures; the man who threw like lightning; who . . . who . . . who . . .

Got rocked.

In the first play-off start of his career, Clemens was battered for five runs in the first three innings of an 8-1 loss. His fastball, clocked at 95 mph, was plenty hard but all over the place. His breaking stuff was feeble. The high-octane refusal to lose that had made Clemens great during the regular season was now the cause of his doom. Clemens wasn't merely excited for the play-offs. He was pumped! He wanted to throw the baseball 200 mph! Blow a hole through the catcher's mitt!

In a pattern that would last throughout his career, Clemens followed up a horrible start by conceding nothing.

Roger, was it your elbow?

"No."

Roger, was it the cold weather?

"No."

Roger, did you just not feel right?

"I felt fine."

"He could've been overstrong," McNamara said. "He had six days off. That's a lot of time."

The thought was relayed to Clemens.

"No," he snapped. "I love to be too strong." Clemens, livid with himself, wasn't so thrilled with his manager, either. McNamara left him in for an exhausting 134 pitches, most coming after the game was out of hand. "What am I gonna do," McNamara asked, "throw in the towel?"

As he had repeatedly done before, Clemens was able to convince himself that the bad performance wasn't really so bad. Four days later, with the Angels leading two games to one, Clemens eagerly returned to the mound for game four in Anaheim. "I expect to dominate," he said. "After my last start, anything less than that would be disappointing."

What few fans knew was that, on the Red Sox flight from Boston to California following game two, Clemens had experienced an allergic reaction to the menthol in cigarette smoke, hacking so much that other passengers had been asked to extinguish their butts. When the pitcher arrived at Anaheim Stadium for his start, he was a mess. His nose was a faucet and his skin a lizardly shade of green. Generally animated before taking the field, he slouched by his locker and hoped for the best. When passers-by asked if he was OK, Clemens nodded glumly.

"But Roger always got going once he grabbed the ball," says Boyd. "He could be sick, sad, dying, whatever. Give him that ball, and the bad all goes away."

Clemens was good. Really good. Starting on three days' rest, he took a five-hit 3-0 lead into the ninth, looking as untouchable as he had in the regular season. Through the first eight innings, no Angel reached third base, and nine had struck out. "People forget how fantastic he was that day," says Dan Shaughnessy of *The Boston Globe*. "He was at his best." Yet after Clemens gave up a leadoff home run to Doug DeCinces to start the ninth, forced George Hendrick to ground out to third, then allowed back-to-back singles, McNamara, an erratic handler of pitchers, replaced him with Calvin Schiraldi, the former Longhorn whom Boston had obtained from the Mets during the off-season.

The result was disastrous. As had been the case at the University of Texas, Schiraldi struggled in a big spot. He surrendered two runs in the ninth, and two innings later California's Bobby Grich singled in the game winner. Schiraldi walked off the field, sat in the dugout and bawled. Now down three games to one, the Red Sox looked done.

"It's like we were on our deathbed," Clemens said, "and the preacher had to come read us the last rites." The obituaries were being written, the names of scapegoats marked in blood. McNamara would be flogged as a choker. Schiraldi would be dismissed as a bust. And Clemens would be labeled as "great—but not *quite* ready."

And then, defying history and logic, the doomed-to-choke Boston Red Sox fought back. Down to the last strike in the top of the ninth inning of game five, outfielder Dave Henderson hit a two-run homer off Donnie Moore to give Boston a 6-5 lead. Though the Angels tied the game in the bottom of the inning, Henderson won it in the 11th with a sacrifice fly. "One minute we were dead, and the next minute the Angels were dead," says Marty Barrett, Boston's second baseman. "The way I saw it, after Hendu hit that home run there was no way the Angels could come back. It broke their spirit."

As Barrett predicted, the Red Sox returned to Boston and dominated game six, 10-4. The following afternoon, a man spotted Angels slugger Reggie Jackson as he was strolling through the aisles of the Paperback Booksmith on Boylston Street.

"Hey Reggie, what's going to happen tonight?" he asked.

"We're gone, man," Jackson replied.

Pitching on three days' rest for a second straight outing, Clemens overwhelmed the Angels, allowing four hits over seven innings in Boston's ALCS-clinching 8-1 win. Because baseball historians remember the California-Boston series for Henderson's heroics and Moore's lapse (and, tragically, his suicide three years later), Clemens' excellence goes overlooked. "Anyone who questioned Roger's heart or courage had no idea what they were talking about," says Hurst, who afterward used a bottle of champagne to lather his friend's hair. "Roger was all about guts and courage. He carried us to the World Series."

FOR A NATION CLAMORING for a so-called Dream World Series, the Red Sox come-from-behind ALCS triumph was a gift from the baseball gods. For the first time in seven years, the clubs with the two best records in the game would meet for October supremacy. It was the miracle Mets against the miracle Red Sox. Dwight Gooden versus Roger Clemens. Keith Hernandez and Gary Carter versus Wade Boggs and Jim Rice. Two baseball cities, separated by a mere 210 miles, that hated each other. "The Athens and Sparta of baseball," said *Sports Illustrated.*

With a baseball-best 108 wins, as well as a dramatic six-game NLCS triumph over the Houston Astros, New York was favored by the experts. "We were both teams," says Boyd, "that knew how to overcome every type of adversity."

Boston opened the World Series on a high note, taking game one at Shea Stadium 1-0. Clemens tried cheering his team on but spent much of the time inside the clubhouse battling the flu. He was sapped of energy, lacking appetite, hot as a sauna, sweating profusely—and the game two starter against Gooden.

Few contests in World Series history had been accompanied by more hype. Though Gooden was by now engaged in a devilish battle with drug addiction, to New York's faithful he remained the beloved "Dr. K." Shea Stadium's 55,063 seats were filled, and those unable to snag tickets lined the parking lot with barbecues and portable televisions.

Unfortunately, both pitchers faltered. In his defense, Clemens—coughing up phlegm and shaking with the chills—looked as if he were dying. Over four and a third innings, he walked four and allowed three earned runs. Gooden was even worse, allowing eight hits and six runs in five sloppy innings. Boston won in a romp, 9-3.

The Red Sox had come to New York hoping to split the first two games. Instead, they won both.

NEW YORK FLEW TO Fenway and took the next two games, beating up on Boyd and Nipper, respectively. But when the Red Sox again pounded Gooden in game five, lighting him up for nine hits and four runs over four innings, Boston was on the verge of its first world title in 68 years. Hurst, who went the distance while holding the Mets to two runs in the 4-2 game five triumph, had emerged as Boston's surprising Fall Classic hero. And now, following five days of rest, it was Clemens' turn. Having posted what he considered to be a "sort of so-so" postseason, Clemens relished the chance to close out the Mets at Shea Stadium. "This year has been grueling on me," Clemens said. "I feel I have met the challenge. Now I have one more. This is the biggest game I've ever pitched. I think we're all going to be keyed up."

Through four innings Clemens was nearly perfect, yielding no hits and walking only one in the crisp 52-degree New York night. The Red Sox took an early 2-0 lead off of Mets starter Bobby Ojeda, and the damage should have been significantly greater. Over the course of the evening, Boston would strand 14 runners.

The Mets tied the game at 2 in the fifth, and on their bench players were starting to gain confidence. Hernandez, the Mets first baseman and a veteran with a keen eye for midgame trends, noticed that Clemens' fastball was flattening. "Look," he told teammates. "The guy is starting to lose it." Having logged 254 innings during the regular season plus another 27 in the postseason (his previous high had been 216 in 1984), Clemens was justifiably exhausted. Through the first three innings, 25 of his pitches were clocked in excess of 94 mph. Over the next three innings, the total dipped to three. "We needed to jump on Roger," says Ed Hearn, the Mets backup catcher. "He was hittable."

Yet somehow Clemens kept the Mets at bay. In the top of the seventh, with Boston runners on first and third, Evans hit an RBI grounder to second, handing Boston an important 3-2 advantage.

Though Clemens was struggling, the Mets weren't laying a hand on him. He was an unfamiliar pitcher with uncommon guts, and even if his fastball was starting to dip into the low 90s, New York's hitters still approached the plate with excessive caution and respect. After he retired the Mets in order in the bottom of the seventh, Clemens returned to the dugout, where McNamara greeted him. "Roger," he said, "I need to know how you're feeling right now."

Through seven innings, Clemens had thrown 135 pitches, limiting the Mets to four hits and two runs. While facing Mookie Wilson with one out in the seventh, however, he had torn a fingernail on his right hand. He was bleeding from both his index *and* middle fingers and could no longer throw a competent slider.

"Skip," Clemens said, "I can still go."

McNamara looked his ace up and down. What else was Roger Clemens going to say? Of course he thought he could still go. He *always* thought he could still go. McNamara, though, had other ideas.

"There's no way Roger wanted out," says Dave Stapleton, the backup first baseman. "I've heard a lot of lies about game six and that Roger asked McNamara out is one of them."

"Roger absolutely did not ask out of that game," says Barrett. "I was right there, and I can swear for a fact that he didn't. But Roger was young and respectful of authority, and he didn't say, 'I want to finish' either. He left it up to John McNamara."

With a runner on second and one out in the top of the eighth, McNamara sent Mike Greenwell, a rookie outfielder, to the plate to pinch-hit for Clemens. Just 23 years old and petrified, Greenwell struck out on three pitches.

The rest is baseball lore. The Red Sox brought in Schiraldi, the ex-Met, who surrendered the tying run in the bottom of the eighth, only to be saved by Henderson's two-run home run in the top of the ninth. Boston held a 5-3 lead in the bottom of the ninth, and the Mets' first two hitters, Wally Backman and Hernandez, made easy outs. Beneath the stadium, members of New York's equipment crew were busy wheeling dozens of bottles of bubbly into the Boston clubhouse, hanging WORLD CHAMPION BOSTON RED SOX T-shirts and hats in each locker stall. A scoreboard operator accidentally flashed CONGRATULATIONS RED SOX! across the Jumbotron.

Then Gary Carter singled up the middle. Kevin Mitchell, who moments earlier had been inside the clubhouse booking a flight back home to San Diego, blooped a single to second (with his fly open, no less). Third baseman Ray Knight, who had committed a throwing error to allow the Red Sox to take the lead, singled to center, scoring Carter and sending Mitchell to third with the potential tying run.

Throughout the previous inning, Clemens stood alongside Nipper in the bullpen, laughing and joking and even taking the time to sign an autograph for a security guard. As the Mets mounted a rally, he continued to whisper the same words, "It's OK . . . it's OK . . . just one more out . . . it's OK."

Now, however, it wasn't OK. Schiraldi was pulled, and into the game came right-hander Bob Stanley. He stood on the mound and stared down Wilson, the Mets' free-swinging outfielder. By now Clemens was sitting by himself, his palms rubbing together in prayer.

With the count 2-2, catcher Rich Gedman flashed the sign for Stanley to throw his palmball to the outside portion of the plate. Stanley nodded, reared back and let loose a pitch that fluttered . . . fluttered . . . fluttered, then—*snap!*—broke inside, past Wilson and Gedman and back behind the plate. Mitchell charged home with the tying run. The game Clemens had mastered less than an hour earlier was now tied.

Following two more foul balls, Wilson bounced the most famous slow roller in baseball history. As the ball approached Bill Buckner, the 36-year-old first baseman hung back, bent down, reached with his glove and . . . *nothing*. The baseball rolled between his legs and into right field. Knight charged home with the winning run.

For the next 20 minutes, Clemens sat in front of his locker, numb. He had given his all, and it wasn't enough. Two nights later, Boston's fate as chokers was confirmed yet again. The Red Sox lost game seven, 8-5.

Clemens couldn't leave New York soon enough. After the final game, Jack Rogers, Boston's traveling secretary, was standing in the Shea outfield when he was hit on the head with a beer bottle. "Baseball like it oughta be!" Clemens screamed toward the near-vacant upper deck. "They throw golf balls out of the stands and now this. This place sucks. They ought to blow the whole place up."

With the exception of Woody Booher's death, it was the lowest moment of Roger Clemens' life.

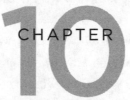

A Legend in Bloom

In the weeks and months after the World Series, the heartbroken Roger Clemens tried to move on. Unanimously winning the Cy Young Award didn't hurt, nor did becoming just the fourth pitcher to capture the American League Most Valuable Player trophy. To add to the good tidings, on December 4, 1986, Roger and Debbie were gifted with their first child, a boy named Koby Aaron Clemens. (The *K* is a nod to Roger's favorite letter—the symbol for "strikeout.") Standing at the hospital bedside of his wife, Roger was giddy. "I'm gonna tie the baby's right hand behind him and let him be a left-hander," he said. "I think they're in demand." A few days later, Roger ordered 100 Koby Clemens baseball cards, which, under CAREER HIGHLIGHTS, read, "In the year 2005, he stars at the University of Texas in baseball, beats Arizona State for the national title and catches the winning TD pass to beat Oklahoma, 21-14, in the Cotton Bowl."

Yet the harder Clemens tried to expunge the final moments of the 1986 season from his mind, the more he fumed. He could deal with falling to a team as good as the Mets. He could even accept, begrudgingly, having been removed from game six of the World Series. "Mac was doing what he thought was right," he told reporters. "It's not easy being a manager."

What Clemens could *not* deal with, however, was the tidbit that McNamara had told the media in the immediate aftermath of game six: That Roger Clemens had *asked* to be removed from the game.

Asked!? Bloody fingers be damned, Roger Clemens had never asked to be removed from anything. Yet there was McNamara, informing those who doubted his game-handling abilities that he had wanted to leave Clemens in; that there was no way in hell he would have willingly removed his best pitcher from a World Series game of that magnitude; that Clemens had—what's the best word?—*requested* to come out.

"The decision was definitely all Mac's," Clemens said. "He makes the decisions here."

To those who had come to know McNamara during his time in Boston, the shifting of blame was hardly a surprise. Though popular with a handful of Red Sox veterans, the 54-year-old skipper was a guarded, crotchety man who trusted few people outside his tight ring of coaches and friends. Upon being hired by the Red Sox, McNamara owned a lifetime major league record of 751-805 and had been fired three times. He saw himself as one of the geniuses of the game, and anyone who dared question his moves or motives was, in his eyes, a buffoon. "Everybody thinks he can do your job," he snarled. "Everybody."

So when the press asked about Clemens' departure from game six, what was he supposed to say? That he was wrong? No way. Not McNamara's style. He would blame his ace before taking any personal responsibility.

Clemens was livid. "Did McNamara tell you that he's a drunk?" he later asked television announcer Tim McCarver in an unsubstantiated off-the-air rant. "Did he tell you that he had the clubhouse guys fix him a drink in the fifth inning? That he was completely clueless?"

Upon reporting to spring training, Clemens' mood hardly improved. Because he had slightly more than two years of major league service, Clemens was required to pitch one more season before becoming eligible for arbitration. Hence, while Yankees first baseman Don Mattingly, the MVP *runner-up,* was being awarded a $1.975 million salary via arbitration, Clemens was forced to accept Boston's offer of $500,000—a mere $160,000 raise from 1986. "We decided to renew Roger's contract at a figure we think is fair," Lou Gorman, Boston's general manager, said at the time. "This is fair."

On March 6, shortly before he was scheduled to start Boston's exhibition opener, the furious Clemens bolted from camp without a word to the press. "Starting tomorrow, our offer to the Red Sox will increase by $1,500 a day," said Randy Hendricks, Clemens' agent. "I'm tired of reading the Red Sox have the hammer. Other people have hammers, too."

What frustrated Clemens wasn't necessarily the paltry contract offer but that the Red Sox had lied to him. During the off-season, Clemens, his agents and Gorman had agreed to a one-year, $1 million contract that left all sides smiling. Yet when Peter Ueberroth, baseball's commissioner, learned of the agreement, he called Gorman in a tizzy. "Lou, I'm reading that you're going to pay Roger Clemens $1 million," said Ueberroth. "Please tell me it's not true."

"That's right," said Gorman. "I shook hands and made a deal with the man."

A lengthy pause.

"Well, Lou, I'm ordering you not to give him $1 million," said Ueberroth. "You can't pay him more than $500,000. Not a penny more."

"But Pete," asked a stunned Gorman, "what am I supposed to do here?"

Over the previous two years, baseball's ruling class had colluded to drive down wildly escalating salaries. Whereas once upon a time free-agent stars such as Lance Parrish, Tim Raines and Bob Horner would have drawn competing bids from dozens of clubs, they were

now largely being ignored. Raines, the reigning National League batting champion, received a single offer—a $100,000 raise to return to
Montreal. Horner, one of the game's great power hitters with Atlanta,
was so insulted that he bolted for Japan's Yakult Swallows. Of baseball's 33 free agents from 1985 and '86, 29 returned to their old teams
without having received multiple offers. "Clubs are working together,
making fewer dumb financial decisions, signing fewer multiyear contracts," Toronto GM Pat Gillick told Ueberroth at the general managers' meetings.

"Be honest with each other," Ueberroth responded. "Exchange information."

Clemens was stung by Gorman's take-back and crushed when—in
an effort to defend its actions—the team compared Clemens to Bret
Saberhagen, the 1985 Cy Young Award winner for Kansas City, whose
lazy work habits had resulted in a mediocre follow-up campaign. "That
pissed me off pretty bad," Clemens said. "I don't appreciate hearing
those things."

On March 11, five days after he walked out, Clemens sent Debbie
and Koby back to Houston with plans to follow soon. "I'll tell you
this," he said. "They definitely picked the wrong person to make an
example of." That afternoon, the team announced that it would fine
its ace $1,000 per day until he returned to camp. The move, intended
to scare Clemens, instead angered him further.

At a press conference from his Houston office, Hendricks, sitting
alongside his client, became one of the first people to publicly call baseball's bluff. He cited an "overall plan orchestrated out of New York City
that says, 'We're going to hold down the salaries of all young players
irrespective of their performance' . . . if Roger can be knuckled under
and signed for a relatively low contract, every young professional that
shows up to negotiate for the next five years will be told, 'Why should
you get a large raise? Roger Clemens did not, and he won the Cy Young
and MVP award.' "

In the Red Sox clubhouse, players were well aware that the team had screwed Clemens over. More than on most clubs, Boston veterans generally trusted the owners. When there had been a threat of a players strike in 1985, Bobby Ojeda, at the time a 27-year-old pitcher, stood up during a team meeting and screamed, "Fuck the owners! The owners don't give a fuck about us!" He had been shouted down by older teammates. Now, however, the question in the clubhouse was a good one: If Gorman is willing to treat a reigning 24-game winner like this, how will he treat . . . *me?* "I guarantee you, everybody on this team agrees with [Roger]," said pitcher Al Nipper. "He's just doing what he thinks is right."

By March 20, Clemens was back home in Texas, throwing batting practice to Spring Woods' varsity team, taking daily four-mile runs and demanding a two-year, $2.4 million deal. To the world, he appeared resolute. In his head, he was tormented. Unlike most ballplayers, who viewed spring training as one long, sweat-engulfed nightmare, Clemens lived for the regimentation and detail. He liked the feel of perspiration trickling down his forehead, of the Florida sun beating on his back. He wanted to run endless wind sprints, then take a five-mile jog through the unpaved side streets of Winter Haven. He missed the chorus of "Man, you work hard" and "You're gonna kill us." Clemens lived for the regular season, but he *fed off* of spring training.

And now, thanks to the greed of multimillionaire owners, he was in Houston, pitching to pimply 17-year-olds.

If the pitcher and his agent believed the public would have sympathy for a 24-year-old man *forced* to take $500,000, they were badly mistaken. "When a baseball player talks about principle, it's hard to get sympathy," said Kirk McCaskill, a California Angels pitcher. "It's hard for people to understand because of the money." Sure, over the previous three seasons baseball's attendance had risen by 16 percent. And sure, baseball's licensing revenues had skyrocketed by more than 150 percent, to $450 million. And sure, the man driving down his salary—in this case, Red Sox general partner Haywood Sullivan—was über-rich. But throughout the sporting universe, where to many fans and pundits a half-million dollars sounded like a lottery bonanza, Clemens was yet another greedy athlete. Wrote Scott Ostler of the *Los Angeles Times:* "Would someone please tell this kid, who has exactly one good big-league season, that all he has to do is win 15 games this year and he'll get an automatic $1 million minimum in arbitration next season, and so on, up into the stratosphere? Is that such a bad deal, Roger? Can you suck it up for one year, scrape by on half a mill?"

Finally, alarmed by the media attention being given to the Clemens–Red Sox battle, Ueberroth intervened to help reach a settlement nobody was happy with: $650,000 in 1987, $1.5 million in 1988. On April 4, 1987, Clemens returned to Winter Haven and rejoined the organization.

Barely a month had passed since he left, but in that time period Clemens had changed dramatically. He would pitch for the fans and for his teammates and for the love of the game, but—come day's end— he would pitch mostly for himself.

ON APRIL 11, FOLLOWING a single exhibition start, Roger Clemens made his 1987 debut, allowing four runs over four innings in an 11-1 loss to Toronto at Fenway Park. It was his earliest departure from a game in nearly two years.

Those Red Sox loyalists who hoped the 1987 season would be a natural continuation of the magical '86 run were disappointed. The Red Sox who took the field to defend the American League pennant were a splintered group, still tormented over the way the previous year had ended. "It hasn't been much fun," said Don Baylor, the team's designated hitter. "Last year when we won, the Red Sox were 'we.' Over the winter it was completely different. It was 'This guy didn't catch that ball,' 'This guy didn't throw the right pitch.' All of a sudden everything was 'I,' and that's not the way you do things."

When an exasperated McNamara held a team meeting for players to express their gripes openly, nary a word was spoken. "I guess," Baylor said afterward, "the differences are still there."

Although Clemens declared himself in tip-top shape, the results told a different story. After 12 starts, his record sat at 4-5, and while his 3.07 ERA ranked sixth in the league and his 84 strikeouts fourth, he was merely a very good pitcher—not the Rocket. His fastball was unpredictably tailing left and right. His newest pitch, a split-fingered fastball that was supposed to look like a heater, then drop, was hanging up in the zone. The umpires were squeezing him, his conditioning was so-so, and the hometown fans—still agitated by the holdout—were ambivalent. Clemens blew a 9-0 lead to the Yankees and a 7-0 lead to the Angels. Against the Twins on June 1, Clemens gave up seven earned runs, including a career-high three homers. "He doesn't have the control he had, that's the problem," said Marty Barrett, Boston's second baseman, after the game. "That, plus the fact that hitters aren't going for his high fastball. And we just haven't scored runs for him."

By early July, the Red Sox—done in by an aging roster and the ghost of Mookie Wilson—were 39-43 and eleven and a half games out of first, and Clemens was 7-6. McNamara, who was in charge of selecting the American League pitchers for the All-Star team, left his ace off, denying him of a $300,000 bonus. It was hard to argue. "He's 7-6," said Gorman. "If he were 17-5 that would be a different story."

Clemens recovered to have a 12-3 second half, but with the Red Sox clubhouse in turmoil and the bullpen a pit of mediocrity (the team recorded a league-worst 16 saves) and McNamara's pep talks largely ignored, Boston plummeted to fifth place in the AL East, 20 games behind the champion Detroit Tigers.

It was an unhappy time to be a Boston ballplayer, and Clemens—still stung by the contract negotiations—was unhappier than ever. At home he enjoyed playing with his infant son, and on the road he relished the companionship of pals such as Nipper, Bruce Hurst and Oil

Can Boyd. But he hadn't endured losing like this in years. What was it Randy used to say? That winning was contagious. Well, so was losing. While Clemens continued to run and lift with a prize fighter's intensity, older teammates packed it in. Where was Bill Buckner's heart? Dwight Evans' drive? Where was the rooting for one another? The shouts of encouragement?

Where were the Boston Red Sox of old?

One of the few highlights (and oddest moments) of the Rocket's season came on Friday, September 4, when he appeared in the Plymouth Room of Boston's Lafayette Hotel to—according to a press release—"discuss fashion tips and 'How to Score with Your Wardrobe This Season.'" According to Lois Frankenberger of the Jordan Marsh department stores, Clemens represented the company's "All Star Team '87—a group of sports figures who have achieved a personal style most admired by fashion experts." That two of Clemens' wardrobe staples were weathered jeans and cowboy boots mattered not. For two hours (and a $5,000 appearance fee, plus free clothing), he signed autographs and looked pretty.

The remainder of the season, though, was ugly. With the Red Sox languishing in fifth place, Gorman waved the white flag, trading Buckner to California, Baylor to Minnesota and Dave Henderson, the '86 play-off hero, to San Francisco. By August, the lone reason for fans to head out to Fenway was to watch Clemens. In his final start of the year against Milwaukee, Clemens tossed a complete-game two-hitter, striking out 12 in Boston's 4-0 win at Fenway. The triumph made him the first AL pitcher to have back-to-back 20-victory seasons since Tommy John in 1979–80. "I'm trying to win the Cy Young," he said afterward, "and I didn't want to leave any doubt in anybody's mind."

By finishing 20-9 and leading the league with seven shutouts and 18 complete games, Clemens reinforced his status as baseball's best arm. Just a year earlier, people had been asking whether he or Dwight Gooden would be the next mound superstar. Now, with the Mets right-hander having missed a portion of the season after failing a drug test, there was no question. Clemens captured 21 of 28 first-place Cy Young votes. "It's gratifying because it puts me in a class with people I looked up to," he said. "[Sandy] Koufax, [Denny] McLain and [Jim] Palmer. I felt I beat the Cy Young jinx. A lot of guys have gone by the wayside after having a good year. Now maybe I have a chance to do something nobody's ever done and that's win it three times in a row."

ON THE AFTERNOON OF May 30, 1988, the telephone rang in the small visiting clubhouse at Anaheim Stadium.

"Roger," said one of the equipment guys, "it's for you. Sounds sort of important."

In the immediate hours before his starts, Clemens habitually hid from the world. Teammates knew to leave him alone. Reporters tip-toed by. If you were a clubhouse attendant who needed to, say, lean in and pick up his dirty shorts, well, you didn't. Once, while preparing for a start in Oakland, Clemens knocked over an elderly reporter. He failed to apologize, oblivious that the collision had even taken place. "I could walk right by my mother, and she'd be yelling in my ear, and I wouldn't even notice," he said. "I've got my mind on something else."

But this was a special circumstance. On the other end of the line was Debbie Clemens, calling from their home in Texas. "Roger," she said, "I've gone into labor."

In the course of the previous few weeks, Roger and Debbie had discussed what would transpire should this happen while he was at the ballpark. The resolution was obvious: He would immediately drop what he was doing and come home. No fuss, no debate, no questions asked. Through the first two months of the season, as the Red Sox struggled to keep pace in the loaded AL East, Clemens was as master-ful as ever. He entered the night with a 7-2 record and 1.80 ERA; so overpowering that, upon being asked whether anyone would match his 31-win season of 1968, former Tigers ace Denny McClain replied, "Roger Clemens, that's who." In other words, the Rocket had earned the right to take a night off—especially for the birth of his second child.

Yet now, approximately an hour before his 12th start of the season, Clemens looked deep within himself, debated the priorities of family versus baseball—and chose baseball. "I'm going to pitch," he told his wife. "And as soon as the game is over, I'll be there."

The baby, a boy named Kory Allen Clemens, was born later that day, healthy and without complications. Through the years, Debbie Clemens has been asked about that moment, and she maintains that her spouse made the proper call. The pitcher's decision was even lauded by Richard Justice of *The Washington Post*, who praised Clemens' guts, determination and dedication by writing, "It was the best of times, it was the worst of times, but when it was over, the legend of William Roger (Rocket) Clemens had grown a little more."

"He's amazing," Rich Gedman, Boston's catcher, told Justice. "He's got a fire inside him like I've never seen in anyone else in my life." Indeed, Clemens' showing against the Angels was phenomenal. Despite being, in Clemens' words, "distracted," he struck out nine in a complete-game 5-2 Sox triumph. Yet although the moment certainly emphasized Clemens' rugged approach to the game, it also hinted at something else: a superstar's unparalleled self-centeredness. "The guys who are not egomaniacs would have gone home, because they can get outside of themselves and know the right thing is to be with their wives," says Pat Jordan, the former minor league pitcher and noted sportswriter. "But the egomaniacs cloak their egos with 'I can't let my team down' or 'I owe it to the organization.' Which is another way of answering the question: What would you rather do, pitch a baseball game or watch your wife go through labor?"

Immediately after the game Clemens' trip to the airport was delayed so that he could explain his decision to the assembled media.

"Sure, I'd like to have left," Clemens told Dave Strege of the *Orange County Register*. "But I owe it to the team. We've been struggling, and anything I can contribute, that's my job." The scenario was eerily similar to an episode that had taken place 14 years earlier, when Steve Garvey, the Los Angeles Dodgers' first baseman, missed the birth of his daughter, Krisha, in order to play in game two of the World Series against Oakland. When a nurse asked Cindy Garvey whether she wanted to watch the game, she launched into a tirade. "I'm just coming out of anesthesia—the nurse is putting on the TV," she later recalled. "I screamed at her to shut it off. Hell, he didn't come to watch me. I could have died in childbirth, and my man wouldn't have been there."

"I've seen it happen a million times," says Jordan. "An athlete reaches a certain level of success, and his ego takes off."

Those who know Clemens well pinpoint the start of the ego explosion to the week of the 20-strikeout night of 1986, when the fat kid from the Dayton suburbs officially became a star. A couple of days after that game, Clemens offered every Boston player and coach an autographed photograph of his record-setting 20th strikeout. The gesture, while commendable on the surface, begs the question: What type of person presents a signed picture of *himself* as a present?

Throughout the 1987 and '88 seasons, Clemens increasingly referred to himself as "Rocket" and "Rocket Man" during interviews, an offputting third-person usage. (Never a fan of Clemens, third baseman Wade Boggs instead called him "Mr. Perfect.") Especially bizarre was his insistence that his offsprings' names begin with the letter *K*. When Debbie told her husband that she liked "Coby" for son number one, Roger's response was, "Great! And we can spell it with a *K!*" Upon learning his wife was pregnant again, Roger immediately scouted out *K* names. (He settled on Kevin Anthony but Debbie didn't like it, so the couple went with Kory Allen.) As the years passed, the couple's two additional children—boys named Kacy and Kody—would also be branded with a *K*. "If you want to make the argument that we're talking about one egomaniacal motherfucker, look at the four *K* names," says one of Clemens' major league peers. "Who does that?"

As Jordan would later write of Clemens in a piece for *The New York Times Magazine:*

> A French dilettante once said, "I am such an egotist that if I were to write about a chair I'd find some way to write about myself."
>
> Clemens's egotism is more childlike and innocent. He doesn't realize that he sees himself as the center of his small universe, at the center of every story he tells . . .
>
> Everyone is a bit player in Clemens's universe, even his beloved mother, Bess, who reared him and his five siblings mostly without a father. She left her first husband when Clemens was a baby, and her second husband died when Clemens was 9. Bess has been fighting emphysema for years. "She has her good days and bad," Clemens says. "I only hope she can hang on to see me go into the Hall of Fame."
>
> Clemens assumes everyone's pleasure revolves around him. . . . He says he hates to miss a start because that might deprive his fans, especially young boys, from the pleasure of seeing "the Rocket Man punch out 20." The Rocket Man is his nickname. He sometimes autographs his book "Rocket Man" or "Roger 'The Rocket' Clemens" and then adds a list of his awards.

When the Clemens family purchased a Porsche, Roger insisted on a CY-MVP vanity license plate. When Clemens ate out at a restaurant, he would look around, hoping someone would recognize him. (Then, when he was recognized, he would audibly complain about the lack of privacy.)

Strangely, Clemens' blooming ego was a boom to his pitching. Even as he became consumed with his own accomplishments (the family's Texas home doubled as a private Roger Clemens museum, overloaded with displays of game balls and autographed photographs), an arrogant Clemens was a dogged Clemens. Not only did he believe himself to be the best, he wanted to stay there. During the offseason, Clemens had added a half inch to each thigh by working religiously on a leg machine in his garage. He arrived four or five hours before games he wasn't starting, delving into a regimen of film study, fly-ball shagging, wind sprints and stretching. "He was the most intense, most competitive guy I'd ever played with," says Rick Cerone, a Boston catcher in 1988–89. "The first game I ever caught him, the first guy for Detroit gets a single and the second guy homers. Well, the third guy comes up, and Roger fires a ball over the top of his head and starts screaming, 'This shit is going to stop now!' And it did."

For the injury-plagued Red Sox, however, Clemens' drive wasn't nearly enough. At the 1988 All-Star break the club was 43-42 and nine games behind Detroit in the AL East. "All things considered," McNamara said, "I'm very happy to be one game over .500."

That quote—optimistic mediocrity—proved to be McNamara's noose. Over the objections of Lou Gorman, Jean Yawkey, the team's co-owner, fired her manager four hours before the Sox were scheduled to face Kansas City to start the season's second half. Boston's players were thrilled. Lee Smith, the team's new closer, routinely griped about the way McNamara used him, and young players such as Mike Greenwell, Todd Benzinger and Jody Reed had been pining for his dismissal for weeks. Nobody was more giddy than Clemens, who had never forgiven his skipper for selling him out in the press after game six of the 1986 World Series.

Boston's new manager was Joe Morgan, a 57-year-old Walpole, Massachusetts, native who had hit .193 in 88 career major league games before beginning a lengthy minor league coaching career in 1966. Morgan finally stuck in the bigs in 1985, when he was named to

McNamara's staff, and through the first half of the '88 campaign he was quite content coaching third base. "Nobody really thought of him as the next manager of the Red Sox," says Gorman. "But we needed someone."

Morgan debuted on July 15 at Fenway, and the Sox swept Kansas City in a doubleheader. Boston went on to win 12 straight (24 straight at home) and 19 out of 20, and suddenly the city was caught up in "Morgan's Magic."

"It was funny, because Joe was just this good ol' boy," says Cerone. "Yet everything he touched turned into gold. He couldn't do wrong."

By August 3, Boston and Detroit were tied for first. Morgan's club was hailed as the lovable scrappers from Beantown, rallying behind a native-son skipper and a bunch of fresh-faced kids such as Reed, Greenwell and Ellis Burks. Yet at a time he should have been carrying his ball club, Clemens' output was perplexing. On August 14, he endured the worst outing of his career, giving up eight runs in one and a third innings in Detroit's 18-6 demolition at Fenway. It was his third straight loss, and Boston's 24-game home winning streak was kaput. "The Boston Red Sox aren't upset about falling farther behind Detroit in the American League East," wrote Ben Walker of the Associated Press. "They're too worried about the question all of New England is asking: What's wrong with Roger Clemens?"

As the Red Sox surged toward the division title behind the starting pitching of Mike Boddicker and Bruce Hurst, Clemens imploded, enduring a 1-6 stretch through much of August and September. Prior to his mystifying downturn, Clemens was 15-5 and leading the league in ERA, shutouts, strikeouts and complete games. Boston finished 89-73, winning the AL East by a single game, but Clemens was miserable. He pouted. He moaned. He passed on going out with teammates, instead sitting in his hotel room or lifting weights. His numbers (18-12, 2.93 ERA) looked great on paper but were deceiving. Wrote Shaughnessy, "Strange as it sounds, Clemens has been Boston's fourth-best starter in August and September. That's like thinking of John Lennon as the fourth-best Beatle."

In Boston, reporters were wondering aloud whether Clemens was hurt, slumping, distracted—or merely folding in a tight pennant race. Fans booed him. Boston was a city of heart and drive and grit, but where was *Rah-jah*'s heart and drive and grit? "With Roger, there was always a lot of piling on from people," says Shaughnessy. "When he didn't pitch well, there was no place to hide."

The Red Sox faced Oakland in the American League Championship Series, and after the A's beat Hurst in game one at Fenway, it was up to Clemens to shut down the best lineup in baseball.

For six innings, Clemens was the Rocket of old, striking out eight and holding a 2-0 lead. With a runner on first and no outs in the top of the seventh, Clemens stared down at Jose Canseco, Oakland's right fielder and soon-to-be AL MVP. Canseco liked heat. Clemens threw heat. Canseco was all about power. Clemens was all about power. Canseco never backed down. Clemens never backed down.

Clemens threw an 0-2 fastball over the plate.

Canseco cocked his bat.

Boom!

The ball went far into the Boston sky, finally landing in the netting above the Green Monster. Game tied, 2-2. Four batters later, Mark McGwire singled home the go-ahead run, and Boston lost 3-2.

Another play-off start, another play-off disappointment for Roger Clemens. With two more wins, Oakland swept the Red Sox to advance to the World Series.

Once again, Boston fans were left wondering about their ace. Was he a savior or just a great pitcher with questionable fortitude?

Most important, was he a winner?

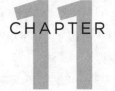

CHAPTER

11

Baggage

His intentions were righteous.

Really, they were.

Roger Clemens wanted his teammates to be treated with respect and dignity by an organization that, all too often in the late 1980s, seemed to view its employees as chattel. He wanted the families of players to be given tickets for the upper box seats close to the dugout, not the grandstand behind home plate. He wanted a security guard for the family room, parking for wives, a telephone in the home clubhouse (as opposed to the pay phone in the concourse). In short, Roger Clemens wanted Major League Baseball players to be treated like Major League Baseball players.

"Roger stood up for us," says Tom Bolton, a Boston pitcher. "He wasn't the official player rep, but he took it upon himself to fight our battles."

That, more than anything, is how Clemens found himself staring into a TV camera on the afternoon of December 5, 1988, sitting alongside Channel 5's Mike Lynch for a highly publicized two-part interview. Had he been, say, Marty Barrett or Ellis Burks, Clemens would have used the airtime to tell funny stories or praise Fenway Park or discuss the migratory patterns of Mediterranean bluefin tuna.

Instead, he vented.

In a rambling ode to the dangers of speaking before one thinks, Clemens went off on everyone, from Red Sox fans to the owners to his teammates. His furor was sparked by Bruce Hurst's imminent departure to San Diego as a free agent and how little the Sox had done to keep him. "There are some things going on there in Boston that make it a bit tough as far as on your family," he said. "Travel, road trips and carrying your own luggage around isn't all that fun and glory."

Wait. Had a man about to sign a three-year, $7.5 million deal complained about having to carry his own luggage? To suggest the session didn't go over particularly well is the greatest of understatements. "[The interview]," wrote Jack Craig of *The Boston Globe*, "exposed nature's revenge in giving Clemens a weak mind to go with a strong arm."

Boston's fans were livid, overloading the Red Sox switchboard the following morning with one "To hell with Roger Clemens" call after another. "When I saw that Clemens on TV last night, it was the first time in my life that I wanted to throw something through the set," said Dan Coughlin of Dorchester, a Sox fan for 50 years. "I wouldn't want my grandchildren to be like him. What kind of role models are these guys?"

Will McDonough, the *Boston Globe* columnist who had nicknamed Clemens "the Texas Con Man," teed off:

The average person does not think it is a hardship to wait four hours in an airport for a plane when you are getting paid big money to do it. The average person does not think it is a hardship if a player's wife does not have a seat where she can see the mound or give her husband a kiss on the way off the field. The average person does not think it is a hardship if the team does not provide a place for the wives to park. The average person makes a living and doesn't bring a spouse to work. If your wife is going to be a distraction at the game, let her stay home. You are getting paid thousands per game to be on the mound pitching the best you can without distractions.

The backlash stunned Clemens. He was just trying to stand up for his guys. Yet in a follow-up televised interview intended to make amends, Clemens again placed his cleats squarely in his mouth. "These things just need to be taken care of, and, again, I'm not going to go into it, but that's what bothers me, too," he said, rambling on for several minutes. "If somebody, you know . . . I don't . . . ah, and it's something I'm going to have to take care of myself, but I don't appreciate reporters writing about my family. And somebody's gonna get hurt one time doing that. I don't have a problem saying that. I don't care what somebody writes or says about me, but now when they start talking about my wife or my kids, somebody's gonna get hurt and it's not gonna be me, because I don't appreciate those things 'cause, again, I'm the one doing the job of trying to perform a service. And again, I'm very serious in saying those words because that means something to me."

Uh . . .

Though nobody seemed 100 percent certain what Clemens was talking about, it didn't sound good. He made additional efforts in the coming days to repair his image until, at the urging of his agents, he stopped talking. By then, however, he was no longer Boston's golden boy. All professional athletes are allowed to make certain mistakes—to drop a ball or miss a practice or even curse out an overzealous coach. Clemens, however, had stepped over an uncrossable line. As the nation battled an increasingly deteriorating economy, Clemens was whining about the hardscrabble life of a baseball player. "Nobody," says Dan Shaughnessy, "wants to hear that stuff. Especially in a city like Boston."

Was Clemens the ingrate writers like McDonough made him out to be? No. Though plenty cocky, Clemens was, simply, a man who knew how to do one thing very well but struggled in most other areas. His baseball traveled 96 mph, but his quotations went up and down, left and right. His mind thought one thing, his tongue and lips said something entirely different. He often stared at reporters with the vacant gaze of a seven-year-old boy in an adult-level spelling bee. The Rocket heard the questions, understood most of the words, yet just couldn't get out what he wanted to say. Clemens loved pitching at Fenway Park. But when it came time to transform his feelings into eloquent words, he was at a loss. The baseball diamond was his medium of choice. The English language was not.

For Clemens and the Red Sox, 1989 did not go smoothly. The team finished third with an 83-79 record, and the pitcher compiled a 17-11 mark and 3.13 ERA. For most major leaguers, the statistics would have suggested a career year. Not Clemens, who found that everything he touched turned into excrement. He promised to throw an opening-day no-hitter versus Baltimore but gave up four runs in a Red Sox loss. The *Boston Herald* fired him as a guest columnist. An anonymous teammate told a writer, "Clemens, is he on the team? We hardly see him. He comes and does his work, but it's not like he's even on the team." Pat Santarone, the Baltimore Orioles groundskeeper, told *The Baltimore Sun* that, in 21 years on the job, the only player he had ever had trouble with was Clemens. Joe Morgan fined Clemens for leaving the stadium before the completion of a game. Greenwell ripped the team's pitching staff, and he and Clemens squared off in the clubhouse.

"Just get your fucking hits!" Clemens screamed.

"Fuck you!" countered Greenwell.

"No, fuck you!"

Clemens even had it out with one of his boyhood idols. On April

30, he started against the Texas Rangers and their ace, 42-year-old Nolan Ryan, at Arlington Stadium. In the top of the fourth inning, Ryan threw a fastball that nailed Jim Rice's shoulder. In the dugout Clemens stood up and screamed. "All right, you want to play that, we'll play that!" Staring at the ground, Ryan raised his head and flashed his serial-killer glare directly at the young pitcher. Frightened, Clemens froze. He was humiliated and uttered not another word.

Oh, and the Red Sox lost.

BY NOW, ANY WARM, fuzzy feelings about Roger Clemens were gone.

The media found him to be guarded, unfriendly and, quite often, full of it. Boston's fans questioned both his fortitude and his awareness of their existence. Teammates often wondered where he was. "Roger earned the right to act a certain way," says pitcher Greg Harris. "But you still have to be there for your team." He remained one of the American League's two or three best starters, but the luster had been lost. Over the previous two seasons, Clemens had tried to incorporate his curveball and slider more prominently into the repertoire. The result was a better-rounded pitcher, but also a pitcher prone to occasional blunders. He was, at last, hittable.

In these tough days, there was one person Roger Clemens had always turned to: His older brother.

The years had not been kind to Randy Clemens. He was 35, unemployed and in the midst of a life implosion. Though Randy's downfall had started in college, it gained momentum during the 1985–86 prep basketball season, when Troy High School, finally exhausted by the yelling and the ranting and the embarrassing behavior, fired him. Two incidents sealed his fate. The first stemmed from an ongoing conflict with Tom Dunn, the school's girl's basketball coach, concerning usage of the school's gymnasium for practice time. Following several heated exchanges over a few weeks, Randy snapped. Surrounded by the girls' *and* boys' teams, he lit into Dunn. "Get your team out of the fucking gym before I kick your fucking ass!" he screamed. "I fucking mean it!"

The second incident occurred during a game at Springfield South, when a referee made a series of iffy calls against Troy. "Randy thought he could work the officials like Bobby Knight, and this guy wasn't having it," says Larry South, a Troy assistant coach. "They went back and forth, and Randy—who always had to be the biggest, toughest man—starts moving toward the ref at half court. It looked like they were going to fight."

Suddenly, from the top of the wood bleachers stormed *the* Roger Clemens, in town to visit his brother. The Rocket hurdled the scorer's table, charged the referee and jabbed a finger toward his chest while pushing Randy aside. "Roger was out of his mind," says South. "He'd flipped, and he looked like he was going to do something violent."

Officials from both schools intervened, but it was apparently too late for Randy Clemens.

First, he was ejected.

Then, come season's end, he was canned.

"His reputation was tattered," says South. "Nobody was going to hire him after that."

For most of his life, Randy's world had revolved around basketball. He knew he was destined to become a big-shot coach, that it was merely a matter of time before someone came to Troy, recognized his genius and offered him a Division I contract. With his dismissal, however, the dream was over. He would never coach again. Now the father of a son, Marcus, and a daughter, Jessica, Randy eventually moved his family to Lakeland, Florida, where he worked managing a sporting goods store. But warm weather and the idea of a fresh start proved illusory. Randy was devastated when his wife, Kathy, packed her belongings, grabbed the children and left for good. "She was tired and fed up and finally couldn't take anymore," says Carolyn Gray, Kathy's sister. "Randy lived in this secret world of drug abuse, where he became an embarrassment. She spent years trying to hide his problem from us, but by those last few years it was pretty obvious. Randy was really, really bad." According to associates, "bad" understates Randy's cocaine use. "I don't think he was a bad guy," says Gray. "But the drugs turned him into something devilish."

The only thing Randy could cling to was his younger brother. Without Roger to serve and support and brag about, what was Randy but a washed-up has-been jock? He threw himself into Roger's career, negotiating his brother's first big-league contract and—once Roger hired real agents—hanging on as a "representative."

During Roger's holdout before the 1987 season, Dan Shaughnessy of *The Boston Globe* tried to reach him for comment and couldn't. He tried to reach Roger's agents and couldn't. So he drove to Lakeland and knocked on Randy's door. Though nobody from Roger's side was supposed to comment, Randy commented. "If Lou [Gorman] wants to get nasty about this, Roger will demand to be traded, and I don't think they want a mad Roger Clemens around," he said. "This is just going to be a knock-down, drag-out fight. Roger is extremely serious about this. He does not want to be made an example of. He told me he's going to sell his house as soon as possible. He means business."

Roger had said nothing of demanding a trade, let alone selling his house. He just wanted a fair deal. It was one of the last times Randy Clemens would ever be quoted in a newspaper article in relation to his brother.

Not that Roger cut Randy off completely. Not yet, at least. He was still Roger's boyhood hero, still the big brother who had taught him how to compete and work and win. They spoke regularly on the telephone, and though Roger was certainly aware of Randy's battles with drugs, the topic was never broached with teammates or coaches. "I had no idea about that," says Dennis Boyd. "None at all."

One can only imagine what this was like for Clemens, especially when Kathy and the children moved from Florida to Texas to be closer to Roger's mother, Bess (who would help with child care). It was the darkest secret in the already private life of a baseball superstar, and it ate Roger up.

Perhaps that's part of the reason why, come 1990, he seemed more angry, agitated and reclusive than ever. During baseball's 32-day lockout from February 15 to March 18, most franchise players spoke out on behalf of the cause. Not Roger, who skipped out on the Boston Baseball Writers Dinner and refused to return calls from the *Globe* and *Herald*. Even when the impasse ended, Clemens maintained an air of defiance, wearing uniform number 14 in honor of the departed Jim Rice (Clemens was furious that Boston hadn't re-signed the slugger) and treating the media as if they were grime beneath his thumb. He felt that the press had been excessively hard on him the previous season and he no longer owed time to these "rats" (his word) who infested the clubhouse. "The same press that sat on my lawn, came into my house and played with my kids turned on me," he said. "I've been paraded as a spoiled athlete. I'm not a spoiled athlete, I'm a human being."

In 1990, Clemens waged his personal battle against, well, everyone. He kept track of those who had questioned his fortitude and strove to shove it down their throats. There was a newfound rawness to the man, a disconcerting intensity that overwhelmed opponents and worried teammates and coaches. Following a three-hitter at Milwaukee, Clemens lingered in the trainer's room and the shower as reporters waited to speak with him and teammates boarded the bus for the airport. "If that were me," one player groused to Jack Rogers, the team's traveling secretary, "you'd be pulling me out of there by my ears." Around that same time, Clemens walked off the team's charter flight when he decided the delay was too long. His teammates were livid— especially when Clemens got Rogers banned from road trips. When Clemens demanded that media no longer be allowed on the team bus on trips to and from the airport, the Red Sox complied. "His ego was very, very big," says Joe Hesketh, a Red Sox pitcher. "I love Roger. But I can't lie about it. He could be a pain."

Clemens opened the year by compiling an 11-2 record and 2.60

ERA, and his command had never been better. There were pitchers who threw harder and there were pitchers with sharper control, but in 1990 nobody mastered both with such aplomb. "All you could hope for as a hitter was that Roger would hang something up in the zone," says Billy Jo Robidoux, a Red Sox first baseman. "The problem was, that season Roger never hung something up in the zone. Everything was fast, hard, precise."

Even when Clemens didn't have his best stuff, he refused to settle for an off night. Shortly after being knocked out by the Orioles in the second inning of his June 18 start, he could be seen running the streets outside Memorial Stadium—sprinting, jogging, sprinting, jogging. Should he have been inside, rooting on his teammates during a 7-2 loss for which he was largely responsible? "Yes," says Hesketh. "But when you saw someone at that level of greatness working *that* hard, it sent a very profound message to the rest of us. If Roger Clemens takes his work that seriously, so should we."

If Clemens' 1986 dream season was a 99 on a 1-to-100 scale, this was a 98.5. He entered the All-Star break with a league-high 12 wins (he made the team but, suffering from a dead arm, did not pitch), and Boston sat a half game in front of Toronto in the AL East with a 46-36 mark. Whereas past Boston juggernauts had been powered by right-handed hitting, these Sox were all about pitching. At 12-4 (and an astonishing 9-1 following Boston losses), Clemens was headed toward his third Cy Young Award, and Mike Boddicker (11-4) and Greg Harris (7-3) were solid complimentary starters. Clemens captured his 20th win with a 9-2 drubbing of Cleveland on August 30, reducing his major league–low ERA to 1.95 and increasing his strikeout total to 198. He completed the month with a 6-0 mark. "We're talking about a guy who comes around every 25 years," said Bill Fischer, Boston's pitching coach. "How many are there? Whitey Ford in the late '50s and early '60s. Nolan Ryan. Bob Feller in the '30s and '40s. Koufax. Drysdale. I mean, you can count them on two hands, probably."

The Red Sox were on fire. Clemens was unhittable. The city, still simmering over the Rocket's comments from 1989, was beginning to forgive.

And then the bottom fell out.

Wrote Shaughnessy in the September 6 *Boston Globe:* "Your real estate taxes have been doubled. Your mother-in-law is moving in for good. Your daughter has a date with the lead singer of 2 Live Crew. The teachers' union in your hometown has hired Jerome Stanley. And now for the really bad news: Roger Clemens has a shoulder injury."

Clemens missed 25 days in the heart of the August pennant race, with his Red Sox fighting Toronto for a postseason berth. "He was the one guy we couldn't afford to lose," says Dennis Lamp, a Boston reliever. "And he was gone." Boston went 9-13 without its ace, allowing the Blue Jays to reduce the deficit from six and a half games to one. Making matters worse, the Red Sox were distracted by nonstop will-he-or-won't-he reports of Clemens' return. One day, he was almost ready. The next day, he was on his baseball deathbed. During Clemens' time away, Jim Palmer, the sports broadcaster and Hall of Fame pitcher, reported that the Red Sox ace had been playing 18 holes of golf shortly before telling WBCN radio that he was unsure whether he'd be back by season's end. What the hell was going on?

By the time Clemens finally returned to the mound for a September 29 matchup with Toronto at Fenway Park, Boston was one game up with five to go. Over six innings, Clemens struck out five, walked two and gave up four hits and no runs. Boston's 7-5 victory was the biggest of the season—an all-but-official death knell for the spunky Blue Jays, who would wind up finishing two games back.

"If Roger Clemens told me he could walk on water, I'd probably believe him," said Fischer. "There's probably nothing he can't do, including driving a tank or flying a plane.

"The man," Fischer said, "is a pitching God."

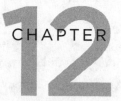

CHAPTER 12

Unraveling

His name was Joseph, he was Italian and he was doing life for murder.

That's pretty much all Terry Cooney remembers now about the man who changed his life. At the time, more than 40 years ago, Cooney was running the physical fitness program at the Sierra Conservation Center in Jamestown, California, when Joseph pulled him aside and said, "Why don't you get out of this depressing line of work and do something fun?"

"Fun?" thought Cooney. "What the heck is that?"

An Oregon College of Education dropout who had spent much of his adulthood aimlessly wandering—serving in the Marines, then working as a railroad switchman, then selling Pontiacs and classified ads—Cooney often wondered what it would be like to have passion for his job. To actually look forward to going to work in the morning.

"There was an announcement on the radio during the Game of the Week," Joseph the Murderer said. "They're looking for people to go to Florida and train to be umpires. You should do it."

Hmm . . . maybe the con was onto something. Cooney had spent several years officiating in one of Fresno's city baseball leagues, and the gig always brought him joy. The close plays. The drama of the late innings of a tight game. "Really, I loved umpiring," he says. "So I listened to Joseph and gave it a shot. What did I have to lose?"

Seven years later, on April 8, 1975, Cooney was positioned alongside third base in Cleveland Stadium, working a game between the Yankees and Indians. Sports historians remember it as the day Frank Robinson became baseball's first African American manager. Cooney remembers it as the start of his first full season as a major league umpire.

"I loved everything about the job," says Cooney, who would go on to work one World Series, three American League Championship Series and two All-Star Games. "The travel, the restaurants, the camaraderie, the people. I know some umpires who got very nervous before each game, but I never did. I looked forward to it."

He was especially looking forward to game four of the 1990 ALCS, when the Oakland A's would be trying to complete their sweep of the Boston Red Sox en route to their third straight World Series. Like any umpire worth his weight in dirt, Cooney was a guy who loved working home plate for the great matchups. Oh, it was fine to officiate, say, Baltimore's Bob Milacki versus Chicago's Greg Hibbard on a cold, damp Tuesday evening in April. But give Cooney Frank Viola pitching against Nolan Ryan, or Mark Langston locking horns with Teddy Higuera, and he was in heaven.

On the afternoon of October 10, 1990 at the Oakland–Alameda County Coliseum, Cooney was in the clouds: On the biggest stage in the biggest game beneath the brightest spotlight, Boston's Roger Clemens versus Oakland's Dave Stewart. Two 20-game winners, two Cy Young Award favorites, two battlers.

"How can't you get excited for that?" says Cooney.

In the 11 days since his return against Toronto, Clemens had been acting erratically. Irritated one moment, sedate the next, jumpy, confused, animated, obnoxious. By his locker at Fenway he had hung a nameplate reading POSSESSED/REBEL, and who could argue? On Tuesday, October 2, Clemens slammed his right fist into Joe Morgan's door after arguing that, when the team inevitably clinched the division title, the media should be kept out for 30 minutes (as opposed to 15, a league rule). The ensuing bruise had left the Red Sox concerned that he might not be able to start game one of the ALCS against the free-swinging, power-packed Athletics.

Clemens did start, and he pitched well (six innings, four hits, no runs), but the A's, led by Stewart's stellar eight innings of work, beat up on Boston's bullpen in a 9-1 rout at Fenway. They won the next two games too, receiving superb pitching from starters Bob Welch and Mike Moore and ample production from a lineup featuring Rickey Henderson, Jose Canseco and Mark McGwire. Before the series began, there was little doubt that Oakland was the superior team. Even Clemens knew it. What he could not swallow, however, was the behavior of Oakland's players, who strutted through the first three games as if they were the '27 Yankees. "The showboating was really an issue with Roger," says Tom Bolton, a Boston pitcher. "He saw how those guys were always pumping their fists and doing goofy high fives, and it really got to him."

Clemens came even further unhinged. After his game one start, he left without speaking to the media—a fineable offense. During the second game, he screamed at home-plate umpire John Hirschbeck and taunted Welch, the Oakland starter and a recovering alcoholic. "What are you drinking now?" Clemens yelled. "Are you drinking milk, you pussy?" When Morgan requested that he calm down, Clemens chewed the manager out. "I worry about Roger," said one teammate, "because he always seems ready to detonate."

Oakland's Harold Baines, an 11-year veteran, approached Clemens at one point and said, "Roger, man, calm down. What's the big deal?"

"The big deal," Clemens screamed, "is that we haven't won a World Series since 1918! That's the fucking big deal!"

There have been numerous theories to explain what transpired on that Wednesday afternoon in Oakland, when Roger Clemens started game four and went cuckoo. *Roger was upset because his wife caught him with another woman in his hotel room* (not true, teammates say). *Roger was loaded up on some sort of mood-altering steroid* (not true, teammates say). *Roger's body was taken over by aliens* (a possibility). "Roger was just overly hyped up," says Mike Marshall, a Boston outfielder. "He knew we had to win, and he was trying to do anything. Plus, he was pitching against Dave Stewart."

Indeed, if Clemens had a nemesis, it was the man known as "Stew." Unlike the legions of other starting pitchers who cowered at the sight of the Rocket, the 33-year-old Oakland ace relished the opportunity to face baseball's best. He was 6-1 lifetime against Clemens and 3-0 with a 1.65 ERA in 1990. "People thought I got geared up to face Roger, but I really didn't," says Stewart. "You want to know why I did well against him? Because Roger knew if he hit one of my guys, I'd hit two of his. It was a special two-for-one deal, and it got to the point where Roger stopped backing guys off the plate against us. His intimidation factor was gone."

Stewart found Clemens to be arrogant and overstuffed with fake bravado. "I didn't hate Roger," says Stewart. "But did I want us to kick his butt? Of course." Clemens found Stewart to be haughty and condescending. "What makes Dave Stewart so good," he said, "is that he has eight guys behind him that could be on the All-Star team."

On the morning of the game, Clemens made an emotional phone call to Rich Gedman, his longtime catcher, who had been traded to Houston in June. With his voice quivering, Clemens told Gedman how badly he was missed. "You know Rich," he said, "I wouldn't be here, pitching today, if it weren't for all you did for me as a catcher." Later that afternoon, Clemens intentionally rammed his right shoulder into

Boston Herald photographer Jim Davis, who was leaning against the rear of the batting cage.

In the moments before the first pitch, John Marzano, Boston's backup catcher, approached Dick Berardino, the bullpen coach. While warming up, Clemens had launched a pitch into the stands, where a gaggle of fans had been taunting him. "Roger seems really hyper today," Marzano said. "Something ain't right." When Clemens exited the bullpen, he was grabbed by Mike Boddicker, Boston's number two starter. "Roger, you've gotta calm down," he said. "I want to pitch in this series again."

Calm down? *To hell with calming down.* If his teammates weren't willing to take back this series, Clemens would do so himself. He decided every strikeout would be followed by a celebration. The first K would be sealed with a finger-to-the-throat gesture. The second K would be capped by Clemens' right hand turned into a pistol. *Pow! Gotchya.* He would blow smoke from the gun—Charles Bronson in spikes and stirrups.

The game started with Stewart holding the Red Sox scoreless in the top of the first. As he had done 32 times in 1990, Roger Clemens proceeded to emerge from the Boston dugout. Only he didn't look like Roger Clemens.

Surrounding his mouth was a brown Fu Manchu beard, neatly trimmed but—for the normally clean-shaven Texan—unusual. Clemens had considered shaving off the left half of the goatee, just to freak the A's out. His shoes were adorned by the fluorescent green faces of two plastic Teenage Mutant Ninja Turtles—one on each spike. Back home in Texas, everyone in the Clemens household had a Turtle alter ego. Koby, three and a half, was Raphael, and Kory, two, was Donatello. Clemens chose Shredder.

One more detail: Under each eye Clemens had applied a thick coat of eye black.

"That's the only time I've ever seen a pitcher wear eye black," says

Dana Kiecker, a Boston right-hander. "I was sitting next to Marty Barrett in the dugout, and I said, 'I wonder how long Roger's going to last today.'"

The first inning went as planned for Clemens, who retired the Athletics in order. When Boston failed to score in the top of the second, the A's again came to bat. This time, Clemens struggled. After getting Baines to pop up, he allowed back-to-back singles to Carney Lansford and Terry Steinbach. McGwire reached on a fielder's choice, scoring Lansford with the game's first run. "Roger looked sort of lost," says Boddicker. "He wasn't the usual Roger."

The next batter was Willie Randolph, Oakland's second baseman and the weak link in an otherwise formidable lineup. Since coming to the A's in a trade from Los Angeles in mid-May, Randolph had hit just .257 with one home run and 21 RBIs. At age 35 and with a slowed bat, he was the type of player Clemens expected to blow past with relative ease. Instead, he struggled. Randolph worked the count to 3-1, and Clemens' fifth pitch was a high, inside fastball.

As Randolph began his trot toward first base, Clemens sulked. "I was looking down at the dirt . . . and I was kind of shaking my head," he said later. "And then I looked back and I saw the umpire's throat guard moving, and I said, 'You know, I'm not shaking my head at you.' And then he continued to say something back at me very loudly, and I said, 'I'm not shaking my fucking head at you.' The next thing I know, I was gone."

Good story. But not entirely true.

Cooney and his fellow umpires were fed up with Clemens, who had spent much of the series' first three games barking from the Boston dugout. So now Cooney was barking back. "Are you shaking your head at me?" he yelled at Clemens. "Are you? Just throw the ball up here, and I'll call the balls and strikes." Umpires are supposed to defuse heated situations, not throw gasoline on a flame. But instead of walking away or offering a simple "Nope," Clemens reacted. "I'm not fucking talking to you!" he said. "Just keep your fucking mask on!"

He then launched into an epic tirade, calling Cooney "a gutless cock-sucker" and a "motherfucker" while screaming, "That pitch was right down the fucking middle." (It was—but about a half foot high.)

Standing 60 feet, 6 inches away, with his mask still on, Cooney tossed Clemens from the game with a dramatic, over-the-top punch in the air. Clemens seemed perplexed until second baseman Jody Reed said, "Roger, you've been thrown out." *Bam!*—Clemens snapped. He charged Cooney, pushing Jim Evans, the right-field umpire, to the side. From the bench, Marty Barrett, Boston's reserve second base-man, tossed two orange Gatorade containers and a white plastic trash bucket onto the field.

"I'll be totally honest," says Jeff Gray, a Boston right-hander who pitched two and two-thirds innings that game. "If I were Terry Cooney, I would have done the same thing. Roger was usually so unflappable and in control, but for whatever reason he was sort of crazed that day. I've never known why."

Stewart believes he knows. Having pitched for 16 seasons in the majors, Stewart says he can recognize the difference between a man ready to perform and a man ready to go home. And Clemens clearly wanted to go home. "He got himself thrown out of that game on pur-pose," says Stewart, whose A's went on to win 3-1, then lose the World Series to the Cincinnati Reds. "Terry Cooney asked him to repeat what he said three times, and Roger never once altered the anger of his statements. He knew the end result would be his ejection, but he kept saying it. There was so much at stake for Boston in that game, and Roger did everything he could to get thrown out. To me, it was obvious. He didn't have good stuff, he was getting hit, there was a lot of pressure. So he found a way out of the situation."

ROUGHLY ONE MONTH LATER, Dr. Bobby Brown, the Ameri-can League president, fined Clemens $10,000 and suspended him for the first five games of the 1991 season.

Baseball's Players Association immediately appealed the decision, arguing that umpires had become excessively confrontational. The case was handed to Fay Vincent, the 52-year-old commissioner.

"We had a hearing, and it came down to one question," says Vincent. "Did Roger Clemens call Terry Cooney a motherfucker."

Vincent pauses.

"Weighty issue," he says, chuckling. "Very weighty."

Vincent, Roger and Debbie Clemens, Terry Cooney and a handful of representatives from the players' and umpires' unions gathered in Vincent's New York City office the following April. Gene Orza, the MLBPA associate general counsel, brought along a lip reader from the New York Society for the Deaf. "My name is Deborah Copeland," the woman said, "and I can tell what people say from reading their lips."

"Are you deaf?" Orza asked.

"Yes," Copeland said.

"So if I show you a tape of the incident, you can tell me what was said?" Orza asked.

"Yes," said Copeland. "I can."

Orza whipped out a tape of the game, recorded by a CBS camera located behind home plate. He played the Clemens-Cooney incident, sans sound. Everyone in Vincent's office watched in silent bewilderment. When it was over, Vincent turned on the light.

Orza stood up. "M'am," he said, "did Roger Clemens utter the word 'motherfucker' during that video?"

"No," said Copeland. "He never said 'motherfucker.' 'Motherfucker' did not come from his mouth."

"So no 'motherfucker,'" Orza asked again.

"No 'motherfucker,'" Copeland replied.

"Thank you."

Vincent had to stop himself from laughing. Was this what three years of Yale Law School had resulted in?

"The stenographer was a little lady straight out of *Little House on the Prairie,"* Clemens later said with a chuckle. "She couldn't believe what she heard. The poor old woman's hands were shaking. I'm thinking, 'I hope *Little House on the Prairie* makes it.'"

Upon composing himself and hearing the various opinions, Vincent reached a verdict: Though Cooney had indeed unnecessarily instigated things, Clemens had crossed a line when, upon being thrown out, he had verbally *threatened to kill the umpire.* The exact words: "I'm going to find out where you live and come after you this winter."

"So Roger lost the appeal," says Vincent. "Not for what he did, but for what he said. You can't kill umpires. It's just not allowed."

Early the following season, Vincent awkwardly, cautiously, approached Clemens before a game at Fenway. He assumed the Boston pitcher was still mad and didn't quite know what to expect. "Hey, Mr. Commissioner!" said Clemens. "How are you doing?" He extended his hand toward Vincent.

"Roger," Vincent said, "I thought you might be angry with me."

"Angry?" said Clemens. "No, you vindicated me. I can deal with the suspension. I just wanted to clear my name. You showed I didn't start it."

ALTHOUGH CLEMENS WAS CONTENT with Vincent's ruling, the city of Boston was becoming increasingly disenchanted with its star.

Yes, loyalists were upset by his apparent allergic reaction to big games, by his implosions when the heat was on and the Sox needed him most. In eight postseason starts, Clemens had won but once.

Yet worse than the failures were the lies. By now, it was clear to all those covering the Red Sox (and reading about the Red Sox) that Clemens was *challenged* when it came to telling the truth.

Had he taunted Bob Welch for his alcoholism?

No, said Clemens.

Yes, said reality.

Had he cursed at Cooney?

No, said Clemens.

Yes, said reality.

"He lied nonstop during our hearing," says Cooney. "It was disgusting."

Had Clemens blasted Red Sox fans in past interviews? Had he threatened members of the media? Had he stormed off of a team charter? Had he . . . had he . . . had he? Countless times, Clemens said no. Countless times, reality said yes. Clemens told people he had been drafted by the Twins out of high school. Not true. Clemens told people he had played basketball at Texas and that the Seattle Supersonics and Boston Celtics had both been interested in his services. Not true.

"He was a liar, plain and simple," says Sean McAdam, who covered the Red Sox for *The Providence Journal*. "Roger was as full of shit as any athlete I've ever seen in my career. He said whatever worked for him, whether it was truthful or not. Reality didn't matter for Roger Clemens in any way, shape or form."

Despite an astonishing 21-6, 1.93 ERA season that saw him place second to Welch in AL Cy Young voting, Clemens' reputation had taken a serious hit. His allies in the Boston media were down to one or two, and friends in the clubhouse were vanishing as well. Clemens was increasingly deemed by those around him to be unstable "He was erratic," says Hesketh. "A great guy usually, but erratically behaved." In some circles, the pitcher had even become a punch line. The Pressman Toy Corporation contacted him to be a spokesperson for a new board game, "Read My Lips," that called for players to try to decipher phrases mouthed silently by their partners.

More than ever, Clemens needed a friend.

Once again, he turned to Randy.

On the night of January 18, 1991, the Clemens brothers, along with Craig Godfrey, Roger's brother-in-law, attended an Andrew "Dice" Clay concert at the Houston Summit. Afterward they went to Bayou

Mama's Swamp Bar, a 20,000-square-foot dance club in the city's up-scale Galleria section. "It was a cool place where people went to chill," says Alonzo Highsmith, the Dallas Cowboys running back who was at the club that night. "Definitely not a spot people went looking for trouble."

In the early morning hours, Randy got into a heated altercation, screaming at a salesman named Ellis Lee Herron Jr. and spilling his beer on a female patron. According to one witness, Randy actually pushed the woman hard enough that she fell to the floor. When Louis Oviedo, an off-duty police officer who was working that night as a security guard, attempted to arrest Randy, Roger allegedly jumped on his back and wrapped his neck in a choke hold. "It was an all-out brawl," a bar employee told *The Boston Globe*, "and Clemens was right in the middle of it." Witnesses said Roger had been drinking. Roger said he hadn't. When Oviedo attempted to arrest Roger, Randy alleg-edly punched the off-duty officer.

"Roger didn't know who this guy was," Highsmith says. "He wasn't wearing a police uniform. Roger was moving in to protect his brother, which anyone would have done."

Roger was arrested for hindering an apprehension, Randy for ag-gravated assault. Both were detained for 12 hours in a nearby jail. "When I walk into a place like [Bayou Mama's], everybody knows I'm there, so somebody has a chip on his shoulder or thinks I'm a tough guy," Roger later said. "Now I got people coming at me everywhere." When the media caught wind of the incident, Clemens—still licking the wounds of his ALCS meltdown—found himself plastered across front pages nationwide. That he would eventually be found not guilty of hindering Randy's arrest mattered not.

He was a marked man.

NOW 28 YEARS OLD and about to enter his eighth big-league season, Roger Clemens was no longer a naive, innocent country boy just hoping to pitch well and help the team win. He was an ornery, arrogant, deceitful country boy just hoping to pitch well and help the team win.

He talked of his "great respect" for Lou Gorman, the general manager, but made it clear he considered the man to be an out-of-touch buffoon. Asked by Dan Shaughnessy of *The Boston Globe* to cite literature he particularly enjoyed, Clemens' response was telling: "I sit and do books like Dave Winfield's," he said.

Over the winter the Red Sox signed Clemens to a four-year, $21.521 million (a nod to his uniform number) contract extension, making him baseball's first $5 million man. As part of the agreement they asked that he curtail his misdeeds and start behaving as a team leader. Down from his locker came the POSSESSED/REBEL nameplate, replaced by one reading, simply, ROCKET. "I'm going to change some things," he told *The New York Times* in a piece headlined "Clemens Works on New Pitch (Maturity)." "I've always led by example. I know we have to be tougher and better than everybody else because of where we play. But you're going to see a kinder, gentler Roger Clemens."

On the mound he was once again majestic, going 18-10 with a 2.62 ERA and winning his third Cy Young Award for a Boston club that finished 84-78 and seven games behind Toronto. "Nobody could touch him," says Wayne Housie, a Red Sox outfielder. "I used to take BP against him, and every ball he threw moved up and down and all over the place. He wasn't hittable." As ordered, Clemens tried to make more time for teammates. Whereas in recent years he had placed a wall between himself and younger players, now he was opening up. One could approach the ace and ask a question. Maybe even two questions. He would shag balls in the outfield and join in the locker room banter. "Roger never went all out to help, but you could see the effort was being made," says Mike Gardiner, a 25-year-old Boston starter. "[Rookie pitcher] Kevin Morton and I were feeling our way with the team, and Roger would talk to us, tell us the things he saw. He helped me with my pregame routine, as far as warming up without throwing so much beforehand. It was very valuable."

Most noticeably, Clemens preached work ethic. He roped other pitchers into long runs along the Charles River and two-hour weight sessions, laughing giddily as, one after another, they rushed to the nearest bathroom to vomit. At home, he kept a room filled with six exercise machines and a freezer reserved solely for his ice bags. "I always thought Dave Stewart was the hardest worker in the world," says Matt Young, a journeyman starter who came to Boston in 1991. "But nobody I ever played with worked as hard as Roger." During spring training, Clemens would run between three and four miles immediately before a start, then do 50 to 70 pickups (a backbreaking drill involving sliding along a line while lifting baseballs from the ground) between innings. His weekly sit-ups numbered into the thousands, and he strengthened his fingers by flexing them in bowls of uncooked rice. "You've gotta pitch tired!" he'd tell teammates. "You've gotta pitch mentally and physically fatigued, so you can handle the situation during the regular season when the games count." Clemens kept notebooks on every opposing hitter, pitcher and umpire. (He even took notes on his teammates, assuming one day they'd be opponents.) Dan Petry, the 13-year veteran who was finishing out his career with Boston, still recalls Clemens' eight-mile midnight jog *after* a game. "I'd seen a lot of things," Petry says, "but nothing like that."

The same could be said of Clemens' newest pitch, a split-fingered fastball that he had been tinkering with over the past few springs. The idea had first popped into his head after the 1986 season, when Mike Scott, at the time the Houston Astros ace, showed off his grip at a charity golf event. Clemens worked tirelessly on the splitter until the ball fell completely under his spell. "It's a violent pitch and it has to be thrown violently," Clemens said. "I had to strengthen a variety of different muscles and tendons in my hand and arm to be able to throw the pitch effectively."

When implemented correctly, "Mr. Splitty" (as Clemens nick-named the pitch) looks exactly like a fastball, then—*woosh!*—drops from waist to knees at the last possible moment. In other words, hitters sitting on Clemens' fastball were in trouble. How well did it work? With his splitter diving off the plate, Clemens threw 30 scoreless innings in April. "That thing," said Kirby Puckett, the Twins star outfielder, "should be illegal."

CLEMENS' EFFORTS TO REFORM his behavior and live up to his $5 million commitment didn't last. In the aftermath of a disappointing 1991 run, Lou Gorman, the Boston GM, fired Morgan and promoted Butch Hobson, who had spent the past season managing the team's Triple A club in Pawtucket. A 40-year-old former Sox third baseman, Hobson looked like a rugged Paul Newman. He played quarterback and safety for Bear Bryant at the University of Alabama, and in 1978 started at third for the Sox despite loose bone chips in his right elbow. He committed 43 errors but earned enduring respect. "Between pitches he adjusted the chips," Don Zimmer, his manager, once said. "Sometimes he didn't get them back in time, and he couldn't throw. He was tough."

In Boston, Hobson didn't inherit a mess—so much as a stuffed-to-the-brim garbage dump. Shortly after Hobson named Carlos Quintana his starting first baseman in late February, the ballplayer broke his left arm and right foot in a car crash (he would miss five months and never live up to expectations). Jack Clark, the team's washed-up designated hitter, delighted in taking shots at managers and teammates, and by spring training Mike Greenwell, the star outfielder, was already ripping the organization. Mo Vaughn, Boston's top prospect, needed to shed an extra, oh, 30 pounds. "These guys don't need a hitting coach," said Richie Hebner, the team's former hitting coach. "They need a shrink."

For Hobson, the most awkward development involved Clemens, who, without consulting with his agents, his general manager, his new manager or his teammates, failed to show up for the first day of spring training. Then he failed to show up the next day. And the next day. And the next day. And the next day. And the next day. And the next day. And the next day. For eight full days, as Boston's pitchers and catchers went through the mindless motions in Winter Haven, Clemens remained in Houston. He practiced with his high school baseball team. He trained with Chuck Norris. He played plenty of golf. He worked a charity event as a celebrity bartender at the Velvet Elvis Pub. When asked that night why he wasn't with his teammates, he replied, "For what? So I could be standing around spitting sunflower seeds?"

Clemens refused to call the Red Sox, turning Hobson into the least powerful man in Boston blue and red. The manager spoke longingly of his plans but didn't even know whether they should include his ace. Sounding like a 16-year-old girl hoping to be asked to the junior prom, he told the *Boston Herald*, "I expect a call tonight . . . I want that call." Teammates, once openly supportive of Clemens, turned on him. A red carpet, leading from the clubhouse door to Clemens' locker, was taped to the floor. A balloon was tied to his stool, alongside a note reading WELCOME BACK, WE MISSED YOU. Another sign, nearby, read, REMEMBER THE GOLDEN RULE: WHOEVER HAS THE GOLD MAKES THE RULES. On a picnic table located in the center of the room, someone placed an empty milk carton with Clemens' picture taped to the side. The caption read, HAVE YOU SEEN THIS PITCHER?

"He brings attention on himself that's not needed," said Clark. "Maybe he had things to do back home. Well, so do I. I didn't want to leave my family either."

When Clemens finally arrived on the morning of March 2, a swarm of reporters and TV cameras stood ready. He walked into Hobson's office and, without prompting, apologized.

"That's all I needed to hear," Hobson said, extending his hand. "Now let's get to work."

Clemens changed into a warm-up outfit, took the field at Chain O' Lakes Park and began jogging laps. Hobson, who wanted to establish a dialogue, ran beside him. Yet for reasons nobody has ever rightly determined (Clemens was absentminded; Clemens was cold; Clemens was deep into the Color Me Badd groove), the pitcher refused to remove his Walkman headphones from his ears. The Boston media gleefully dubbed the incident the "Day One Emasculation of Daddy Butch."

"That wasn't a good moment for Roger, Butch or any of us," says Gorman. "I think a lot of what Roger did was misunderstood by the media. But not all of it. He wasn't *that* likable of a guy. Oftentimes, it showed."

Stung by their criticisms, Clemens once again ignored teammates. "Roger was Roger," says Ken Ryan, a Boston pitcher. "As a young player, he wasn't the easiest person to approach. It's not like he wouldn't talk at all, but if you needed anything substantial or worthwhile, you first had to show that you were worthy in his eyes." Clemens' main foil was the press. One day he was talking. The next day he wasn't talking. He was rude and snarky and proprietor of a long memory. "Roger was an easy guy for the media to go after and attack," says Leigh Montville, a *Sports Illustrated* writer and former *Globe* columnist. "He would always do these strange meltdown things that automatically made him look foolish. What was the press supposed to do, ignore him? But Roger didn't like the coverage, and he let everyone know about it."

Finally fed up, the city's press corps declared an unofficial war on Clemens. If he wanted to treat Boston's writing establishment like shoe-bottom crud, the favor would be returned. McDonough, never a Clemens supporter to begin with, ripped the "Texas Con Man" with a gleeful (and strikingly unprofessional) regularity. The harshest blow came from Bob Sales, sports editor of the *Boston Herald*, who had a tabloid mentality befitting his place of employment. "Our readers came to our paper to be entertained," says Sales. "We wanted to be accurate and have standards, but at the same time we wanted to have some fun. Roger was someone we could definitely have fun with."

Having complained about the *Herald* "misinterpreting" some of his statements, Clemens considered cutting off the paper's reporters. "I said, 'Fine,'" says Sales. "You want to be that way, we'll be that way."

The result was "The World According to Roger," a regular feature in which the *Herald* would run Clemens' quotations in transcript form, without cleaning up the verbal gaffes. "Roger was a runaway train when he talked," says Steve Buckley, a *Herald* columnist, "and every time he opened his mouth it was like a snowball rolling down hill. And the snowball would hit a twig and go a different route." "The World According to Roger" first appeared on March 8, 1992, following Clemens' spring debut against Milwaukee:

WINTER HAVEN, Fla.—Excerpts from Roger Clemens' comments yesterday following his three-inning, four-run spring debut:

"I'm just really fatigued out there. I'm panting pretty hard and that's the way I want to be. It makes me concentrate on my arm . . . just everything. I was really fortunate [the first-inning grand slam] happened, it made me concentrate. These guys . . . they were bearing down. I was working on a lot of form . . . I think all the balls were in the middle of the plate."

"I don't think it's a big deal. I don't worry about it down here. I'm pretty much seeing dugout to dugout. I'm just happy to go back to concentrating like I did before."

"After I got the bases loaded and [Rob] Deer hit the bomb, we changed that [windup] real quick. So much for that."

"We won't have a chance to sweat when we get up North

with the flurries and the drizzle . . . but I'll be ready to go nine by that time."

Clemens was not amused. He lashed out against the *Herald* and threatened to never again speak with the newspaper's reporters. "Yeah, right," replied Sales. Tony Massarotti, the *Herald*'s first-year Red Sox beat writer, explained to the pitcher that he had nothing to do with "The World According to Roger," though he was forced by his editors to funnel quotes to the copy desk for the next day's edition.

"It included stutters, stammers, pauses, with the sole purpose of embarrassing him," says Massarotti. "I was too young and inexperienced to say anything, but I thought it went too far."

Led by the bumbling Hobson, the Red Sox were a mess. They finished in last place with a 73-89 record. "That team never came together," says Herm Winningham, a Red Sox outfielder. "Roger was supposed to be the leader, but he was never around to lead. You'd just never see him. When I first came up with the Mets, you'd watch Mookie Wilson and George Foster and even Darryl Strawberry help guys out and show them the ropes. That wasn't Roger's way, and we were pretty divided. It wasn't a good year to be a Red Sock."

Clemens put together another stellar season, finishing 18-11 with a 2.41 ERA and making the All-Star team. But he continued to keep the press at arm's length. In the June 19 edition of the *Herald,* George Kimball wrote about a 70-year-old woman who had once asked Clemens to sign an autograph for her grandson, who suffered from Down syndrome. Clemens had supposedly refused the request, and the boy died—in her words—"never learning that his hero had feet of clay."

When Clemens heard of Kimball's piece, he flipped. In the course of an average day at the ballpark, the pitcher signed at least fifty autographs. Unlike teammate Wade Boggs, the superstar third baseman who walked past fans with a regal haughtiness, Clemens was usually quick to whip out a Sharpie. He signed for kids, he signed for adults, he signed for the overly aggressive, he signed for the placid, he signed for the professional collectors. He certainly signed for the handicapped.

On the day the grandmother approached, Clemens probably missed her. In a crowd of screaming fans, how hard would it be to overlook a bent-over senior citizen? "Roger was not a mean-spirited person," says Young, the Red Sox pitcher. "We all have faults, but he was not cruel."

On the evening of July 18, Clemens was about to address the assembled media following his 1-0 shutout of the Twins when he spotted Kimball toward the rear of the 20-person crowd. He began to take questions, then stopped midsentence. "Hold on a second, y'all," he said. "I'll spend all night here talking to y'all individually if I have to until this lowlife leaves. I'm not saying a word until he leaves."

Kimball was stunned. "What's your problem?" he asked.

"No!" Clemens yelled. "I'll never talk to you again! Get out of here! That's the lowest blow! I've been here eight and a half years and that's the lowest blow I've ever had since I've been here! I can take articles on the field, but you're horseshit! Take off!"

Clemens was now screaming. All other activities came to a halt. "You're a horseshit lowlife, and it's obvious by the way you take care of yourself!" he said. A nice man and seasoned wordsmith, Kimball was portly, with a bushy beard. "Take a hike!" Clemens said. "Get your dead ass out of here! I'm not talking! I'll be more than happy to accommodate these people, but that's a low blow and you know it! I hope you can sleep at night! It's fucking bullshit!"

Not wanting to hinder the work of his peers, Kimball shuffled off. Then—*pop!* He felt something soft glance off his left shoulder. Kimball looked to the floor. It was a Wonder Bread hamburger bun. "Did Roger Clemens just throw a bun at me?" Kimball thought. "Did he ju—" *Whiz!* Clemens launched another bun, this one past Kimball's right ear. Then another one—also a miss. "It's fucking bullshit and you know it!" Clemens shrieked. Tony Pena, Boston's catcher, pushed Clemens away. Clark, the veteran designated hitter, urged Kimball to leave. "Please, just let it go," Clark said. "He's close to losing it right now."

Shortly thereafter, with Kimball gone, Clemens explained to the media that the article in question had blamed him for the boy's death. The piece, though harsh, did nothing of the sort.

"Roger," someone asked, "did you actually read it?"

Clemens rubbed his cheek.

"Well, no," he said. "Not exactly."

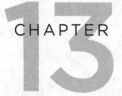

CHAPTER

The Ladies' Man

On March 18, 1993, the Boston Red Sox were in the midst of their first spring training at City of Palms Park in Fort Myers, Florida. Unlike Winter Haven, a numbingly dull town where excitement came in the form of McDonald's and a night of *Star Trek* reruns, Fort Myers offered Boston's players a bevy of activities. There were movie theaters, a bowling alley, chain restaurants, miniature golf.

The Bridge.

That's where Roger Clemens and a handful of his Boston teammates were this particular night—one of Fort Myers Beach's hottest bars, where the reggae was played loud and live and the drinks were tropical and served in funky glasses with cherries and miniature umbrellas. Located on the shoreline, patrons could access The Bridge via foot, car or—if one was feeling particularly nautical—water. "I remember Roger arriving on a boat with some teammates," said Jennifer Sirbaugh, who was at the bar that night. "I found him to be extremely arrogant and insufferable. But Mindy was taken with him."

By "Mindy," Sirbaugh is referring to one Mindy McCready, her 17-year-old friend, roommate and former coworker at Melons, a Hooters knock-off a few blocks away in Fort Myers.

In an ocean of drunks, how could Roger Clemens not notice Mindy McCready, what with her tight pants and hourglass figure and flowing blond locks? A local girl who lived with her mother, Gayle, just a few miles down the road, McCready often came here to sing on open mic night. In the pre–*American Idol* era, she dreamed of using music to escape a horrid home life—of packing up her stuff, moving to Nashville and becoming the next Tanya Tucker. "There was a desperation to leave the life that I had known and hated so much in Fort Myers," she once said. "You can't always 'get there' on ambition alone. There has to be something a little stronger. And there's nothing stronger than a desperate person."

Her life was, in many regards, a clichéd country song. Born to an abusive father, Tim McCready, and his ill-suited wife, Mindy was a few months shy of two years old when Gayle had her reciting the Gettysburg Address, the Twenty-third Psalm and the Pledge of Allegiance to anyone who dared sit on the family's sofa. On long drives, Mindy would sing "Old MacDonald Had a Farm" into a brush or imitate the way Farrah Fawcett shook out her hair on *Charlie's Angels.* Her first official performance came at age three, when she crooned a religious tune at a nearby Pentecostal church. Her idol was Sandi Patti, the operatic-voiced gospel star.

The oldest of three siblings, Mindy was 11 when her parents divorced. She was immediately designated cohead of the household, in charge of cooking, cleaning and making all the beds while her mother worked as an ambulance driver. "I was given the choice to act like a child or grow up and be responsible," she said. "Anybody would rather play with Barbies than vacuum the house, make the beds and cook dinner, but that wasn't an option." Obsessed with finding a new husband, Gayle would doll her daughter up and drag her along to the clubs and singles bars. That Mindy was a young teen never seemed to be an issue. She had the body of an 18-year-old and handled her whiskey better than most adults. "Mindy has some hollow scars in her soul from her youth," says Thom Schuyler, a Nashville songwriter who worked with McCready. Wrote Laurence Leamer in his book *Three Chords and the Truth:* "Gayle was not out here looking for a night's dalliance. She pushed the leering lounge lizards and make-out artists away and sat waiting for Prince Charming to arrive. As for her daughter, she didn't bring the 14-year-old Mindy to introduce her to romance but to make it easier for Gayle to sit there."

As Gayle fell into and out of love with an endless stream of men who would begin as "my dream boat" and invariably end as "my scumbag ex-boyfriend" (she married a United Airlines pilot named Thomas Phelan when Mindy was 15, divorced him after two years and married again), Mindy was miserable. She ran away from home multiple times, only to return after a couple of days. She had her first boyfriend when she was 14—he was three years older and allowed Mindy to move in with his family. When the relationship ended, she quickly took up with a 26-year-old police officer. Mindy was 15 but told him she was 18. Upon learning of the relationship, Gayle stormed the sheriff's office. "Do not let him come to my house again," she screamed, "or I want his job!"

All the while, Mindy was becoming a drinking, smoking, sexually active wild child—as well as a karaoke bar junkie. "Her girlfriends pushed her forward, daring her to sing," wrote Leamer. "Mindy sang Trisha Yearwood songs and Crystal Gayle songs and Reba songs and Wynonna songs. The audience applauded but no more than they did for others who came forward to sing the recorded background music. They did not notice her."

Clemens noticed. He wanted to meet her. He *had* to meet her. Although he had spent the first few years of his career remaining loyal to his wife and children, marital fidelity among major league ballplayers is nearly as common as blind relief pitchers. During the 1990 season Clemens finally gave in. Still socially awkward and verbally clumsy, he lacked the game of his smoother teammates. One night, for example, Clemens went out with some fellow players to the Palace nightclub in Saugus, Massachusetts. He approached one of the waitresses, a 25-year-old bombshell named Barbara Leslie, and stammered, "What would you do if I tried to kiss you?"

Leslie barely flinched. "What would your wife say if you tried to kiss me?" she hissed before walking off.

To those who knew him, Clemens was thought to be the one player who *wouldn't* cheat. Inherently straitlaced, he had enough trouble looking women in the eye, let alone moving in for the kill. Why, he had just built a 13,000-square-foot house on a three-acre plot outside Houston. The facility was intended to ward off the outside world from Clemens and his family. "I don't know whether it's a phobia or not," he said. "But I have a hard time dealing with a lot of people I don't know around me." Though very few ballplayers actively spoke of their wives to the press, Clemens was effusive in praising Debbie. They seemed to be not only husband and wife, but good friends. "He loved her, and he loved his kids," says Dennis "Oil Can" Boyd. "I don't care what anyone says. Roger was a good husband."

Yet here he was, in a grimy bar, lusting after Mindy McCready, who said she was 18 but was really just 17. "She had a fake ID, so nobody ever questioned her," says a longtime McCready acquaintance. "She was a regular part of that scene."

That night, after flirting and drinking together, Clemens whisked McCready away on his boat, eventually winding up at the Sheraton in downtown Fort Myers. According to a close confidant, McCready said they had sex together for the first time that night. If so, she was 17 and Clemens was 30. Based on Florida Statute Section 794.05, which states that "a person 24 years of age or older who engages in sexual activity with a person 16 or 17 years of age commits a felony of the second degree," their assignation constituted statutory rape. Clemens could have faced up to 30 years in a state penitentiary.

In Clemens' (thin) defense, he probably believed McCready to be of legal age—though barely. Early that morning, as McCready slept in the hotel bed, Clemens rose, placed a $100 bill for taxi money on the night table and quietly exited. He had to get back to his family's apartment, where Debbie and the kids likely awaited. Though he left Mindy a phone number, Clemens never expected to hear from her.

A couple of days later, he found a white envelope on the stool near his locker. The return address read M. MCCREADY. Clemens ripped it open and found his $100 bill, along with a note. "I didn't want the money," she wrote. "I wanted you."

Clemens called later that day and saw her again by week's end.

The three-time Cy Young Award winner officially had a mistress.

THOUGH HE WAS STILL considered an elite player, Clemens' 1993 season was the worst of his career. He posted his first sub-.500 record (11-14), and his ERA ballooned to a Tim Birtsas–like 4.46. In late March, Lou Gorman had given him a $5.7 million contract extension, thus ensuring that the Rocket would remain a Red Sox starter through the end of 1996. "I think once I shut it down in Beantown, that's it for me," Clemens said at the time—his first of more than two dozen ensuing retirement declarations over the course of his career. ("I'd like to play until the year 2000," he told *USA Today* a few weeks later. "I will not see 40. I'll be seeing my kids grow up by then.")

Clemens began the year with a 3-0 record and 1.48 ERA, then realized the Sox would be adequate and seemed to give up. While on the disabled list in June with a strained right groin muscle, he somehow found the time (and good health) to compete in the Canon Greater Hartford Open Celebrity Pro-Am golf tournament alongside Billy Andrade. As he approached the 17th hole, a spectator yelled out, "It really looks like he's on the disabled list over there! How's the groin feeling?"

Clemens smirked. "This," he said, referring to his golf swing, "is easy."

Whereas Clemens had once devoted 100 percent of his energy to pitching, he now seemed distracted and disinterested. When the team traveled to Minneapolis for a series with the Twins, he was fined by Butch Hobson for staying out into the early-morning hours with teammate John Dopson (perhaps Hobson would have never known, were Clemens not bitten on the hand by a mixed terrier in the process). He followed the path of thousands of poorly advised athletes by entering the restaurant business. Clemens lent his name and time to "Roger Clemens Sports World Wood Roasted Chicken," a chain whose first storefront opened in Warwick, Rhode Island. (The eatery twice changed names, first to Roger Clemens Flame-Roasted Chicken, then to Roger Clemens' Cafe Boston. After three years of mediocre cuisine and cash receipts, Clemens' restaurateur days ended with a whimper.) He went one month without a win and in an August 21 home start against the Indians was booed mercilessly. "Roger wasn't the pitcher I remembered," says Frank Viola, a Boston starter. "He lost some zip on his fastball, and his head wasn't totally into it."

"Roger didn't pitch that well, but it wasn't all his fault," says Tony Fossas, a Boston reliever. "You put a good quarterback on a bad team, and he'll be a bad quarterback. Our players weren't very good, so neither was Roger." On September 30, Jack O'Connell, the *Hartford Courant*'s esteemed baseball writer, named him to his annual All-Overpaid Team, alongside traditional dogs such as Melido Perez and Vince Coleman. Five days later, in Mike Shalin's Red Sox report card for the *Herald*, Clemens—usually an automatic A—was handed an F. Wrote Shalin, "If Joe Schmo goes 11-14, Joe Schmo gets a C–. But Clemens is Clemens."

And Clemens wasn't very good.

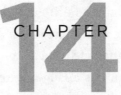

CHAPTER

The Devil and Dan Duquette

The savior arrived, only he looked nothing like the saviors Red Sox fans had come to know and love (and then, inevitably, hate and boo). In these parts, a savior looked like Ted Williams— tall and strapping, with a freckled face, suntanned arms and a confident smile that reassured men and wooed women. He looked like Fred Lynn, bat twirling in the air, patiently waiting for that inside fastball to turn on. He looked like Jim Rice and Dewey Evans and Wade Boggs and, heck, even Roger Clemens.

He did not look like . . . *this.*

On the afternoon of January 27, 1994, the new savior of the Red Sox was brought to town and introduced at Fenway Park. Just 35 years old, he wore uncomfortably large glasses, a slightly oversized suit jacket and a tie featuring disjointed images and designs. Whether the words emerging from his lips were happy, sad, excitable, comical or statistical, the expression on his face—*Did someone here pass gas?*—rarely changed.

Dan Duquette meant business.

He was Boston's new $2 million general manager. Just three years removed from their last division title, the Red Sox had fallen off a cliff. Their record, 73-89 in 1992, had been a similarly unacceptable 80-82 in 1993. Their roster included 15 players 30 and older, and their barren farm system was a laughingstock among rival scouts. Manager Butch Hobson, loved by all, respected by none, had been a dreadful hire. Lou Gorman, the outgoing GM, was a nice man with funny stories and unrivaled integrity, but the age when player transactions were consummated over a handshake and a few cold ones was over.

Born and raised in the western Massachusetts town of Dalton, Duquette had long dreamed of this day, of becoming a Somebody—with a capital S—in Boston baseball. As a fifth-grader he had been kicked out of class for smuggling a transistor radio into school to catch the opening game of the 1967 World Series between the Red Sox and the St. Louis Cardinals. As a solid sophomore catcher at Wahconah Regional High School, Duquette had handled three pitchers—Jeff Reardon, Chris Kirby and Jerry Erb—who would be drafted by major league teams. Though significantly better in football than baseball (he played linebacker at Amherst College), his love was reserved for the small white ball. "I've always felt I could [be a general manager], and I thought I was prepared," he said at his introductory press conference. "Actually, I should be honest—this is what I intended to do since I was 18, when Lenny Merullo told me at one of his Scouting Bureau tryout camps that I wasn't going to make it in the major leagues."

As a college senior, Duquette met Paul Ricciarini, a scout with the Blue Jays, and asked, "How do I get into your business?"

Ricciarini was taken aback. "Are you sure—with your education—you want to do this?" he asked.

"I'll scout," said Duquette, "I'll work in an office, I'll file reports . . . anything."

His intellect and tenacity landed him a gig as assistant scouting director with the Milwaukee Brewers, and in 1986 he was promoted to scouting director, drafting such players as Gary Sheffield, Darryl Hamilton, Greg Vaughn and Jaime Navarro. In October 1987, Duquette was hired by the Montreal Expos to be the club's director of player development, and in September 1991 he was named the team's seventh general manager. "Dan looked to be everything you'd want in a general manager," says Tony Massarotti, the Red Sox beat writer for the *Boston Herald*. "He was innovative and creative and smart and savvy, and he knew how to find good players. But . . ."

For all his undeniable intellect, Duquette was as warm and cuddly as a holding cell. Unlike Gorman, who had told Boston's players that his door was always open, Duquette looked at the Red Sox roster and saw chips. Not names, not personalities, not men with feelings and families, but chips. Move one, get two. Get three, move four. Some chips were old and scratched up, others were new and shiny. But, come day's end, they were all merely pieces of plastic, to be shuffled here and there as Duquette saw fit. "When Dan got to Boston, the first thing I told the other players was, 'Boys, watch out,'" says Joe Hesketh, a Red Sox pitcher who was in Montreal with Duquette. "He was a soft-spoken guy, but when he did things it was to everyone's dislike. He wasn't really human. He was more like a computer."

When Duquette assessed the Boston roster, he saw a team in dire need of a makeover. In Montreal, the Expos relied on youth, speed and vigor to surpass expectations. These Red Sox, by comparison, were dull, plodding and overpaid.

One didn't have to be an IBM programmer to know Clemens, now a 31-year-old veteran, was the type of man Duquette was pinpointing when he said, "We're going to bring in younger ballplayers in their prime years . . . we have a number of players on the downside of the curve." As Montreal's general manager, Duquette had made his name with a series of bold transactions, including dealing three nobodies to the Reds for closer John Wetteland and snagging pitcher Pedro Martinez from the Dodgers for second baseman Delino DeShields. But Clemens possessed the two key traits of an untradable chip: He was overpaid and underperforming. "The idea of having a pitcher of Clemens' talent is exciting," Bob Watson, Houston's general manager, said at the time. "But I couldn't afford him."

Accustomed to Boston executives tiptoeing toward his locker with prideless deference, Clemens was taken aback when the new GM routinely walked by without saying a word. Before games, Duquette would stand behind the cage in his neatly pressed shirt and slacks, watching batting practice with his arms crossed, his gaze icy. Whereas Gorman fancied himself a fan as much as an executive, Duquette fancied himself an architect. Players came and players went. Why get attached? "It wasn't personal with Dan," says Massarotti. "It was business. I doubt he was out to get Roger. But it wasn't in his nature to go up and give him a hug." Roger's wife, Debbie, gave birth to the couple's third child, a son named Kacy, and shortly thereafter the older boys, Koby and Kory, flew to Boston to spend a week with Dad. Roger brought his two sons to the park, dressed them in little Red Sox uniforms—and was told that one of Duquette's new policies included not allowing children on the playing field or in the clubhouse before games. Clemens was dumbfounded.

The strike-shortened 1994 season was a strange one for the Rocket. He infuriated Duquette by again showing up late for camp but pitched significantly better than he had the prior year, ending with a 9-7 mark and ranking second in the American League in ERA (2.85) and strikeouts (168). Yet with the Red Sox, who finished 54-61, out of contention from the start, younger power pitchers such as Montreal's Martinez and Seattle's Randy Johnson were capturing the attention of the national press corps. Clemens was old news. Stale news.

Having seen many of his peers vanish into retirement, Clemens began thinking more seriously about capitalizing on his fame while it lasted. Along with the sagging wood-roasted chicken market, he instructed his agents to find as many endorsement deals as possible. Yet by now Clemens was known to be difficult and obtuse, and there were few opportunities for him to earn extra income. He appeared in a series of Food and Drug Administration advertisements to make the public aware of new nutrition labeling laws (the other major celebrity in the spots was Curious George, the cartoon monkey) and had so-so deals with Reebok and Upper Deck trading cards. But he didn't need to hire anyone to answer his phone. "His persona is so negative, no advertiser wants to go near him," said Brandon Steiner, a sports marketing expert. "He is one of the best pitchers in baseball but has no endorsements, even though he's never been involved with drugs or alcohol. Turning his demeanor around would help."

The confounding factor in Clemens' persona was that, despite Steiner's take, he wasn't a prototypically evil guy. This was no Barry Bonds, scowling his way through life. This was no Steve Carlton, ranting about the 12 Jewish bankers atop a hill. Was he the most approachable Boston player? Hardly. But when members of the Red Sox went out for dinner after away games, Clemens almost always whipped out his credit card and declared, "This one's on me, fellas." He organized golf outings for the pitchers, reserving and paying for rounds at some of the nation's finest courses.

"And any time we were on the road, Roger made sure the wives were taken care of," says Jeff Russell, a Boston reliever. "If there was a concert in town, he got tickets and limos for the wives. He took us all to a Metallica concert. And even though I hated Metallica, I loved him for doing that sort of thing. Beneath the guard, there was a big heart within Roger."

With his mother, Bess, a cigarette smoker for 35 years, suffering from emphysema, Clemens agreed to star in an antismoking commercial sponsored by the Massachusetts Department of Public Health. "Last year they called me off the field three times in the ninth inning, and I thought it was my mother's last breath," he told the press. "Smoking totally deteriorated her lungs. I'm going to tell the kids, the teenagers, that it's not cool to do that."

Rough on the outside, Clemens was surprisingly empathetic when it came to illness. What with their sculptured physiques and high-flying, highly compensated lifestyles, many professional athletes fail to even consider the downtrodden. Not Clemens. Beneath the radar of teammates and reporters, he often left Fenway for a jog around the city, only to detour at Children's Hospital Boston, where he would spend hours with sick patients, signing balls and telling stories. "He was there more often than anyone would ever believe," says Wally McDougal, the team's assistant equipment manager. "It hurt Roger to see those kids, and he wanted to help. Not for the attention. Just because he cared."

One day, Clemens arrived at the hospital to visit a young boy who was dying of cancer. Told Roger Clemens was here to see him, the patient sat up in his bed, only to frown when the Red Sox ace entered the room.

"You're not Roger Clemens," he said.

"Sure I am," countered Clemens. "It's me."

"No it's not," said the boy. "You don't even look like him."

"Wait here," Clemens said. He sprinted from the room, down the hallway, out the front door and up the street to Fenway. Clemens hustled into the clubhouse, put on his white Red Sox uniform and returned to the hospital.

"Oh!" squealed the boy. "It is you!"

"Who else does that sort of thing?" asks Steve August, Boston's traveling secretary.

Years later, when August's father, Bill, was dying, Clemens told him to call if he needed to talk. When Bill finally passed, August telephoned his friend. Debbie answered the phone. "Roger's not here, but you have to give him a ring at his mom's house."

"No," said August, "I'm sure he's busy. I don't want to bother him."

"Steve," Debbie said, "do it now. He'll want to talk to you."

Over the next one and a half hours Clemens offered August his love and support. "He told me about all he went through losing his father, and the strength it takes to handle everything," says August. "I'll never forget that."

Toward the tail end of 1993, Dan Shaughnessy, the hard-nosed *Globe* columnist, was devastated when his seven-year-old daughter, Kate, was diagnosed with leukemia. Shaughnessy had earned much of his salary ripping Clemens over the years, and the pitcher-writer relationship was a frosty one. Roughly two weeks after Kate's diagnosis, however, an enormous package arrived at the front door of Shaughnessy's Boston home. The return address said, simply, R. CLEMENS, KATY, TEXAS. "Even the UPS guy was curious what was in there," says Shaughnessy. "We had no idea."

Opening the box, Kate squealed with delight. Inside was an enormous stuffed white teddy bear, along with an autographed baseball. Fifteen years later the animal, christened "Clementine" by Kate (now 22 and a recent college graduate), remains a fixture in the Shaughnessy household. "It certainly didn't change the way I covered Roger," says Shaughnessy. "But it said something about him that he could separate what a person does for a living from who he is as a person. I was touched."

IN JANUARY 1995, ROGER and Debbie Clemens went on a week's vacation to Honolulu, where they ate, swam, read, danced—and renewed their wedding vows.

It was Roger's idea, a token romantic offering to his lovely wife but also a telling glance into his mind's inner workings. By this point, Clemens' affair with Mindy McCready was well established, and he was known to have had other dalliances on the major league circuit.

Yet much like the serial killer who cheerfully shows up for work each day at the post office, Clemens had (and still has) an uncanny ability to compartmentalize these parts of his life. He could hit three batters in the head and incite a massive brawl, then moments later praise the clubhouse pot roast and baked potatoes. He could walk five in one and two-thirds of an inning, then tell the assembled media that he had thrown the ball well. He could sleep around while reaffirming his commitment to his beloved bride.

For nearly all of his life, Clemens' sole focus was baseball. That's what Randy, his older brother, had demanded, and the result was a physically fully formed adult who had missed out on much that life had to offer. The teenage Clemens had never really known of puppy love, of running wild with his friends, of spring break trips to Cancún. He was a sports cyborg, instructed to throw as hard as possible as often as possible. But Clemens was inexperienced in the ways of the world, and he knew it. Sometimes, he told teammates, it'd be fun not to be a ballplayer, to just be a normal guy with normal plans and normal worries. To be unexceptional. This isn't to say that Clemens is introspective. He's not and never has been. (Says Tyler Kepner, who covered Clemens later in his career for *The New York Times*, "I don't think he ever thought introspection would serve a purpose.") But Clemens is human, and his background resulted in certain inescapable flaws.

Hence, while other major leaguers bemoaned the strike that canceled the 1994 World Series and carried over into the following season, Clemens, Boston's player representative, seemed to feel as if he were released from shackles. Finally, here was a free pass to spend time away from the ballpark and indulge his cravings. For the first time since signing with Boston a decade earlier, Clemens abandoned much of his grueling fitness plan and lived it up. He traveled to Hawaii; played golf several times a week; served as a celebrity judge on *Star Search;* attended Super Bowl XXIX, between the 49ers and Chargers in Miami, and the NCAA men's basketball Final Four in Seattle. "Baseball is at a standstill," he excitedly told the *Orlando Sentinel* in January, "but I'm doing *everything*."

When the strike finally ended in early April 1995, the Roger Clemens who reported to Boston's spring training facility in Fort Myers, Florida, had changed in three noticeable ways.

First, he sported a new haircut that Karen Guregian of the *Boston Herald* described as "a cross between Marcia Clark and Billy Crystal." (This was not a compliment.)

Second, he was unusually open and reflective with the media, telling a pack of reporters, "If we win this year, you will not see me back here. If we win a World Series, I have nothing left to prove." Usually an overzealous (and, to some, annoying) braggart when it came to his own fitness regimen, Clemens now admitted that he was tired of waking up at 6 A.M. to run five miles, that he'd rather play golf.

Which helps explain the third change: Clemens looked fat.

Perhaps "fat" is too strong. He was pudgy. Beefy. Plumpish. John Kruk–esque. He reported at 234 pounds, nearly 20 pounds heavier than his usual playing weight, and was scratched from his first exhibition start with a strained calf (the immortal Gar Finnvold took his place). To Duquette, he was the picture of a fading veteran on the express train to mediocrity. Even though the team's new manager, the gregarious Kevin Kennedy, sang Clemens' praises, Duquette knew the truth: Clemens wasn't quite a has-been, but his days of winning 20 games or another Cy Young Award were over.

That opinion was only reinforced when, on April 22, Clemens was diagnosed with a muscle strain in his right shoulder that would keep him out until early June. To Clemens, this was merely a setback. But Duquette, who took pride in knowing when a player's better days had passed, viewed injuries to veterans as evidence of a weathered body's vulnerability.

Clemens' return to the Red Sox was mixed. His 10-5 record was certainly impressive, and his down-the-stretch excellence (5-0, 1.95

ERA from August 7 through September 6) proved to many that his best was still awfully good. But if Duquette had learned one thing during his ace's absence, it was that Boston was a pretty strong club—with or without Clemens. The Sox won the AL East with an 86-58 record, earning a matchup with the 100-win Cleveland Indians in the American League Divisional Series. Kennedy named the Rocket his game one starter, hoping the man who had once inspired fear in opposing hitters could still muster his inner Nolan Ryan.

In his first year as Boston's skipper, Kennedy viewed the start in a simplistic baseball context—a great pitcher trying to win an important game. But there was more at stake.

Wrote Will McDonough in *The Boston Globe:*

This is prime time, when the true greats of baseball separate themselves from the pack. The real big guys play at the highest level in the biggest games.

Roger Clemens should want this.

When he said at the beginning of the season that he hungered for another chance at a World Series with the dream of bringing a world championship to Boston, he never imagined he would be in the position he is in now.

But it's here . . .

If Clemens wants to make the Hall of Fame for sure, his chance is now. He has not been great in the postseason. He has started eight games and won just once. That is not the stuff prime-time players are made of.

Was Clemens a prime-time player? He opened the game against Cleveland with three no-hit innings but fell apart in the sixth, as Boston nursed a 2-0 lead. A two-out walk to Omar Vizquel kicked things off. *No big deal.* A hit-and-run single by Carlos Baerga moved Vizquel to third. *OK, still two outs.* Albert Belle followed with a two-run double. *Well, at least the game's tied*. Eddie Murray stroked an RBI single. *Oh, boy*. Like that, the lead was gone. Boston lost 5-4, and the Indians swept the series.

"For one reason or another," wrote Ken Rosenthal of *The Baltimore Sun*, "Clemens hasn't gotten it done."

Duquette was thinking the very same thing.

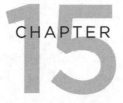

CHAPTER

War

I n the winter between the 1995 and '96 seasons, Roger Clemens—now, at 33 years old, officially an aging pitcher—turned to coaching.

No, he hadn't retired from the majors. Clemens was the pitching coach for the Houston Red Sox, a select Little League travel team of 9- and 10-year-olds whose backup second baseman was a freckle-faced boy named Koby Clemens, age 9.

To the regional TV stations, this was a slam dunk of a feature—local baseball superstar makes nice with the kiddies. To newspapers, it was an easy-answer space eater for a slow news day. CLEMENS PITCHES IN FOR KIDS, read the headline in the April 1, 1996, *Patriot Ledger* in Quincy, Massachusetts. Who could resist big, tough, burly Roger Clemens turning soft and sappy around the tykes?

Regrettably, Clemens wasn't soft and sappy. He was, instead, every Little League coach's worst nightmare—a wealthy, loud, arrogant blowhard who trumpeted his opinions to all. This hardly made him unique among major leaguers who coach their children—the crazed competitiveness that translates into professional stardom does not turn itself on and off like a stoplight. But on Houston's youth baseball fields, it did make him a major pain in the rear.

Vaughn Bacon, coach of the little Sox, has long refused to bash Clemens. He was, after all, the Rocket—the best baseball player anyone in these parts had ever seen. And yet . . . "Roger wanted Koby to play more than he probably deserved to play, and he let me know it," says Bacon. "Koby was younger than the other boys. I had to be fair. But I understood where Roger was coming from."

Bacon understood, not because Clemens was an eager parent who wanted his son to succeed. He understood because Clemens had spent large wads of cash to snag his underage son a prominent spot on the club.

Thanks to Clemens, every member of the Houston Red Sox had three sets of uniforms (home, road, alternate)—all neatly embroidered, all sleeveless, all the class of the USA Select League. Every member had three or four pairs of new Reebok cleats, a new batting helmet, a new aluminum bat and new socks. "Roger wanted bang for his buck," says Bacon. "I can't really blame him."

He brought a similar sense of entitlement to Fort Myers for spring training. Entering the final year of his contract, Clemens would have been smart to arrive in tip-top shape and with some newfound humility. For the first time ever, opposing organizations would soon be debating whether to throw free-agent money his way.

Instead, he was portly (Will McDonough of the *Globe* nicknamed Clemens the "Pillsbury Doughboy") and brash. "The whole incredible work ethic thing was a little overstated," says one former teammate. "Roger didn't put in the same effort that he had in the past, and it showed. He wasn't as athletic, he wasn't as built, he wasn't as determined and he didn't throw as hard. He became this guy who started nibbling at the plate instead of just rearing back and throwing heat. One day Roger asked me if I thought he was doing something wrong. I said, 'Yeah, you're pitching like a human being.' He was getting older. It happens to us all."

Clemens was taken aback when Duquette signed Mo Vaughn, the team's 28-year-old first baseman and reigning AL MVP, to a three-year, $18.6 million deal while leaving his future undecided. Sure, Clemens liked and respected Vaughn, but who was the real star here?

Publicly, Clemens told the media that he was happy with the $5.5 million he would make in 1996 and that the most important thing was winning. "I'm getting paid really nice, and I'm not concerned about a contract." he said. "The contract is not my main focus." But why didn't the GM fawn over him the way Lou Gorman had? Why wasn't he running personnel decisions by his ace? Clemens had a bunch of ideas for returning Boston to play-off glory. Instead, Duquette was turning the Red Sox into a beer-softball-league team, signing robotic, immobile boppers like Kevin Mitchell and Jose Canseco to patrol the outfield corners. "Roger was very frustrated," says Reggie Jefferson, an outfielder–first baseman. "A lot of starters on our team stopped showing up on time for batting practice, and our defense was terrible, and Roger wondered what in the world was going on."

If any Red Sox fan still believed in his ace's greatness, he surely came away from the 1996 season disillusioned. Clemens began the year 0-4 with a 4.17 ERA in his first six starts, went 3-0 in his next five starts, then endured a 1-7 slump that sealed his fate with Boston. Duquette believed in building a team around young, driven, dogged players— not fat, indifferent, fading whiners. When asked by *The Boston Globe* to assess Clemens' decline, a National League scout said, "His fastball isn't what it used to be. There were times in 1986 when he could throw it 97 miles per hour consistently. Now he throws it in the low 90s. . . . He's not dominating anymore."

Duquette agreed. "I'll tell you what Felipe Alou once told me in Montreal," he said. "When you're a young player, the manager is in charge of your career. When you establish yourself as an everyday player, then you're in charge of your career. But when you're at the end of your career, you're back in the hands of management."

Even more noteworthy than Clemens' physical decline was the emotional distance he placed between himself and the club. For all his arrogance through the years, Clemens wanted to win. *Needed* to win. He would scream at opposing players from the dugout and berate umpires and try to will the Red Sox to victory. He wasn't simply one of the guys. He was *the* guy.

Now that had changed. As Boston battled the Texas Rangers at Fenway Park on April 25, Clemens urgently darted from dugout to clubhouse on three or four different occasions. Was Debbie pregnant? No. Was his mother sick? No. Was Randy in trouble again? No. Sotheby's was holding a John F. Kennedy auction, and he had to phone in his bids for JFK's irons and woods. (His top bid, $121,000, fetched neither, but Clemens would eventually buy one of the former president's pens for $165,000.) What did it say about the pitcher's interest in the game? About his priorities?

On the night of June 8, Clemens, holding a 2-1 lead against the Brewers at Fenway, was pulled in the eighth inning. Instead of sticking around and rooting for his team, he stormed into the clubhouse, dressed and left Fenway well before the game's end. His frustration over a season gone bad had been building. The next day he met with the *Globe*'s Dan Shaughnessy and launched into a nonsensical rant. "I know it's the fastest I've ever left the park," he said. "I had to put the defroster on in the car because the heat from my arm was causing the windows to fog up. I'm not going to bury anybody in public. I've never done that. But it's very disheartening. I don't mind getting beat, but you can't get out-hustled like we did. That's what's driving me crazy and makes me want to tear somebody . . . it just gets me so upset.

"We go hard for two and a half hours and then get beat in the last 30 minutes of a game because of a lack of concentration. That's when you tighten up the holes, and that's why we're losing. For some reason, the focus isn't there. For some reason, it's hard for some of these guys to concentrate. It's something I can't understand."

Boston's players were incredulous. If anyone was guilty of being a poor teammate, it was Clemens, who seemed to show up later and later before games and never took blame for a poor performance.

BY 1996, MINDY MCCREADY was a full-fledged country star, with a Top 10 hit, "Ten Thousand Angels," and a rapidly growing number of male fans. McCready had left Fort Myers for Nashville two years earlier, with little more than a demo tape and a truck. Now, at age 20, her debut album was on its way to selling 2 million copies, and her belly button ring (shocking by country music standards) made her the talk of the industry. "At the time there were people in the business who considered her to be the full package," says Jay Orr, the former country music writer for the *Nashville Banner*. "She could sing, she had the looks and she had a song that everybody knew. She wasn't ground-breaking, but she was very big."

Although McCready would date a conga line of famous boyfriends, ranging from the actor Dean Cain to Khaled al-Fahd, a prince of Saudi Arabia, her true love was reserved for a faraway baseball player. McCready and Clemens regularly spoke on the phone, and featured prominently in her Nashville home were several photographs of the two of them, locked arm in arm. Clemens told McCready that he loved her, that they would one day be together. He flew her to be with him on the road, bought her expensive gifts. Even when McCready was briefly engaged to Cain, who starred as the Man of Steel in TV's *Lois & Clark: The New Adventures of Superman,* she carried on relations with Clemens. "Mindy told everyone about it," says a McCready friend. "She considered Roger to be her boyfriend."

In McCready, Roger had involved himself with the anti–Debbie Clemens, who had recently given birth to the couple's fourth child, a boy named Kody. Well mannered and fiercely disciplined, Debbie ran the Clemens household like a drill sergeant, dropping off this son at football practice, that one at a friend's house. She managed much of Roger's promotional affairs from the family home in Houston, played golf with friends semiregularly, spent time at the gym and worked on various charities via the Roger Clemens Foundation. She was safe and secure and decent—but lacked the adventure of a young sexpot like McCready. Clemens was looking for action on the side, and he found the right woman. "I've had some teammates in the past who just couldn't hold it together," Clemens once said. "They were extremely talented, but they just had too many distractions in their life off the field that they couldn't handle. And that's one of the reasons I've been successful in my career—I've got a team of All-Stars backing me up everyday."

In other words, thanks to Debbie's diligence, Clemens had time for Mindy.

ALTHOUGH KEVIN KENNEDY MANAGED the team to a solid 85-77 mark in '96, it was yet another disappointing season for the Red Sox, who finished in third place, seven games behind the Yankees and three behind Baltimore in the Wild Card race. Clemens' 10-13 record was slightly misleading (his 257 strikeouts led the league, and he was backed by terrible outfield defense), but he was far from the ace of just a few years ago. Save for one glorious moment—a 20-strikeout game against the Tigers on September 18 that tied his own major league record—his output oozed mediocrity. "Clemens was still awfully good," says Darren Bragg, a Boston outfielder. "But I think he was frustrated."

As he looked around the clubhouse, Clemens surely noticed that he was surrounded by aging and adequate players. What he also noticed was that the one older player who seemed to be getting bigger,

stronger and *better* was Jose Canseco, the 31-year-old slugger in his
second year with the team. Though he roamed the outfield like a
one-legged emu, Canseco's 34-inch KC Slammer bat seemed to be
spring-loaded. In just 96 games and 360 at-bats in '96, the injury-prone
Canseco had 28 home runs and 82 RBIs and elicited enough *oohs* and
aahs to make an otherwise unmemorable Boston season memorable.

Based on the reputations of both men, Canseco was the type of
teammate Clemens loathed. The Rocket was a traditionalist; he believed there was a right and a wrong way to approach the game. In his
initial 10 years as a major leaguer, first with Oakland, then with Texas,
Canseco was all wrong. "The problem with the A's," he once said,
"is all they care about is winning." Canseco posed after home runs,
talked trash to opposing players, seemed to work harder at becoming
a Grade-B celebrity (like Dennis Rodman, Big Daddy Kane, Vanilla
Ice and many others, he had his turn with Madonna) than a Grade-
A superstar. He owned mansions in Miami and Oakland, a 42-foot
Cigarette boat, a 1-900-234-JOSE phone line, where fans could hear
his daily updates for $2 for the first minute and $1 for each additional
minute. On the cover of the 1995 *Red Sox Yearbook,* Canseco posed in
a black tank top, arms folded, biceps popping (wrote Mark Newman
in the *Sporting News,* "It looks less like a team yearbook than, say, the
latest issue of *Playgirl*").

Yet beneath the image, Clemens found Canseco to be something
of a baseball soul mate. Both had spent many years enveloped in the
spotlight, both loved golf, both were thought to be on the downside of
their careers. And both would do whatever it took to survive.

Long before Tom Verducci wrote his groundbreaking steroids
story, "Totally Juiced," in the June 3, 2002, issue of *Sports Illustrated,*
Canseco was revolutionizing the game by spreading the word about
the power of performance-enhancing drugs. Once an unexceptional
180-pound outfielder at Coral Park High School in Miami, Canseco
was selected by Oakland in the 15th round of the 1982 amateur draft,

mostly as a nod to one of the team's veteran scouts, Camilo Pascual. In his first year of professional ball, playing in the Pioneer League, Canseco hit just two home runs in 28 games. The following season, in 93 games of Class A ball, he hit 14 homers. Then, in 1984, he started injecting steroids into his body. Wrote Canseco in his autobiography, *Juiced,* "I wanted to become faster, stronger, better, more powerful than any other athlete."

By September 1985, he was in the majors with the A's, and the following year, he totaled 33 home runs, 117 RBIs and 15 steals en route to winning the American League Rookie of the Year award. Within the tight-lipped world of the major leagues, Canseco served as the first walking, talking, breathing, *hitting* pro-steroids billboard. In Oakland and then in Texas, he told anyone and everyone that steroids and human growth hormone could turn even an average ballplayer into Babe Ruth. Now, in Boston, he was spreading the exact same message. To the media, Red Sox players praised Canseco's talent and dedication, even though his secret formula for success was well known within the clubhouse. "I still remember the first conversation Jose and I had about steroids," says Mike Greenwell, the veteran Boston outfielder. "I think I had just gotten my third hit of the day, and Jose said, 'Dude, I sure wish I could hit like you.' And I said, 'Yeah, but I wish I had your power.'"

That's when Canseco smiled, flexed a bicep and said, "Greenie, if you come down to Miami after the season we can work on that." Later, on the bus ride to the team's hotel, Canseco elaborated. "A lot of my power comes from steroids," he told Greenwell. "And your power can come from it, too. It's all over the place."

Greenwell wasn't interested. "Just didn't seem right," he says. "I believe in integrity."

So, once upon a time, did Clemens. When he was winning 20 games and Cy Young trophies, the idea of cheating was anathema to him. You won by outworking every other player; by spending two hours in the weight room; by running more, studying more, lifting more. "When I was with Pittsburgh, the pitchers would run sprints," says Tim Wakefield, the veteran knuckleballer. "But Roger took it to the next level. He never bragged, and he wasn't big on talking about himself or what he did to prepare. He just did it."

But now Clemens was experiencing two disconcerting developments: (1) As his 34th birthday approached, he was finding that hard work alone wasn't enough, and (2) Canseco's chemical enhancement had turned the slugger into a stud.

During rounds of golf and lengthy flights and bus rides, the two men discussed the ins and outs, ups and downs, pro and cons, of performance-enhancing drugs. When done wisely, and in moderation, Canseco assured Clemens, there was no risk. He could juice up and be as dominant as ever. He could turn back time and once again be the Roger Clemens of 1986.

The Roger Clemens.

AS BOSTON'S 1996 SEASON drew to a close, a divorce between Clemens and the organization seemed increasingly likely. On September 18, Clemens told the *Boston Herald* that he was mentally preparing for his Boston tenure to end, and a week later the agents Randy and Alan Hendricks advised their client to not pitch in the regular season finale, for fear of injury. "I don't know what the big deal is," Clemens said. "It's a no-brainer. It's the business of the game."

Naturally, he knew what the big deal was. With his 20-strikeout masterpiece against Detroit on September 18, Clemens had tied Cy Young for the Boston franchise record of 192 career victories. He was a Beantown icon, and even if the team was mathematically eliminated from the race, Clemens had to make that one last start.

On September 28, 1996, Clemens took the Fenway Park mound for the final time as a member of the Boston Red Sox. With his wife and sons in the stands, he went seven and two-thirds innings, striking out 10 in an otherwise meaningless 4-2 loss to the Yankees. When he was removed from the game by Kennedy, the entire Boston infield converged at the mound to wish him well. In the visiting dugout, Yankee players applauded respectfully. Clemens walked off the field to a standing ovation, then returned seconds later for a two-minute curtain call that reduced the stoic star to near tears. He scooped some dirt from the mound as a keepsake.

"A guy walks off the mound after the way he has performed, and it's tough to take," said Vaughn. "Regardless of whether we win or lose, it wouldn't make any difference. What is important is the time spent and the energy, the years I've known him.

"No one understands what goes on on the field in the games—not the fans, not our families. This is a champion, a warrior who goes to war for us all the time. You have to respect that, respect the effort. And Roger Clemens exemplified that."

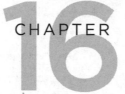

CHAPTER

Twilight

Dan Duquette was right.

That needs to be stated clearly, because for far too long the Red Sox general manager has been branded a fool, a jerk, an ice king. As Roger Clemens' baseball life went agelessly on, as he gobbled up additional Cy Young Award trophies, as he pieced together an unprecedented—and, as it turns out, unnatural—career revival, Duquette was roundly dismissed as, in the words of Joe Hesketh, the former Boston pitcher, "a man with absolutely no clue."

"Who was Dan Duquette?" says Mike Gardiner, a Boston pitcher who had also played under the GM in Montreal. "He was a non–baseball guy who thought himself smart enough to tell a baseball guy when he couldn't perform anymore. He was a person who couldn't even look you in the eye when you entered a room. Forget him."

It is true that Dan Duquette was the rudest and most arrogant baseball man most of Boston's players had ever dealt with. Unlike the majority of general managers, who strove to have open relations with their players, Duquette merely glanced at you as if you belonged alongside a nugget of dog excrement beneath his $1,500 loafers. He was guarded, curt and snide.

But forget him? How could you?

Dan Duquette, after all, was right about Roger Clemens.

Dan Duquette was right.

Toward the end of the 1996 season, Clemens told Howard Ulman of the Associated Press that he would gladly return to the Sox, but only if the team offered a four-year contract. The Rocket's reasoning: He would like to relocate his family from Texas to Boston during the season as long as he could be assured of geographic stability. The sentiment was deceitful. Clemens had never loved the city of Boston; he certainly felt no loyalty toward its obnoxious fans and cold, calculated denizens. No, what he wanted was a large contract offer, so that other franchises would present him with even larger contract offers.

Wrote Mike Barnicle in a *Boston Globe* editorial:

> Face it: If Clemens had not once been able to consistently throw a baseball 95 m.p.h. past men with bats in their hands, he would be wearing bib overalls and sitting on a milk crate at the open door of a trailer somewhere, brushing his tooth while shooing flies away from his head.
>
> The man is a complete dope. You would not for a single second—even with his guaranteed contract—want your child to grow up to be like Roger Clemens: selfish, spoiled and seriously deficient in character.

Duquette offered a four-year, $22 million deal that he knew the pitcher would reject. Behind the scenes, he told confidants that Clemens was lazy and past his prime, a pitcher with too many years on his birth certificate and too many miles on his right arm. When John Harrington, Boston's CEO, protested, Duquette argued that here, finally, was a chance to rebuild the franchise. Clemens' contract, attitude and mediocrity had held the team down for years. "If you check the book," Duquette said, "Roger has not performed at that 200-inning level like he did early in his career." Duquette's take was dead on. By all indicators, Clemens was a pitcher on the downside of his career. Or, to use Duquette's stinging word, in his "twilight." How was he to know that Clemens, once the hardest worker in baseball, would soon follow the lead of Jose Canseco and indulge in performance-enhancing drugs to save his career? How was he to know that the man who had come to think of Fenway Park as his own little country club would rediscover drive, energy and edginess?

How was he to know?

On December 13, 1996, the same day Boston acquired free-agent outfielder Sam Mack, the Toronto Blue Jays signed Clemens to a three-year, $24.75 million contract (with a $9.75 million signing bonus, an easily attainable incentive for a fourth year and the promise that the franchise would spend the money to surround him with a contending cast), making him the highest-paid pitcher in baseball history. What happened to Clemens' insistence that he would either return to Boston or move closer to his Texas home? What happened to Clemens' promise that he would never pitch for a division rival? What happened to Clemens' I'll-put-my-family's-needs-first blather?

"It was garbage, plain and simple," says Sean McAdam, the Red Sox beat writer for the *Providence Journal*. "He said all these things, but when the dough was placed in front of him, Roger's motivation was clear. It had nothing to do with doing the right thing and everything to do with getting paid. I wouldn't begrudge him for that if he were being honest. But he was a fraud."

THE NEW KING OF Toronto baseball entered the ballroom of the Renaissance Toronto SkyDome Hotel on the afternoon of December

13, 1996, resplendent in his spotless white jersey and ready and willing to lie his tail off.

It had been a whirlwind month, with five teams offering to send private jets to Clemens' Houston home to fly him in for negotiation sessions. "I think he was taken aback by how aggressively they went after him," said Mike Capel, his longtime friend. "He said to me, 'Man, maybe they do understand what I bring to a club.'"

One year earlier, Toronto GM Gord Ash and Alan and Randy Hendricks, Clemens' agents, had engaged in a miniwar over Al Leiter, a starting pitcher who had left for Florida as a free agent after the Blue Jays had invested much time and money in helping him recover from injury. "There were a lot of hard feelings on our part," says Ash. "I wasn't sure we'd be willing to deal with the Hendrickses again. But in a way, Roger served as a peace offering. We needed someone to change the course of our franchise, and they needed a home."

To Clemens, the initial thought of becoming a Blue Jay offered the appeal of an airport toilet. Not all that long before, Toronto had been the center of the baseball universe, having won back-to-back World Series titles in 1992 and '93 while drawing more than four million fans per season. With the players' strike of '94, however, the city's sports loyalists had felt betrayed. A hockey town first, second, third and 100th, Toronto would support its Maple Leafs whether they won the Stanley Cup, finished last in the Central Division or robbed the nearest orphanage. "You'd be in the middle of the game, a pitcher's going through the signs, and all of a sudden a huge cheer would go up," says Kevin Witt, a Toronto infielder. "The Maple Leafs just scored a goal." The Jays engendered no such fanaticism. Their season-ticket base slipped to 22,000 from 26,000 in 1993, and many of the leases to the SkyDome's luxury boxes were on the verge of expiring. "As far as atmosphere," says Tim Crabtree, a Blue Jays pitcher, "the SkyDome gets an F." Among men over 18, the televised audience for Blue Jays games had dropped by more than 40 percent. "This is a one-sport town, and everything else is trendy or not trendy," says Steve Simmons, a columnist for the *Toronto Sun*. "Doug Flutie played here for two years [in the Canadian Football League], and he didn't draw flies. Then he went to Buffalo, started winning and people got excited. We're a very quirky people when it comes to our teams."

Clemens knew Toronto wasn't a baseball hotbed. He knew the Jays were a long way from contending in the AL East. He knew the team's manager, Cito Gaston, was regarded throughout the league as a strategic lightweight. He knew his Texas home was 1,645 miles away. But, hey, *whatever*. The stadium was nice, and the golf courses were plentiful. First baseman Carlos Delgado even agreed to surrender uniform number 21. Best of all, there was the money. "I'm here to win a World Series," Clemens told the assembled media. "I've always enjoyed this city. When we came here for the All-Star Game [in 1991], obviously playing here, my wife and my boys have loved this area. That was the most important factor.

"I know by their first offer that Mr. Duquette put out there, it's in my heart that he didn't really want me back. I'm extremely happy now, and he might say different, but I think deep down he's happy, too."

The Toronto media lapped it up. The Boston media had a field day. BIG LEAGUE ARM, BUSH HEART read the headline in *The Boston Globe*. "Good riddance!" wrote the newspaper's Peter May. Said Nicholas Burns, a State Department spokesman and native Bostonian, "Roger Clemens is not a great American. Roger Clemens will never be able to say what Ted Williams and Carl Yastrzemski could say, and that is: 'We were lifelong Red Sox.' Roger Clemens is a traitor."

In a fawning piece for *Toronto Life* magazine, the writer Jay Teitel used 2,437 words to paint the portrait of a caring, sensitive, thoughtful saint of a man who "has been the epitome of baseball color of a decade" and is void of "exactly that hidden agenda, misdirection or intimidation you have to swallow with so many other star athletes."

In other words, Clemens had found the right place for a guy trying

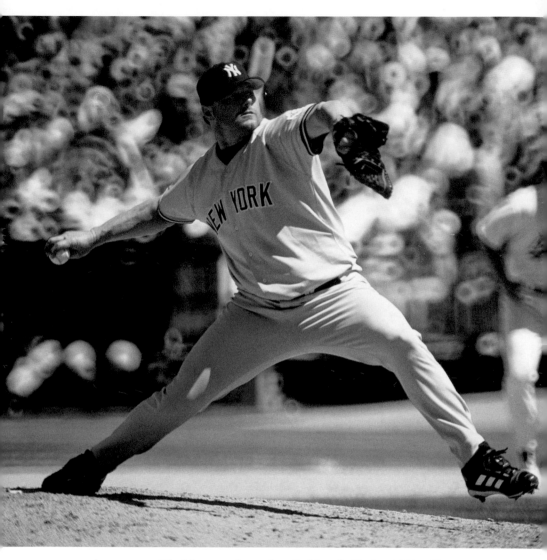

ROCKET SCIENCE Pitching against the Oakland A's in 2003, Clemens displayed his nearly flawless delivery—every movement meticulously planned and endlessly rehearsed. (BRAD MANGIN)

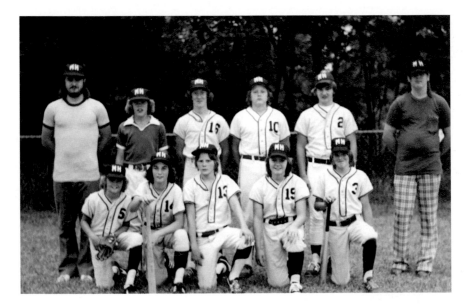

THROWS LIKE A GIRL As a pitcher on his Little League team in 1977, Clemens (number 10) split starts with Kelly Krzan *(front row, second from left)*, the first girl to play youth baseball in Ohio. (PHOTO COURTESY OF MIKE KESSLER)

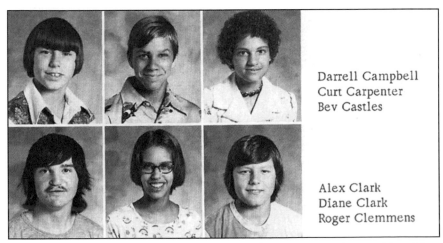

Darrell Campbell
Curt Carpenter
Bev Castles

Alex Clark
Diane Clark
Roger Clemmens

NOT CASTING A SPELL The young Roger Clemens was a forgettable athlete and, judging by the spelling in the 1976–77 Smith Junior High School Yearbook, a forgettable name as well. (PHOTO FROM 1976–77 SMITH JUNIOR HIGH SCHOOL YEARBOOK)

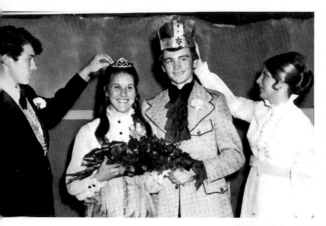

FAST TIMES AT VANDALIA HIGH Randy Clemens and Kathy Huston were the perfect couple at the 1971 Vandalia-Butler High School senior prom— BMOC and his cheerleader queen. (1970–71 VANDALIA-BUTLER HIGH SCHOOL YEARBOOK)

TOP OF THE WORLD Randy was one of Ohio's standout prep basketball players— "He just had it all going on," says a friend. "He was good-looking, smart, a great athlete, well known, popular." (1970–71 VANDALIA-BUTLER HIGH SCHOOL YEARBOOK)

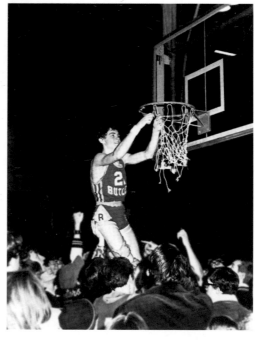

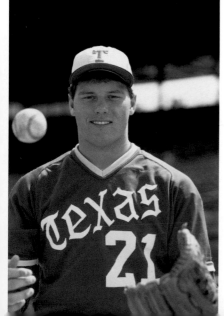

HOOKED BY THE HORNS Clemens wasn't recruited out of high school but improved enough in junior college to earn a scholarship at the University of Texas. (RICH PILLING/MLB PHOTOS)

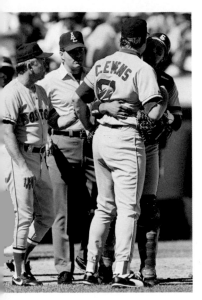

POSSESSED REBEL Clemens had one of the great meltdowns in postseason baseball history in game four of the 1990 ALCS against Oakland. Three months later he was booked after he and Randy allegedly beat up an off-duty cop at a Houston bar. (*Left and below:* BRAD MANGIN)

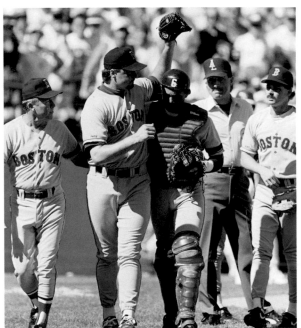

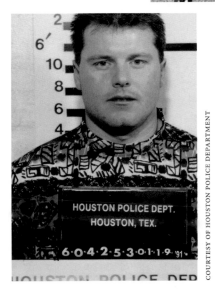

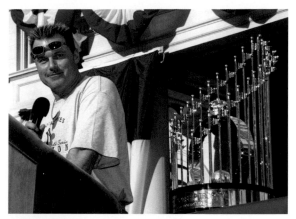

CHOKED UP Clemens was thrilled to be celebrating a World Series Championship with the Yankees in 1999— and delighted that his postseason flops didn't cost his team the title. (JAMES DEVANEY/WIREIMAGE)

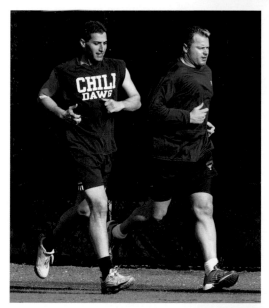

WELL ARMED Andy Pettitte and Clemens became close friends on the Yankees and ardent workout partners; their friendship suffered when Pettitte admitted that he'd used HGH and implicated Clemens. (PETER MUHLEY/AFP)

BROTHERS UNDER THE SKIN Clemens and Jose Canseco seemed like a horrible match, but they found common interests: golf, fitness—and performance-enhancing drugs. (JEFF HAYNES/ GETTY IMAGES)

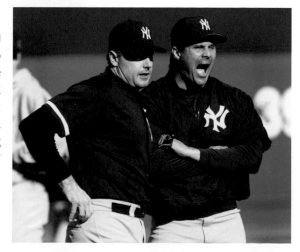

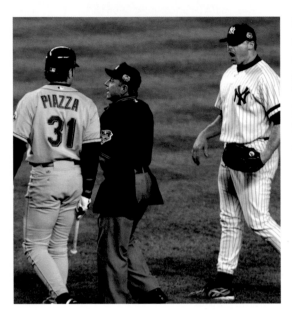

BAT CRAZY Clemens had another epic meltdown against the Mets during game two of the 2000 World Series, flinging a broken bat at Mets catcher Mike Piazza. (DON EMMERT/ AFP)

CITIZEN CLEMENS In the immediate aftermath of the September 11 terrorist attacks, few New York celebrities contributed more time and resources than Clemens. Here, on September 25, 2001, he met with rescue workers before a game. (EZRA SHAW/GETTY IMAGES)

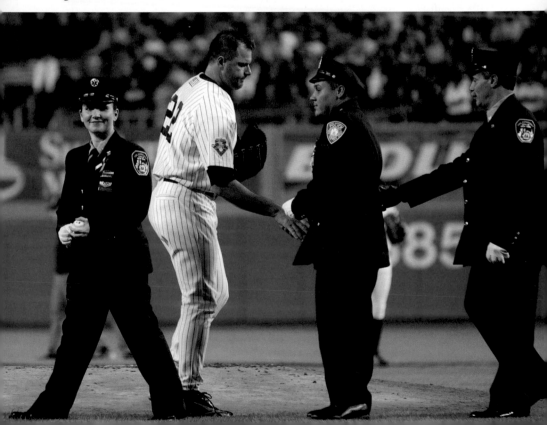

MINOR INDISCRETION Clemens met Mindy McCready in a Florida bar in 1993—when she was 17 and he was 30. Their 10-year relationship was exposed by Clemens' former trainer after Clemens sued him for defamation because of his claim that he'd injected Clemens with steroids. (RON GALELLA/WIREIMAGE)

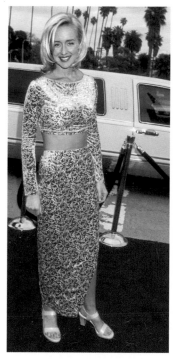

THE K CORRAL Clemens with his wife, Debbie, and their four children *(clockwise from right):* Kory, Kody, Kacy and Koby. (BOB LEVEY/WIREIMAGE)

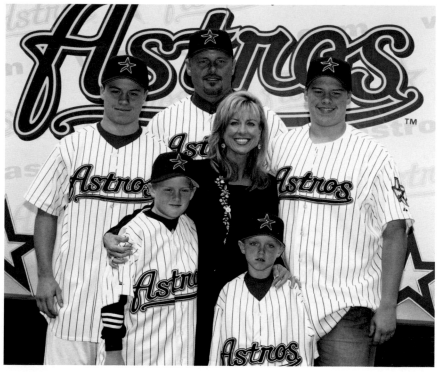

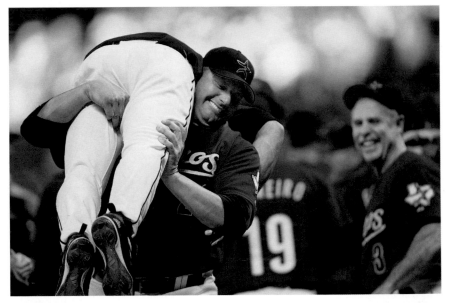

HI HO ROGER When Astros outfielder Chris Burke won the 2005 NLDS against Atlanta with an 18th-inning homer, he got a ride from a giddy Clemens. (DAVID E. KUTHO/SPORTS ILLUSTRATED)

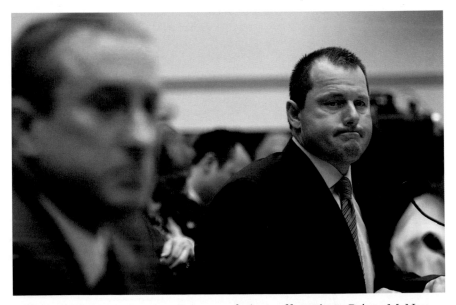

GOING DOWN SWINGING Prior to facing off against Brian McNamee *(foreground)* before Congress, Clemens appeared confident. His blustery testimony, however, was a disaster and put him in legal jeopardy for perjury. (SIMON BRUTY/SPORTS ILLUSTRATED)

to keep his personal life off the radar. He certainly didn't have to worry about the *Toronto Star* or *The Globe and Mail* digging up dirt about Mindy McCready or any of the other women he was involved with. He also didn't have to worry about the second major *scandal* (for lack of a better word) in his life—the rapid decline of Randy, his brother, whose drug addiction was a tightly guarded secret restricted to family members.

Randy's life had turned into a dark tragedy. Divorced from his wife, living here one week, somewhere else the next, Randy had been in and out of drug rehabilitation. On multiple occasions Randy contacted his old Ohio friends to ask for money, never explaining what, exactly, the funds would be used for. "I called him one time when he was with Kathy—they were divorced, but for some reason they were in the same location," says Larry South, Randy's longtime friend. "Kathy sounded scared, and she hung up. Ten minutes later she called me from a pay phone, and she wouldn't tell me anything about Randy or their kids."

Like his old pal, South suffered substance abuse problems, for years battling crack addiction. "It's the only thing you think about doing," he says. "I'd be working on a Monday and thinking about getting my check on Friday so I could buy more crack. I wouldn't wish addiction on my worst enemy."

Roger was at a loss. Family members advised him to let Randy go. "You can't help someone who won't help himself," they said. But for all his flaws, Roger just couldn't abandon kin. He continued to send Randy money and pray that one day God would purge the demons from his body. He wanted Randy to be an uncle to his boys—picnics and bowling and ball games with the entire family. Instead, he looked at Randy—once a strong, powerful man—and saw a spindly, hollowed-out ghost.

"You're talking about Roger's favorite person in the world," says South. "You don't think that damaged him?"

Fortunately for Clemens, nobody knew, and nobody was asking.

Having departed Boston under such hostile circumstances, he arrived in Canada determined to star as Mr. Happy to Be Here. Without prompting, he insisted that Pat Hentgen, Toronto's reigning Cy Young Award winner, deserved to start Opening Day. In exchange for uniform number 21, he bought Delgado a $17,900 Presidential Rolex ("Do you want number 48, too?" pitcher Paul Quantrill cracked). At the behest of the Blue Jays front office, Clemens came to Toronto on January 20 to "test out the SkyDome pitching mound." That he had already made 11 starts at the stadium was no reason to pass on a dreamy photo op. Nor was the fact that, with the NBA's Raptors in the midst of their season, a mound had to be hastily constructed. With roughly 20 reporters, photographers and cameramen gathered around, Clemens donned a Toronto uniform and threw to Blaine Fortin, a minor league catcher who had flown the two and a half hours from his home in Lundar, Manitoba. "That's probably the highlight of my career," says Fortin, who never played beyond Double A. "Early the next morning I was getting phone calls in my hotel room from radio stations. They couldn't find him, so I was next in line."

Upon reporting early for spring training at the Blue Jays' complex in Dunedin, Florida, Clemens felt as if he had entered an alternative universe. After 13 years with the Red Sox, everything was so *different*. The funky uniforms with the bird on the cap. ("It's just so blue!" said Debbie. "I guess it's going to take some getting used to.") The young, humble sluggers such as Delgado and Shawn Green. The fans abuzz at seeing a real-life future Hall of Famer up close. Clemens appeared to be as fit as he had been a decade earlier, bounding from activity to activity with the enthusiasm of a young cockapoo. He even loved his temporary digs, a $350-per-night suite in a nearby golf resort.

By adding a marquee name like Roger Clemens, the Blue Jays considered themselves to be back on the city's sports radar. Maybe local fans were less than enamored by the pitching skills of, oh, Marty Janzen and Woody Williams, but who in their right mind wouldn't come out to see Roger Clemens sling heat?

Answer: Most everybody. The Blue Jays opened at home against the Chicago White Sox on April 1, and despite their bold off-season signing, the game failed to sell out. In a piece that appeared in *The Record* of Kitchener-Waterloo, Ontario, George Holm, the team's director of stadium and ticket operations, dismissed the early apathy. "The problem might be the day," he said. "It's the day after a four-day weekend for most people and I think it's hard to ask people to take that day off, too."

Clemens started the following night, and his superlative 6-1 complete-game triumph was tainted by what even the optimistic Holm would consider an alarming fact: In a stadium that held 49,539, just 31,310 paying customers attended.

Not that anyone could fault Clemens for a lack of effort. In the days leading up to the start, he laid out a plan with team officials that, in his mind, would turn White Sox–Blue Jays into a must-see event. Thinking back to all the Longhorn football games he'd witnessed as an undergrad, Clemens wanted to be introduced like a star quarterback dashing onto the Texas Memorial Stadium turf before a square-off with Oklahoma. Now, as Clemens walked onto the field as a first-time Blue Jay, it was hard not to get goose bumps. "Sirius" by the Alan Parsons Project (the song best known as the Chicago Bulls theme) blasted from the speakers, followed by Elton John's "Rocket Man." Murray Eldon, the SkyDome public address announcer, did his best Michael Buffer by bellowing, "Pitching for your Toronto Blue Jays . . . a 14-year veteran . . . out of the University of Texas . . . *Roooooogggggggeeeeerrrr Clllleeeeeemmmmmmeeennnnns.*"

"I was in the bullpen, and I got the chills," says Crabtree. "That's how cool it was to see Roger take the field that day. It turned the game of baseball into a Hollywood production."

For the first time in his professional career, Clemens was motivated not by money or fame or heroism or victory, but by revenge. Despite his sunny public disposition, Clemens was driven by Duquette's humiliating public snub. Throughout his remarkable major league run, Clemens had acquired a bushel of enemies. He loathed Dave Stewart, despised John McNamara, hated Wade Boggs (a selfish teammate, Clemens believed). But at least those men had all worn the uniform. They knew the euphoria of victory, the devastation of defeat. But Duquette? What right did he have to declare a storied ace washed up? "The worst thing you can do," said Mo Vaughn, the Boston first baseman, "is put a man like Roger in a position to prove something,"

As the season progressed, it became apparent that Toronto's Clemens was better than any Clemens Boston had ever seen. Back to throwing in the mid- to high 90s, only this time accompanied by an otherworldly splitter and his trademark nastiness, he was again unbeatable. He improved to 6-0 with a 14-strikeout gem against the Twins on May 10 (two pitches after throwing a 95-mph fastball over Chuck Knoblauch's head, he drilled the second baseman—whose crime was standing close to the plate—in the right forearm) and took great pleasure as the Red Sox dropped 10 of 11 games to sink to last in the AL East. He followed up with a six-hit beauty against the Indians to go 7-0 and picked up career victory number 200 at Yankee Stadium in a 4-1 win. "It's not just that Roger pitches well," said Joe Torre, New York's manager. "He pitches well even when bad things happen around him. That's the measure of a number one."

Yet, despite becoming baseball's first 8-game . . . 9-game . . . 10-game winner; despite reporters from *USA Today* and *Sports Illustrated* and *The New York Times* and every other conceivable major outlet flocking to the Toronto clubhouse for their requisite "Return of the Rocket" profiles, something about the "Clemens ♥ Toronto" romance seemed contrived. Much of it was due to the mounting sense that Clemens, who had once thought the Blue Jays (11-12 and five games back come April's end) could possibly compete, was unhappy, uncomfortable and desirous of a trade. When the big money had been thrown his way, becoming a Blue Jay had been a marvelous concept. Now, stuck in reality, he was trapped on a bad team in an indifferent market. When confronted by Allan Ryan of the *Toronto Star* in late June, Clemens neither confirmed nor denied his feelings. "It's not working out," he said. "Everybody can see that. But I haven't said anything that would give anyone the idea that I want out."

That was a lie. In fact, Clemens had said something—several things—to friends, family members and even teammates.

"What the hell is going on here?"

"This isn't what I signed up for."

"Are we even trying to win?"

For someone making enough money to clothe and feed Ethiopia through the year 4197, Clemens sure liked to complain. He whined about the clubhouse food and the road accommodations, about the seats on the airplane and the buses. "He was a supernova," says Huck Flener, a Toronto pitcher. "I had never been around that type of star before. He had his own special box for his glove, because he didn't want it to be smashed in the team bag. He had a special suitcase with a glove protector inside. He also changed his jersey every inning, because Roger didn't like a sweaty jersey. So he had 15 jerseys in his locker. The rest of us had two."

Unlike Boston, Toronto is a city of golf courses—beautiful, wide-open green landscapes that seductively call out to the avid links enthusiast. "One of the reasons Roger ended up coming to Toronto is his love for the Toronto-area golf," said Paul Beeston, the Jays president. "He's crazy about the game." Now, playing two or three times per week during the season, Clemens expected every major facility to acknowledge three things:

1. Roger Clemens is great.
2. Roger Clemens never pays for golf.
3. By "never," Roger Clemens means *never*.

So it was that Clemens had a major tiff with the National Golf Club of Canada, which was ranked as the country's 11th best place to play.

The confrontational relationship actually began one year earlier, when Clemens and the Red Sox had come to town for a series with the Jays. Prior to the team's arrival, one of Clemens' agents contacted Marinus Gerritsen, the club's manager, about his client being allowed to play at the private facility. "That shouldn't be a problem," Gerritsen told him. "It's $1,000 for the foursome."

When the Red Sox arrived, Clemens took three teammates to National and played 18 holes. As the group retreated to the clubhouse, Clemens plopped down 10 Red Sox–Blue Jays tickets on the counter. Instead of showing the pitcher the requisite deference, the young employee behind the desk ignored the bribe and handed Clemens a bill for $1,000.

"This must be a mistake," Clemens said.

"No," the kid replied. "Not a mistake. It's what you owe."

With that, Clemens whipped the tickets off the desk and broke out his American Express card.

"I'm sorry, Mr. Clemens," the employee said. "We only take Visa or MasterCard."

Clemens paid with a different card and stormed off. On his way out the door, another young worker—a teen responsible for manning the greens—apprehensively approached the pitcher and asked for an autograph. "Fuck off!" Clemens barked. "Leave me the fuck alone!"

Now that Clemens was a Blue Jay, he compiled a mental list of all the area country clubs that he assumed would swoon over his arrival. He left tickets, signed autographs, posed for pictures—and rarely paid for so much as a Diet Mr. Pibb. When asked his thoughts on National, he teed off. "I used to like that place," he told a writer. "But it's gone way downhill."

Over the course of the season, Clemens' golfing addiction became the talk of the Toronto clubhouse. Clemens played golf in the cold, in the heat, in a light drizzle and in (what felt like) a typhoon. He shot a career-best 70 on the Plantation Course at the Kapalua Resort in

Hawaii, sported a five handicap and was dreadful at putting. Wrote Robert Rodriguez in *Avid Golfer* magazine, "If golf is a gentleman's game, Clemens is the perfect ambassador. He can hold his own on the golf course, as evident in his many pro-am appearances. Clemens has played with the best, played on the best, and works diligently to play at his best." The man who was being paid to lead the Jays on *and* off the field was often late to the ballpark and absent from team meetings. "He'd be off golfing while we were preparing for a game," says one teammate. "It was pretty audacious."

AT THE ALL-STAR BREAK Toronto was 40-43, 14 games behind Baltimore in the AL East. Having already been selected to five American League All-Star teams, Clemens, 13-3 with a 1.69 ERA, was indifferent about flying to Cleveland for another go-around. "This is my sixth All-Star Game and . . . it's . . . very . . . special," he said, mustering all the passion of a DeLonghi toaster salesman. "I can share it with my boys."

Truth be told, Clemens was focused on a contest a week after the so-called Midsummer Classic, when the Blue Jays would travel to Boston for their first time in 1997. Normally allergic to introspection, Clemens had pondered this reunion for a long time. Even though the Beantown court of public opinion had initially found Duquette guilty of jettisoning a legend, Clemens' repeated darts thrown toward the organization had largely turned the town against him. "It's a matter of channeling my emotions," he said beforehand. "It's going to be awkward coming out of the visitors' tunnel and warming up in the visitors' bullpen. But once I get on the mound, I should be locked in."

With both teams struggling (the Sox were 39-49), this was the moment Boston and Toronto sports fans had been waiting for—a game with meaning.

It didn't disappoint.

In an act noteworthy for its sheer classlessness, Boston's organist, a man named Richard Giglio, played the theme to *The Mickey Mouse Club* as Clemens walked to the bullpen for warm-ups. It was a surreal moment—for many Bostonians, the first time seeing their erstwhile god in anything but the familiar red, white and blue. Clemens was loudly cheered and loudly booed when he took the mound for the bottom of the first, and the attendees became even more animated when Nomar Garciaparra and John Valentin, the first two Boston hitters, singled to open the game. When Garciaparra later scored on a fielder's choice, making the score 1-0, Boston fans exploded with delight.

Wrote Steve Buckley of the *Boston Herald:*

Say this about Roger Clemens: Though he never delivered a World Series championship during his days with the Red Sox, he always delivered wonderful theater.

This is an inarguable point, and it makes no difference whether you loved him or loathed him, whether you considered him a hero or a rogue. When he pitched, in victory or in defeat, it was a memorable experience.

Over the next seven innings, Clemens allowed two more hits while setting a Blue Jays record with 16 strikeouts. His fastball, clocked as high as 98 mph, seemed to shoot off electric sparks under the afternoon sun, and his splitter had the Red Sox repeatedly chopping at air. Yet what elevated the event from remarkable to unforgettable was an improbable, only-in-the-movies conversion that took place in the Fenway stands. Much like the final fight scene in *Rocky IV,* when Rocky Balboa goes to Russia, faces Ivan Drago and gradually wins over the once-hostile Soviets with his heart and courage, Clemens' dominance reminded Sox fans of the good ol' days.

When Clemens struck out Garciaparra, Valentin and Vaughn to

wrap up a flawless eighth inning (and end his afternoon of work), he was saluted with a raucous standing ovation from the capacity crowd. As he walked off the field, the noise overtaking any further Disney-themed organ music, Clemens shot an unmistakable glare toward the private box of Boston CEO John Harrington—where Duquette sometimes sat. The intent was clear. "Shit, I don't think there was a person on our bench or in our bullpen who wasn't happy about that," says Vaughn Eshelman, a Boston pitcher. "We were playing against Roger, but we *hated* Duquette." Following Toronto's 3-1 victory, Clemens was doing a TV interview on the field when hundreds of fans came to the railing and chanted, "Roger! Roger! Roger!" As Clemens gleefully tipped his hat, a second chant started up: "Duquette sucks! Duquette sucks! Duquette sucks!"

Clemens flashed a grin and a thumbs-up. Who was he to argue?

CLEMENS PITCHED BRILLIANTLY IN 1997, winning his fourth Cy Young Award by leading the league with 21 wins, a 2.05 ERA and 292 strikeouts. Yet with the Blue Jays finishing 76-86 and 22 games back in the AL East, the attention paid to his dream run quickly faded. The national reporters stopped coming, the attendance never surged, the invisibility of the franchise resulted in as gloomy an August and September as the Blue Jays had ever experienced. "The city was underwhelmed by him," says Teitel. "He won the Cy Young Award, he pitched with courage—but nobody really cared. He was just seen as another hired gun in town for the money."

Indeed, Clemens had made his mark: His was perhaps the quietest dominant season in baseball history.

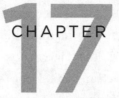

CHAPTER

17

Under the Influence

There was talk.

Not that much talk, admittedly. But one must consider the time period. We were just emerging from the mid-1990s, when "steroids" and "performance-enhancing drugs" were words and phrases reserved for the NFL, the WWF and back-alley gyms with shady characters and crooked needles. Mark McGwire and Sammy Sosa were more than a year away from their historic home-run duel, the Mitchell Report was Mitchell Page's career breakdown in *The Baseball Encyclopedia* and, to 99.9999999 percent of America, Victor Conte didn't exist.

But there was talk.

Not within the media, mind you. Writers and reporters weren't yet up to date on the drug culture of professional sports. Fans had little clue, either. They were happy lapping up the 500-foot home runs and 100-mph heaters.

But there was talk.

Among a growing number of major league ballplayers, Roger Clemens' miraculous 1997 season hadn't been quite so miraculous. It wasn't that a man of Clemens' talents couldn't make the jump from 10 to 21 wins in the span of a year. It wasn't even the anger with which he seemed to pitch—occasionally a wild-eyed frenzy that reminded one of a rabid wolf at suppertime.

No, what was off was the physicality of it all. As the number of major leaguers who used steroids and human growth hormone increased, players started to recognize the signs among their peers. "You just knew," says one former major leaguer. "Guys who had no business being huge and strong were now huge and strong." It was Jason Giambi, once a spindly 190-pound third baseman with minimal pop, reporting to Oakland camp with muscles growing out of muscles. It was Jose Canseco, telling anyone who would listen that he could "hook you up with my guy." It was Ken Caminiti, the Padres' third baseman, with those psycho eyes and fits of rage. It was the hushed conversations, the increased number of "handlers" in the clubhouse, the statistically implausible becoming plausible.

It was the reappearance of a fastball.

Roger Clemens worked hard. But over the course of the 1995 and '96 seasons, his fastball was topping out at 91, 92 mph, and his torso was slowly morphing into that of a bowler. "Roger wasn't throwing the ball quite like he used to," says Mike Greenwell, a Red Sox outfielder. "He still had great stuff, but the velocity was off." Now, less than a year later, the 34-year-old Clemens was built like a sculpted heavyweight and throwing as hard as he had in the mid-1980s. "He got his velocity back," Carlos Baerga, the Mets second baseman, explained in September 1997 when questioned about Clemens' inexplicable revival. Had it been noticeable in the past that Clemens' fastball wasn't up to snuff? Murray Chass of *The New York Times* asked. "Oh yeah," Baerga said. "He might have had a great conditioning program in the off-season. Maybe he was determined to show everybody that he hadn't lost anything."

Despite the overwhelming evidence now available that Roger Clemens was chemically enhanced, he has never admitted to using steroids or growth hormone, and no one knows, exactly, when he first picked up a needle. But here is what we do know: In his final two seasons with Boston, Clemens had engaged in regular conversations with Canseco—his close friend, golfing buddy and teammate—about the benefits of Deca-Durabolin and Winstrol (the drug for which Ben Johnson tested positive at the 1988 Summer Olympics), as well as the methodology of "cycling" and "stacking" steroids.

In late January 1998, Clemens approached Gord Ash, Toronto's general manager, about signing a certain needle-loving slugger to the team's payroll. Having served as the sole bright spot in the Blue Jays' otherwise abysmal 1997 campaign and armed with the guaranteed $24.75 million contract and a Hall of Fame résumé, Clemens was now the Michael Jordan of baseball—a man who said "jump" knowing his organization would immediately leap high into the air. "Did we give Roger special treatment?" says Ash. "Sure. But tell me, what star player doesn't get some leeway?"

The general manager did as he was told, handing the 33-year-old disruptive, past-his-prime, defensively incompetent, injury-prone Canseco a one-year contract worth $3 million. "We are walking into this with our eyes wide open," Ash said at the time. "We know what the history has been here."

That wasn't Clemens' only tinkering. Having fired manager Cito Gaston with five games remaining in the 1997 season, the Blue Jays held an extensive search for a replacement, interviewing such Grade-A candidates as Davey Johnson, Larry Bowa, Paul Molitor and Willie Randolph. But who did Ash and Co. wind up hiring? Tim Johnson, an unexceptional yet bubbly man who had just finished guiding the Triple A Iowa Cubs to a 74-69 mark. Rarely considered big-league managerial timber, Johnson possessed three major attributes:

1. Gobs of boyish enthusiasm. "I'll communicate with each of my players every day," he vowed upon being hired, "even if it's just to say, 'Hi, how's the family?' "
2. He had been a coach with the Red Sox when Roger Clemens was there.
3. Clemens *really* liked him.

ALONG WITH THE ADDITIONS of Johnson and Canseco, the Blue Jays made one more major hire to start the '98 season.

Well, maybe *major* hire is a bit of an overstatement. Through the course of a decade, 15 or so teams will likely change their strength and conditioning coaches, without so much as a mention in the local news. Sometimes it has to do with player complaints, sometimes it has to do with career shifts, sometimes it has to do with management looking for a jolt in productivity. Such was the case in Toronto, where the Jays had been—fitness-wise—underwhelming over the past few years. Geoff Horne, who had held the position for five years, was a hardworking professional with a solid reputation. But with the team struggling in a number of areas, someone had to take the fall. "One of our complaints was that we didn't think we were getting full results out of the position," said Ash shortly after naming Horne's replacement. "We needed a more aggressive personality, someone who would capture the attention of the players. If he could throw batting practice and catch in the bullpen, well, that would be great, too. Brian fit the bill on all three fronts."

Ash was referring to one Brian Jerome McNamee, a little-known New York Yankees bullpen catcher whose name was initially put into play in Toronto by Tim McCleary, the team's assistant general manager. As undergraduate students at New York's St. John's University in the late 1980s, McCleary and McNamee had been friends and baseball teammates.

Born and raised in New York City's Rockaway section of Queens, McNamee was the son of a police officer and dreamed of a future in either law enforcement or (God willing) baseball. An uninspiring natural athlete whose arm and bat speed graded as merely average, McNamee somehow started at catcher for three years at Queens' Archbishop Molloy High School, then played at the collegiate level for the Division I Redmen. "He was a very good baseball player here—really into the game, really loved it," said Jack Curran, Molloy's baseball coach. "And he was a really good player for St. John's." McNamee's greatest achievement occurred on the afternoon of May 27, 1988, when he helped St. John's defeat Stanford, the defending national champion, in the NCAA Northeast Regional at Beehive Field in New Britain, Connecticut. Starting at catcher, McNamee scored a run in the 5-3 victory.

Though McNamee believed himself to be worthy of a professional contract, 176 catchers found themselves selected in the 87 rounds of Major League Baseball's June 1989 amateur draft, and his name was never called.

In 1990, McNamee turned to Plan B, joining the New York Police Department as an undercover officer. For three and a half years, he was one of the best on the force, a fierce, fearless cop who, according to a *Sports Illustrated* piece, boasted "an amazing record for making arrests and who gathered citations for excellence." Among his experiences, McNamee was called to the scene in 1991 when Eric Clapton's son, Conor, died after falling 53 flights from an open apartment building window. Said Tim Lyon, a police lieutenant and McNamee's former partner, "He's probably the best police officer I've ever been around."

Wrote Jon Heyman on *Sports Illustrated*'s Web site:

The thing that Lyon couldn't get over was how hard McNamee worked and how loyal he was. "He was probably loyal to a fault," Lyon said.

McNamee has a history of taking hits for folks . . . Lyon recalled one time [in 1993] when McNamee's female prisoner escaped after he asked a colleague to watch the handcuffed collar while he completed paperwork. Since it was a female prisoner, she was handcuffed outside the holding cell. When McNamee returned minutes later, the handcuffs were still there but the prisoner was gone. McNamee knew the incident would hurt his colleague's bid for a promotion. So McNamee took the hit, knowing he'd suffer only a 30-day suspension. "Brian said, 'It's my prisoner, I'll take responsibility,'" Lyon recalled. And so he did.

In the suspension's aftermath, McNamee left the police force. He received a master's degree in sports science from Long Island University and, thanks to McCleary (who at the time was employed by the Yankees), found $60,000-per-year employment as New York's bullpen catcher and batting practice pitcher.

In three years with the Yankees, McNamee's impact was minimal. He acquired plenty of welts helping reliever Jeff Reardon develop a knuckleball, took a 10 percent pay cut in 1995 (as did most "nonessential" team employees) and served up one BP meatball after another. "He was just a guy," says Rick Cerrone, the Yankees' former media relations director. "'Hello, have a nice day'—that sort of guy. I don't think he made too many personal connections."

Though no longer a policeman, McNamee still behaved like one. He was suspiciously guarded and uncommonly reserved. Jokes didn't come easily, and laughs rarely came at all. He enjoyed the perks of being part of a big-league team but largely kept to himself. When Joe Torre was named Yankee manager before the 1996 season, McNamee was fired. Over the subsequent two years, he worked as a personal trainer for wanna-be jocks and muscle-heads.

When, after the 1997 season, McCleary and the Blue Jays came calling, Yankees who remembered McNamee from his days with the team were stupefied. McNamee as a strength and conditioning coach? Hadn't even entered their minds.

Yet when the Blue Jays players reported to Dunedin for spring training, they were greeted by the anti–Geoff Horne—an ornery man with thick shoulders and sculpted forearms who demanded commitment. Was he the sort of guy players would go out of their way to have a beer with? No. But that wasn't important. McNamee meant business. "Baseball players often talk about their game during spring training," wrote Mark Zwolinski of the *Toronto Star.* "But Brian McNamee . . . has them talking about sit-ups."

Not just sit-ups. McNamee forced players to do hundreds upon hundreds of "double sit-ups." Unlike Horne, McNamee insisted the players engage in conditioning work *after* their baseball drills, so that they would know how to battle through fatigue. He spent extra time with first baseman Carlos Delgado on improving his shoulder muscles, with Canseco on avoiding back spasms.

The one Blue Jay preprogrammed for the McNamee regimen was Clemens. Thirty-five years old and staring down the final stretch of his career, he reported to spring training in 1998 noticeably sluggish and overweight—a startling departure from his first season with the Jays. With McNamee now supervising his conditioning, however, Clemens quickly shed the pounds and reverted to form.

Clemens opened Toronto's season with a seven-inning, two-hit gem against the Twins. (Once again the SkyDome was the EmptyDome, with more than 10,000 vacant seats enjoying the Blue Jays' 3-2 victory.) He suffered a groin strain in his next start, struggled for a few games, then on May 3 held Oakland hitless over six innings in a 7-0 rout. When A's rookie Ben Grieve broke up the no-hitter with a single to start off the bottom of the seventh inning, Clemens received a standing ovation from the sparse Network Associates Coliseum crowd. "I could care less about a no-hitter," he said afterward. "We can't sit back on this. We have to push forward and start winning."

The Blue Jays were 11-17 and in last place in the AL East. Just like the previous season, they were headed nowhere fast.

So Clemens had an idea.

•   •   •

AS CORESIDENTS OF THE upscale SkyDome Hotel, Clemens and McNamee spent a great deal of time together. Though the line between superstar athlete and support staff employee was never fully crossed, the two struck up something *like* a friendship. Clemens told his long, name-dropping tales, McNamee listened raptly. Clemens bragged about the time he struck out 20 Mariners, McNamee nodded with faux fascination. "He has this history and this aura, and you hear all these stories," McNamee said. "But really, he is a very approachable guy and very intelligent when it comes to conditioning and what's right for him." Though McNamee exercised perspicacity when he surmised Clemens to be a typical superstar blowhard, he relished the feeling of sitting alongside baseball royalty. Clemens trusted McNamee, sought out his insight and opinions, bought him dinner and made him feel like one of the guys.

That's why in early June, after the Blue Jays returned from a road trip against the Florida Marlins, Clemens trusted McNamee enough that he felt comfortable asking him to inject him with steroids. For the first-year strength and conditioning coach, this was a disturbing request. From working with body builders, McNamee knew a lot about steroids, growth hormones and other such substances. He was, however, a man who believed in the power of human strength and perseverance, who genuinely felt that a 35-year-old man like Clemens could—with enough regimentation—turn back the hands of time. "Mac loved work more than any trainer I know," says C. J. Nitkowski, a veteran major league pitcher and fellow St. John's alum. "The first year I trained with Mac, I pitched poorly, and I asked him whether I should use [the steroid] Winstrol to maybe help get my speed back. He said, 'You don't need it. You'll supplement, but you'll use over-the-counter supplements.' He wanted me doing it the right way."

But with Clemens, what was McNamee supposed to do? He was 30 years old, supporting two children, and baseball's best pitcher wanted his assistance. Clemens knew that McNamee's one-year-old son, Brian Jr., had recently been diagnosed with juvenile diabetes. Doctors taught McNamee how to draw different types of long-acting and short-acting insulin. "Up until then, I had no experience with needles, other than getting them in me from doctors," McNamee said. " . . . I believe that that's why [Roger] came to me, to think that I was able to do that."

It remains unclear why Clemens approached McNamee following the Florida road trip, but it might have had something to do with his June 8 start against the Marlins. With temperatures in the high 80s and unbearable humidity sucking the life out of all creatures great and small, Clemens struggled, allowing three earned runs in seven innings to a bargain-basement lineup. It wasn't that Clemens pitched poorly; what bothered him was that, as younger teammates seemed to glide through the thick air, he was a lumbering station wagon. "Every other pitch I threw would be released differently," Clemens said afterward. "You'd see a spray of perspiration fly off my hand and wrist. I didn't have long sleeves on to absorb it."

A few days later, McNamee injected Winstrol into the pitcher's buttocks for the first time. The steroid had been obtained by Clemens. So had the needles. McNamee arrived at the pitcher's apartment, had Clemens pull down his pants and bend over. In went the drug. A few days later, on June 14, Clemens started against the Orioles at SkyDome. In one of his worst outings of the year, Clemens lasted just five and a third innings, allowing six hits, four runs and five walks. Afterward, he blamed the poor showing on a painful twinge in his right leg.

Over the next four days, Clemens fretted aloud whether his leg would force him to miss a start. However, when he took the mound at Baltimore on June 19, he felt electric. "I noticed right away that I was very strong," he said, "and my arm was alive and my velocity was dynamite." The Blue Jays lost in 15 innings, but Clemens had been rejuvenated.

McNamee said he injected Clemens between 16 and 20 more times

that season—almost always in Clemens' SkyDome apartment (Mc-
Namee recalled once injecting Clemens in the visiting clubhouse of
Tampa Bay's Tropicana Field—he rushed it, and Clemens wound up
with an abscess on his left buttock), always out of sight of teammates
and coaches. Clemens began shooting up Winstrol every fourth day,
then—fond of the results—upped the frequency to every third day.
The pitcher who had been topping out at 92 mph with Boston a mere
two years earlier was now clocked at 100 mph. Before the injections,
Clemens had registered 10 or more strikeouts on one occasion that
season. Over his final 17 starts, he had 10 or more strikeouts 10 times.

IF YOU WERE A member of the Toronto Blue Jays in 1998 and you
were one of the many players *not* using performance-enhancing drugs,
Roger Clemens' shtick had officially grown stale. Sure, it had been
fun when Clemens initially signed with Toronto, what with all the
hoopla. But now, well into his second season with the team, enough
was enough. Reliever Dan Plesac, a 13-year veteran who cringed at the
allowances the organiation made for its ace, went so far as to name one
of his horses "The 21 Rules" in honor of Clemens' special treatment. It
was far from a compliment.

En route to winning 20 games and his second straight Cy Young
Award, Clemens made it increasingly clear that his interest in con-
tinuing as a Blue Jay was waning. So what if the franchise had given
him $24.75 million, the manager of his choice and his close friend,
Canseco, a job when nobody else would? Toronto, Clemens had decided, wasn't committed to winning. In mid-July, as the trade dead-
line approached and the Blue Jays languished 20-something games
out of first, Clemens had his agents informally request a trade. "When
Roger signed with Toronto, there was a good-faith understanding that
the club was committed to win and Roger wanted to be a part of it,"
said Randy Hendricks, his agent. "And that if that did not appear to

be the case, the Blue Jays would make a good-faith attempt to trade him." Clemens confirmed his agent's words, snidely adding, "This is the same situation we were in last year when management didn't know what they were doing."

But just whose fault was this? Although Canseco was having a statistically eye-popping power season, with 46 home runs and 107 RBIs, his .237 average and 159 strikeouts were inescapable holes in the Toronto lineup. And Johnson, the manager had Clemens all but demanded the Jays hire, was a disaster. Though the team finished a respectable 88-74, veterans tuned out his zippity-doo-dah blather. He was eventually fired after his stories of Vietnam combat (in an attempt to put baseball into perspective, Johnson once told starter Pat Hentgen that he had killed a 12-year-old Vietnamese girl he thought was booby-trapped) were discovered to be fictional. "We actually believed Tim," says Robert Person, a Blue Jays pitcher. "We all chipped in once and bought him a motorcycle as a present. Roger came up with the idea of learning what Marine unit he served in and painting it on his helmet. When we tried finding out, well, there was nothing there." Alas, Johnson had not served in so much as the Cub Scouts.

As the Yankees ran away with the division, posting 114 wins en route to the World Series title, the Blue Jays sputtered along. In the final month, Clemens came to the stadium when he wanted to, failed to show up when he didn't. Even as Toronto somehow sneaked to within five of Boston in the Wild Card race in mid-September, Clemens remained indifferent. When he took the mound, he played hard. Otherwise—*whatever.* "It was a running joke," says Ed Sprague, the team's third baseman.

"Roger lived in the SkyDome, but we'd never see him. We'd say, 'What are you doing? Running the ramps while the game's going on?'"

On November 18, two months after Toronto completed the season, Ash, McCleary and (of all people), Dave Stewart, the recently hired assistant GM and former Oakland ace, flew to Houston to meet with Clemens at his home. The trip was a final effort to pursuade Clemens to return to Toronto—and it represented everything wrong with the Blue Jays–Clemens marriage. "I didn't feel good about that, but I was new," says Stewart, Clemens' former adversary. "We really believed Roger would want to stay with the club, but he didn't. Personally, it didn't bother me, because I always felt like I understood Roger pretty well. He was a great pitcher, but he wasn't really conducive to winning. He had pitched for almost 15 years in the majors, and not once had Roger made a difference in anything having to do with winning for a ball club when it counted.

"So to me, if Roger wanted to leave, let him. Good-bye, farewell, have a nice day. We'll be just fine without you. And probably better."

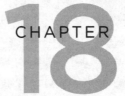

A (Not So) Yankee Doodle Dandy

Roger Clemens officially requested a trade on December 2, 1998, telling friends and teammates that he no longer believed the Blue Jays were dedicated to winning a World Series.

As far as excuses go, it was awfully convenient.

Much like the new home owner who raves about the deal he got, only to later learn he owes $50,000 annually in property taxes, Clemens' excitement over being a $24.75 million Blue Jay faded rapidly. Although he enjoyed the city, Clemens came to bemoan Toronto's overall baseball apathy and its figurative distance from Madison Avenue. A mere one-hour flight from New York City, Toronto could have been Mogadishu, as far as the league's fans were concerned. The Blue Jays annually ranked near the bottom of the majors in merchandising, and any company looking to spend millions on an athletic spokesperson wasn't setting its sights on Canada.

So it was that Toronto GM Gord Ash spent the holiday season shopping Clemens, talking to everyone from Texas and Houston to Cleveland and Anaheim. "I wasn't in a position of strength, because people knew Roger had to be moved," says Ash. "But I figured we could get pretty good value for a pitcher with his resume."

The one team that could most easily afford Clemens was also the one most conflicted about making a deal. Although the defending World Series champion New York Yankees never shied away from adding a big contract, owner George Steinbrenner was still stung by the aftermath of the 1996 season, when he had flown to Houston to meet with Clemens, even pumped iron with the pitcher in his weight room, then fumed as he joined the division-rival Blue Jays. "I like everything [Clemens] stands for," Steinbrenner said in early December. "I did my best to get him and didn't. It was a tough loss for me."

There was also the ol' Hate Factor. Namely, Yankee players *hated* Clemens. Throughout his career with Boston and Toronto, Clemens ranked alongside Baltimore second baseman Jerry Hairston and Cleveland pitcher Jaret Wright as the opponents New York players detested most. The loathing of the Rocket had started in 1991, when he nailed Yankees catcher Matt Nokes with a fastball to the body. Instead of withering in pain, Nokes had managed to pin the ball under his right arm and then throw it back at the mound. "I know it was intentional," Nokes said afterward. "He did it before when I was in Detroit. I hit a homer off him to win a game and he told writers, 'Next game, Nokes is going down.' I went down three times in that next game."

A couple of spring trainings later, after allowing a single to New York's Bernie Williams in a previous at-bat, Clemens unleashed a 95-mph fastball that plunked the earflap of the Yankee centerfielder's helmet. In March 1998, after one of his Toronto teammates was hit by a pitch, Clemens retaliated by grazing Derek Jeter, New York's shortstop, with a chest-high fastball. A few months later, Clemens hit third baseman Scott Brosius in the back with yet another fastball, which led to a bench-clearing brawl. "Those things lingered with us for a long time," says Brosius. "I didn't know Roger, but I really didn't like him. I don't think many of us did."

And yet, this was *the* New York Yankees, a franchise that, under Steinbrenner, craved dominance. If the team had won 114 games in 1998 with a rotation of David Cone, David Wells, Andy Pettitte, Orlando Hernandez and Hideki Irabu, what could it do in '99 with a five-time Cy Young Award winner leading the way?

Ash had intended to deal Clemens by mid-December, but come February he was still looking. Teams were scared off by Clemens' age, as well as word that he would approve a deal only to a franchise that would provide him a four-year extension paying $13.25 million annually.

Finally, with spring training just days away, an exasperated Ash called Brian Cashman, New York's general manager, and told him Clemens *had* to be moved. When Cashman asked for a list of players Toronto would want in return, Ash named three: Wells, long reliever Graeme Lloyd and second baseman Homer Bush. Cashman had to fight to conceal his giddiness.

Steinbrenner, however, was significantly less enthused. Though he would happily part with Lloyd, an effective yet unremarkable major league pitcher, and Bush, the promising 26-year-old speedster stuck behind starter Chuck Knoblauch, he felt a particular kinship for Wells. Rude, abrasive, arrogant and severely overweight, the 35-year-old left-hander was Steinbrenner's kind of Yankee—a beer-swilling, trash-talking gamer who sported an 8-1 postseason record. "If you liked Metallica, tattoos, Howard Stern and post-game beers," wrote Jack Curry of *The New York Times*, "you liked Wells." The pitcher earned his place in Yankee folklore during the 1997 season, when he paid $35,000 for a cap worn by Babe Ruth, then sported it during a start against Cleveland. Wells' status as a Yankee icon was sealed on May 17, 1998, when he threw a perfect game against the Minnesota Twins at Yankee Stadium.

Yet within the New York clubhouse, Wells earned mixed reviews. Teammates liked his competitiveness and bemoaned his obnoxiousness. He screamed at the press and never earned the trust of manager Joe Torre or pitching coach Mel Stottlemyre. "He was such a punk," says Dave Buscema, who covered the Yankees for the *Times Herald-Record*. "Wells went out of his way to treat people like dirt." A couple of hours after Ash had called Cashman, Steinbrenner ordered 30 of the team's advisers to meet at Malio's Steakhouse in Tampa. Famously known for his refusal to listen to others, Steinbrenner was acting completely out of character: quiet, interested, attentive. His heart told him Wells needed to remain a Yankee. His head told him Roger Clemens was too good to pass up. He went around the table, asking each person to vote yes or no. "It was unanimous," said Cashman. "No one could come up with a reason not to make the trade."

Later that night, at 11:42, Cashman called Ash. "Gordie," he said, "we have a deal."

THEY WANTED TO HATE Roger Clemens. They *had* to hate Roger Clemens. To Yankee players, inviting him into their clubhouse was the equivalent of Ronald Reagan having the Ayatollah Khomeini over for Thanksgiving dinner. As both an ace and a headhunter, Clemens had tormented New York for a long time. Why should he be forgiven simply because he was being handed a pin-striped uniform?

"There were a lot of questions about how Roger would fit in with us," says Mike Buddie, a Yankees pitcher. "I was at the game in 1998 when Clemens hit Jeter, and later on I hit [Toronto's] Tony Phillips to even the score. So when I showed up at camp, I was fascinated to see how Roger and Derek would hit it off. Could they coexist? Could they be friends?"

A resounding answer came on the morning of February 26, when Clemens, throwing his first live batting practice as a Yankee, faced a minor league catcher named Jaime Torres. As Clemens stared down Torres, Jeter and Knoblauch approached the cage dressed in full catcher's gear. So locked in was Clemens that he failed to notice the costumes until Knoblauch stepped to the plate wearing the garb. The result was a smile, a tip of the cap and a softly thrown pitch behind the veteran second baseman's back. Jeter, standing nearby, chuckled with delight. "The past is over with," he said. "He's part of the team now. We know it, he knows it."

Unlike in Toronto, where half the players had to be carded before entering a bar, the Yankees were a veteran unit that wouldn't go gaga over the new ace. To standouts like Jeter and Knoblauch, first baseman Tino Martinez and closer Mariano Rivera, Clemens symbolized little beyond a nice upgrade. They wouldn't tiptoe toward his locker seeking counsel or defer to his wisdom. And there would be no surrendering of the number 21, which outfielder Paul O'Neill had worn for six years. Clemens accepted number 12 without a peep. "We were happy Roger was with us," says Brosius. "But we weren't awestruck. We just won the World Series without him."

For most of his career, Clemens had been treated royally. But now, surrounded by 10 players with All-Star résumés and a handful who would one day be considered for the Hall of Fame, Clemens seemed to revert to the chunky kid from Butler Township. No longer the snarling, bullying Rocket, he was once again uncomfortable and somewhat insecure.

Despite predictions of an all-time great team becoming even greater, Clemens' first season in the Bronx was a bumpy one. On the bright side, teammates came to respect and admire the man. He worked hard, showed up early, left late, kept quiet, limited his quotations in the press to dry drivel and oft-repeated clichés and played golf on the off-days. With seven of the club's 10 best pitchers aged 30 or older, Clemens was rarely called upon to offer much beyond the general postgame insight. "Roger didn't say a ton, but that was fine, because he was a genuinely nice person," says Allen Watson, a veteran reliever with the team. "Our spring training lockers were next to each other, which was great to me, because he never sat still for more than three seconds. He was constantly working out, lifting weights, running, icing. What was there to complain about?"

Yet while the Blue Jays were receiving standout performances from Wells (17-10—while wearing the uniform pants left behind by the wide-bottomed Clemens), Lloyd (5-3 with three saves in 74 games) and Bush (.320, 32 stolen bases), Clemens was maddeningly inconsistent for New York.

On opening night at Oakland, he went six and a third innings, allowing three runs and striking out eight in a New York loss. All the right things were said in the postgame interviews (Catcher Joe Girardi: "What we used to face, we saw tonight. It's a lot better on this side"), but there was no denying the mediocrity. Five days later Clemens seemed to make amends, debuting at home against the Tigers by throwing seven and two-thirds innings of shutout ball to earn his first victory. The fans rose in unison as he was removed from the game, and Clemens walked slowly toward the Yankee dugout, tipping his cap. "This," he said afterward, "was a special day. The sun was shining today."

Clemens quickly came to find that New York's followers are knowledgeable, passionate—and brutal. Only five days later, Yankee fans booed Clemens off the diamond after he gave up 11 hits, seven earned runs and three home runs to Baltimore. "We had a great pitcher out there and he had a bad night," said Don Zimmer, who served as the interim manager while Joe Torre battled prostate cancer. "Everybody's human."

Clemens' season played out the way it started. Good start. Bad start. Two good starts. One mediocre start. One nightmarish start. Two good starts. "He still threw hard," says Mike Figga, a Yankees catcher, "but he had to adjust to New York." By the All-Star break he was a misleading 8-3, with a 4.70 ERA. Teammates were intrigued by

Clemens' unconventional rituals. He had the hair on his arms, legs and chest removed on a weekly basis and prior to games coated himself in a malodorous heat balm. (According to *Sports Illustrated*'s Tom Verducci, Steve Donahue, the Yankee trainer, would rub red-hot liniment on Clemens' testicles as part of the pitcher's post-whirlpool routine. "He'd start snorting like a bull," Donahue told Verducci. "That's when he was ready to pitch.") He wrapped much of his body in medical tape to hold everything together. He also wore a plastic mouth guard while he pitched, so that he could avoid grinding his teeth down to nubs. "He pitched and prepared with a linebacker's mentality," wrote Buster Olney in *The New York Times*. "By the time his day in the rotation came around, Clemens was often [overloaded] with adrenaline."

On July 13, he returned to Fenway Park for the first time as a Yankee. The All-Star Game was being played at Fenway, and though Clemens wasn't a member of the squad, he would be honored beforehand in a ceremony for baseball's All-Century team. As each star was introduced by Kevin Costner, the cheers grew louder. From Pete Rose and Johnny Bench to Ken Griffey Jr. and Sandy Koufax, Boston's fans could not have been more gracious.

Until Clemens' name was called. Those in the stadium let their own Benedict Arnold have it, eager to poison what was meant to be a dream night for the Rocket. Yet having returned to Boston as "an enemy" multiple times by now, Clemens was unphased. To the pitcher, it was simply an accepted part of the gig, no more painful than a mild splinter to the thumb. He smiled as he walked onto the field, gazing up at the fans who had once adored him but now wore T-shirts reading CLEMENS SUCKS. If they felt the need to express themselves in such a way, so be it.

Roger Clemens didn't give a damn.

BY LATE JULY, NOBODY was quite sure what was wrong with Clemens—only that something was, factually, wrong with him.

The headlines told the story. YANKS BATS RESCUE CLEMENS read *The New York Times* after Clemens left a game against Texas trailing 5-0. METS BLAST OFF ON ROCKET said the *Newark Star-Ledger* when Clemens lasted two and two-thirds innings against the crosstown rivals. ROCKET BOMBS AGAIN screamed the Bergen *Record* following a four-and-two-thirds-inning disaster against the Angels.

The Yankees had traded for Roger Clemens, only they had wound up with Joey Hamilton. The fire with which the Rocket had pitched so brilliantly for so long seemed to have been left behind in Toronto. Mel Stottlemyre, New York's pitching coach, tried to snap Clemens out of his malaise. "Don't worry about fitting in here," he'd tell him. "Don't feel like you have to live up to an image. Just be yourself." Behind closed doors, the exasperated Steinbrenner began ripping his underlings for endorsing the trade. Maybe Wells wasn't perfect, but he had been the perfect Yankee. Steinbrenner slammed Clemens to Torre and publicly demanded a return to form of "The Terminator."

"I thought we were going to see the Clemens of old," Steinbrenner said. "I'm trying to reason in my own mind what's happening with him."

In a scathing interview with *Playboy*, Wells—pitching adeptly for the Blue Jays—turned the knife. "[Clemens] is not a savior, I guarantee that," he said. "He is a desperate man dying to win a championship. Roger Clemens is going into the Hall of Fame but he is going to go in empty, without a ring. Right now, all I want to do is kick the Yankees' ass. And I want to kick the shit out of Roger Clemens."

Clemens tried increasing his bullpen work and sitting down for lengthier meetings with Stottlemyre. He even switched his uniform number from 12 to 22—a nod to his 12-year-old son Koby, who wore the digits as a second baseman in Houston's "select" Little League.

To the media, Clemens pooh-poohed his difficulties. To others, however, he blamed his slump on the end of his close and personal relationship with Brian McNamee. Without him nearby, Clemens felt lost. He was still able to work hard, still almost certainly able to obtain the performance-enhancing drugs that allowed him to go harder, longer, faster than the younger competition. But Clemens *needed* McNamee's wisdom, his supervision, his skill with a hypodermic needle. When Clemens wanted to know whether he could eat a steak with potatoes, he asked McNamee. When he had questions about a certain drug's impact, he didn't call CVS or Rite Aid—he went to McNamee. Now he was often alone.

The low point of a bad season came on July 31, when Clemens returned to Boston to pitch for the first time as a Yankee. Outside of Fenway, vendors sold T-shirts reading CLEMENS IS A BAG OF SHIT. Fans were handed Old West–styled WANTED posters featuring his face. Clemens lasted one batter into the sixth inning, surrendering five hits and four earned runs in a humiliating 6-5 setback. As he walked off the mound toward the visiting dugout, head down, cap lowered, Clemens was serenaded with a venomous chant of *"Rah-jah! Rah-jah!"*

Fortunately for New York's faithful, the Yankees were too talented for one disappointing pitcher to ruin things. Though a far cry from the 114-win juggernaut of 1998, the '99 team still won 98 games and captured the AL East. Led by Jeter's MVP-caliber season (.349-24-102) and Rivera's 45 saves, New York advanced to its fifth straight postseason.

Clemens, who finished 14-10 with a 4.60 ERA, was now the number three starter, penciled in behind Orlando Hernandez and Andy Pettitte in New York's rotation against the Texas Rangers for the upcoming best-of-five Division Series. In his play-off preview, *Newsday*'s David Lennon called Clemens the "weak link." The *Daily News*' Mark Kriegel went one step further, writing that if Clemens' name were Hideki Irabu, "he might not be on the playoff roster at all."

"When you're that big of a name and you make that type of money, people expect things of you," says Brosius. "I'm not saying that's fair, but it's the way people are. Especially in a city like New York."

Finally, on October 9, 1999, Clemens delivered. With New York leading the series 2-0, he took the mound at Rangers Ballpark in Arlington and overwhelmed the Rangers, who managed three hits and no runs off of Clemens over seven innings. New York won 3-0 behind Darryl Strawberry's three-run homer in the first, and the two enormous monkeys (play-off choker, New York flop) seemed to be removed from his back.

Sort of . . .

Yet while the triumph propelled New York to an AL Championship Series showdown with Boston, critics and fans could not help but note that it had come in a game the Yankees didn't *have to* win, against a mediocre Texas lineup featuring the likes of Royce Clayton and Tommy Goodwin. No, the true test of Clemens' worthiness, of whether he had actually *become* a Yankee, would take place on the afternoon of October 16, when New York, leading 2-0 in the series, traveled to Fenway to face the Red Sox.

As if the moment needed any more drama, Boston's game three starter was Pedro Martinez, the 27-year-old ace who had been acquired by Duquette before the 1998 season to fill the void left by the Rocket. "If you take a Koufax against Marichal," said Rod Beck, a Boston reliever, "this would be something of that magnitude." THE FIGHT OF THE CENTURY read the front page of the *Boston Herald*. The popular Boston bumper sticker for the day: CY YOUNG VS. CY OLD. For Bostonians, Martinez was the anti-Clemens. Smart, bubbly, personable and full of panache, Martinez wasn't the type to brand all of his children with *K*'s or babble in mind-numbing clichés. "We used to joke that Pedro speaks better English than Roger," says the *Boston Herald*'s Tony Massarotti of the Dominican Republic–born Martinez. "Only it wasn't entirely a joke." With a 23-4 record, 2.07 ERA and 313 strikeouts in 213⅓ innings pitched during the regular season, Martinez had established himself as baseball's best pitcher, unanimously winning the AL Cy Young Award.

Upon pulling his SUV into the Fenway players parking lot, Clemens was greeted by curses and taunts. The booing began as soon as Clemens walked to the visiting bullpen. It continued when he strolled to the mound. As Clemens warmed up, the chants began. *"Rahhhhhh-jah! Rahhhhhh-jah! Rahhhhhh-jah!"*

In arguably the biggest non–World Series game of his life, Clemens was brutal. Over two innings, he allowed six hits, two walks and five runs. Overcome by emotion, Clemens tried throwing every ball 150 mph. "He had nothing," Michael Kay, the Yankee radio voice, noted. "I think he's been enveloped by the enormity of the game. He just doesn't have it."

When Torre came out to remove Clemens with no outs and a man on in the third, Fenway's residents responded as if free hundred-dollar bills were descending from the autumn sky. *"Where is Rah-jah?"* they chanted. *"Where is Rah-jah?"* Clemens retreated directly to the club-house, where he threw his glove against the wall in disgust.

IN SPITE OF CLEMENS, the Yankees defeated the Red Sox in five games and advanced to the World Series to face the Atlanta Braves.

Before the Series began, Torre slipped Clemens to the back of the rotation, behind Hernandez, Cone and Pettitte, hoping to dial back the pressure. Like the Texas Rangers, the Braves, winners of 103 games, were no match for New York. The Yankees cruised through the first three games and handed the ball to Clemens under the best possible circumstance: *Win at friendly Yankee Stadium, and the Series is ours. Lose, we still have three more chances.* As Clemens stood on the mound before the first inning, he was approached by Jeter, who patted him on the rear with his glove. "You've been waiting all your life for this," he said. "Now make it count."

Though it was hardly the best he'd ever pitched, Clemens came through. With New York's fans urging him on, Clemens allowed four hits and one run over seven and two-thirds innings, as New York secured an easy 4-1 triumph. He didn't allow a fly ball to an outfielder or a runner past first base until the eighth. For so much of the season, Clemens came off as baseball's Garry Kasparov—cold, indifferent, unemotional. But here he was, clenching his fist and screaming with delight when Jeter made a brilliant play in the sixth; slamming Brosius with a high five following a Brooks Robinson–esque grab in the same inning.

As he walked from the mound midway through the eighth, Clemens gently lifted the cap from his head and waved it to the booming crowd. "Very much needed and deserved," Cone said. "You could tell he needed that." Upon entering the dugout, he was hugged by teammates and coaches. Finally, the man had come through when it counted. Finally, he had a World Series ring.

"Tonight," he said afterward, "I know what it's like to be a Yankee."

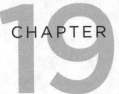

CHAPTER

19

Happiness

This is when the happiness is supposed to begin.

Roger Clemens was, at long last, a world champion. On October 29, 1999, he rode in the Yankees' confetti-coated victory parade down Manhattan's Canyon of Heroes. He looked up at the tall buildings that lined Broadway and marveled at his good fortune. He was fitted for a three-carat diamond ring, featuring a blue stone shaped in the interlocking NY symbol in the middle and a 14-carat white gold NY covered with round diamonds on top. He was lauded for his "gutsy" performance in game four of the World Series, when he had finally pitched like the Rocket of old.

Clemens reported to spring training in the best shape of his career, aided by Brian McNamee, whom the Yankees had hired as an assistant strength and conditioning coach. (To placate Clemens, the team agreed to give McNamee a job—but only if Clemens paid his salary. A giddy Rocket agreed.) Clemens pitched relatively well to open the season, helping the Yankees jump out to a 22-12 start. He had his trainer, he had his fastball and he had his ring.

And, then, silence.

The phone call came on the morning of May 18, 2000. The words hit Roger Clemens hard, like one of his very own 98-mph fastballs to the head.

"Roger, Kathy has been killed."

"Kathy" was Katherine Huston Clemens, Roger's former sister-in-law and the woman largely responsible for turning the baseball player from an awkward, uncomfortable boy into a confident, successful man. When Roger had moved from Ohio to Houston to live with Kathy and Randy, she had been the one who made certain he did his homework; who talked to him about everything, from girls to college to careers; who saw him as more than a vehicle to fortune and fame. "She loved Roger," says Carolyn Gray, Kathy's sister. "And Roger really loved her."

The once-upon-a-time Vandalia-Butler High School prom king and queen had been divorced for more than a decade, yet Kathy was still tormented by Randy and his drug abuse. He often asked her for money and had been in and out of rehab oh, how many times? *Two? Three? Four?* "It hurt Kathy so bad," says Gray. "You could have no idea." A popular third-grade teacher at Holmsley Elementary School in Houston, "Mrs. Clemens" was known for making up stories about the cursive letters and arriving at school with rollers in her hair.

In short, Kathy wanted nothing to do with the world her ex-husband had subjected the family to. Yes, she was once married to a druggie. But why should that ruin her life? Why did it have to haunt her all these years later? Most troubling was what Randy's addiction had done to their two children, Marcus and Jessica. In particular, it was her 19-year-old son who warranted the concern. Coated in tattoos and piercings, Marcus—like Randy—turned to using drugs in his late teenage years. Once, Marcus had come to visit his uncle in Houston, only to be stopped at the front door. "Son, you can come in,"

Roger said. "But first you've gotta take all those metal things out of your body. I don't want my kids seeing you looking like that."

On the night of May 17, Marcus Clemens, now 19, was sick in bed with the flu, and his mother had stayed home at their apartment to care for him. There was a knock on the back door. Kathy looked through the peephole and, not recognizing the men standing there, returned upstairs to her boy. Marcus asked his mother for some Sprite, and as Kathy walked back down to the kitchen, she heard another knock. This time, for a reason that has never been determined, she opened the door.

Five men, ranging in age from 18 to 26, barged into the apartment, demanding to see Marcus. They had come to steal what they were certain would be a large amount of money and Marcus' stash of Ecstacy. Her son still upstairs, Kathy ordered the intruders to leave.

Justin Gore, a 20-year-old wayward drug dealer, whipped out a gun and pointed it at the woman who had once been named Houston's Teacher of the Year. Kathy let out a terrified scream.

Then Gore squeezed the trigger.

"I jumped up as fast as I could and went to the top of the stairs," Marcus later said. "There were two more shots, and I saw her fall." As the intruders ran off, Marcus dashed downstairs, dragging his mother's body into the living room. She had been hit in the head, neck and chest and wasn't breathing. Blood streamed across the floor.

The ambulance came within minutes but nothing could be done. Kathy died en route by Life Flight to Memorial Hermann Hospital. She was 46 years old.

At approximately the same time Kathy's life was ending, Roger Clemens' night was thriving. As she was staring down a gunman, he was facing the Chicago White Sox at Yankee Stadium. As she was being pronounced dead, he was being pronounced alive, having won his fourth game with a beautiful seven-inning, two-run, nine-strikeout masterpiece. As Marcus was describing to Houston police what had transpired in his apartment, Clemens was describing to the *Times,* the *News* and the *Post* what had transpired on his home field. "When we're right as a team swinging the bats, there are not too many holes in our lineup," he said. "That was evident tonight."

In hindsight, it all seemed so . . . vapid. Bernie Williams hit two home runs for New York, Chuck Knoblauch tripled, Jorge Posada stole a base—blah, blah, blah. Who the hell cared? Certainly not Clemens, who was shocked, dismayed, heartbroken by the news. And furious. Not merely at the killers, whom police described as transients who "float from one rave party to another rave party." No, he was furious with his older brother, Randy. When Roger learned the details of the case—the drugs, the violence—he blamed Randy. His brother was the one who had made drugs a part of the family's life. Had Randy died in a drug deal gone bad, well, Roger would have been devastated but not surprised. His life had been heading in that direction for many years. But this was Kathy.

The next day, Roger spoke with Carolyn Gray and her husband, John, who lived in Vandalia, Ohio, near his boyhood home. "Listen, you don't worry about paying for anything involving the funeral or burial," Roger told them. "If it hadn't been for Kathy, I have no idea where I'd be today."

"No," said Carolyn, "she was my sister, and I should . . ."

"Yes," Roger said firmly. "I'm going to handle this. She was your sister, but she was like a mother to me. You have so much to worry about. Let me worry about this."

"As far as I'm concerned," says Carolyn, "Roger can do no wrong in my eyes. I'll always remember the way he was at that time. Always."

On the morning of the viewing, Kathy's family was asked to come to Holmsley Elementary School. Upon arriving, Carolyn began to sob. The sidewalks were coated with farewell messages written in chalk. A banner stretched across a hallway read WE LOVE YOU MRS. CLEMENS and was signed by every student. Carolyn was handed an envelope filled with letters from Kathy's third-graders.

Dear Mrs. Clemens:

I'm very, very sad that you have a new address. But one good thing is I know where it is—heaven. I'm very, very sorry that your wonderful and beautiful life had to end in pain. I guess God couldn't wait to get you in his arms. Maybe he wants to start a school, up in heaven for the younger angels, and he knew you would be the best. Though I can never see you in this lifetime, I can always have you in my hart [sic] and mind. There are also great memories I wouldn't change a bit. I miss you very much.

Love,

Leslie

PS: See you in heaven.

The funeral was held in the chapel at Waltrip Funeral Directors in Houston. An overflowing crowd of family members, friends and coworkers bid farewell to a woman described by her sister as "loving, adventurous, daring, full of life."

Outside the building, a handful of police officers lined the front steps. They were there at the behest of Roger, with one primary directive: If you see Randy Clemens, do not allow him inside.

Somehow, New York's rapacious press corps missed the news about Kathy Huston Clemens. Not a single article appeared in the local newspapers. Clemens kept the information mostly to himself, confiding only in manager Joe Torre and a handful of teammates when he left for the funeral.

As far as Roger was concerned, the relationship with his brother was over. Though it was Kathy who had passed, Randy Clemens— the man largely responsible for creating the Rocket—was dead to him, too.

THE 2000 SEASON, WHICH had began with so much joy, was quickly devolving into a nightmare. Off the field, Clemens struggled to cope with Kathy's death. The endorsement opportunities he desperately craved were few and far between, and his pitching coach, the beloved Mel Stottlemyre, was away from the team while battling multiple myeloma.

With his wife and children back home in Texas, Clemens continued his affair with Mindy McCready, who had recently been dumped by BNA Records due to slumping sales, erratic behavior and rumors of cocaine addiction. He flew McCready to the Yankees' road locations on his private jet and gave her thousands of dollars in cash and gifts. Like a good number of professional athletes, the Rocket had mistresses stashed in several major league cities, all well versed in the details of New York's road schedule. Perhaps his strangest away-from-the-family pursuit came in the form of Charlize Theron, the bombshell South African actress with the 36B-24-36 body and the form-fitting red-carpet outfits.

Clemens had long fancied the starlet, who during the 2002 season came to New York to promote a new film. While eating dinner at Serafina—one of Manhattan's snazziest bistros—an apparently intoxicated Clemens looked up and spotted his Hollywood crush. He approached the actress, introduced himself and asked whether she'd like to join him for a drink. When Theron—who, as a baseball ignoramus, likely had no idea who the pitcher was—declined, Clemens trailed her through the restaurant until a bouncer stepped in his way. "Take one more step," he growled, "and there'll be some real trouble here."

With that, Clemens stopped, looked up as Theron exited through the front door and yelped, "But Charlize, I'd do you right . . ."

Clemens found little more success on the field. In mid-June, Clemens had a 4-6 mark, alternating good and bad starts. He won his 250th career game on May 6 at Baltimore—then got pounded five days later by a Detroit club languishing in last place in the AL Central. He even spent 15 days on the disabled list with a strained groin.

Wrote Bob Klapisch in the Bergen *Record:*

The question is getting closer to a naked cry for help. Repeat after the New York Yankees, who in unison are wondering: what's wrong with Roger Clemens?

The Yankees clubhouse is full of theories, none satisfying, all leading to a possibility so dark, club officials won't even speak about it on the record. And that is, Clemens isn't in a slump, but has instead sunk to a level of permanent mediocrity that will doom the Yankees this summer.

With absolutely nothing going as planned, Clemens told McNamee he would once again like to start using steroids to enhance his game. As had been the case in Toronto two years earlier, McNamee was in no position to argue or demur. So, as before, he began injecting Clemens in the buttocks with testosterone from bottles of either Sustanon 250 or Deca-Durabolin. Unlike the Blue Jays days, when Clemens arrived with the goods himself, this time McNamee was both the administrator and supplier. He bought the drugs from Kirk Radomski, a former clubhouse employee with the New York Mets who in 2008 gained infamy after coming forward as a distributor of steroids to dozens of major league players.

Clemens also had McNamee come to his family's three-bedroom apartment on 98th Street and First Avenue and inject him with human growth hormone, a peptide hormone that stimulates growth and cell reproduction in humans and other animals. Administered properly, HGH can increase muscle mass and protein synthesis, resulting in abnormal strength and speed and—most important for someone of Clemens' age—the ability to recover quickly from physical stress. As most players throughout baseball suspected, the steroid-HGH combination seemed to have done wonders for Barry Bonds, Mark McGwire and Sammy Sosa, all of whom were defying aging while putting up unprecedented numbers.

Clemens' steroid and HGH usage once again directly coincided with his revival. Beginning on July 2, when he mastered the Devil Rays with seven innings of three-hit ball in a 5-2 Yankee victory, Clemens won nine straight decisions and his ERA dropped from 4.76 to 3.30. THE ROCKET IS BACK! screamed a headline from an August 18 story on Salon.com, in which the writer Allen Barra declared, "One of the major comebacks of the baseball season is going on right now, and it's happening in the media capital of the country."

Without the drugs, Clemens had seemed old, stale and nervous. With the drugs, he was the Rocket, throwing high, hard heat while snarling at anyone who dared stand in his way. "His intensity was just insane," says Jay Tessmer, a Yankee pitcher. "Everyone else looked timid by comparison." Clemens received a huge boost on August 7, when New York picked up Jose Canseco, his old steroid guru, off waivers from Tampa Bay. As soon as Canseco joined the team, he, Clemens and Andy Pettitte began regularly working out together. A month later, Clemens pitched one of the most memorable games of his life, entering Fenway Park to catcalls—and silencing the Red Sox offense with eight innings of shutout ball in the 4-0 win. Although the Yankees limped toward the finish, prevailing in the AL East by a mere two and a half games, Clemens charged down the stretch with a 9-2 run. For the first time in two seasons as a Yankee, he was consistently pitching like an ace.

"He's got the body language now," said Torre, "and the attitude that dares people to beat him."

NEXT CAME THE PLAY-OFFS, and Clemens lived up to his postseason reputation, losing the series opener against the A's, 5-3, after surrendering four runs in six innings. Four days later, with the Yankees leading the series two games to one, Clemens was asked to start on short rest, and the results were even more disastrous—an 11-1 pasting that forced New York to fly to Oakland for game five.

The Yankees saved Clemens' hide by winning a dramatic final game and headed into the American League Championship Series to face the Seattle Mariners. After losing the opener, New York dominated the second and third games, with Clemens set to pitch on the afternoon of October 14 at Seattle's Safeco Field.

Though Torre told the media that Clemens had been pushed back to game four because "I wanted to give him an extra day's rest . . . he's older," it was easy to read between the lines: Clemens was not entirely trusted. When asked off the record by reporters what he thought of Clemens, Reggie Jackson, the Yankees' fabled Mr. October, teed off. "I think he's soft," he said. "He'll pitch well today, but only because we're up in the series and he has some wiggle room. Believe me, if we were down two games to one, he'd choke. Because he can't handle big moments. He never has.

"I've always found Roger to be very nervous around me. I think it has to do with me being Mr. October and him being Mr. May."

After New York went down without a run in the first, Clemens took the mound, struck out Stan Javier and Al Martin, then threw a 96-mph fastball near the chin of shortstop Alex Rodriguez, one of the league's best players. The next fastball, also in the high 90s, came even closer, causing Rodriguez to snap his body backward and land on his backside. "Throw the ball over the fucking plate!" Rodriguez yelled at Clemens. From the Mariners dugout, manager Lou Piniella screamed toward the mound. "You wanna do that!" he barked. "You really wanna do that! Because we can play that way, too! Oh, yes, we can!"

In a game that ranks with his two 20-strikeout masterpieces, Clemens allowed one hit while whiffing an ALCS-record 15 in a 5-0 victory. Through six innings, Clemens faced 19 batters, only one over the minimum. Just two balls were hit out of the infield. When Martin finally broke up the no-hitter by doubling in the seventh, there was a brief sag in Clemens' shoulders. He proceeded to strike out Rodriguez and Edgar Martinez, the team's two top hitters.

"Roger was as dominant as I have seen him," said Rodriguez after the game. "He had great velocity, a splitter and a devastating [slider] that was diving, and he didn't throw too many pitches over the plate. I don't care if you are hitting great or you are not, you are just not going to do much."

Three days later, the Yankees beat the Mariners again to clinch yet another trip to the World Series. (Two days after that, Clemens sent Rodriguez's mother a gift basket Yankee wives had presented to Mariner wives. Read the attached note: "I really wasn't trying to hurt your baby.")

This time, New York would be battling New York as the Mets and Yankees squared off in baseball's first Subway Series since 1956.

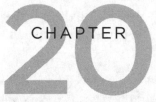

CHAPTER

20

Subway Crash

E very sports superstar has a nemesis.

Goose Gossage could never sneak a fastball past George Brett.

Patrick Ewing rarely got the better of Michael Jordan.

Roger Staubach's Super Bowl dreams were twice dashed by Terry Bradshaw.

And Roger Clemens was regularly manhandled by Mets catcher Mike Piazza.

On paper, it made no sense. Piazza could be a sucker for high heat, and Clemens specialized in high heat. Piazza, a member of the Mets, faced Clemens only twice a year, a clear advantage for the pitcher. Yet leading up to the highly anticipated 2000 World Series, Piazza had a .583 batting average against the Rocket, going 7 for 12 with three home runs. "Oh, Mike owned Roger," says Darryl Hamilton, a former Mets outfielder. "He absolutely owned him."

The saga of the two All-Stars dates back to July 10, 1999, when the

Yankees came to Shea Stadium for the opener of a three-game series. In the midst of a disappointing debut season with the Yankees, Clemens took the mound and was pounded. The big moment came in the bottom of the sixth when, with the game tied at 2 and runners on first and second, Piazza turned on a fastball that he deposited into the left-center bleachers. The Mets catcher was saluted with a standing ovation, and when the noise refused to die down, he popped out of the dugout for a curtain call.

Roger Clemens, Mr. Tradition, *loathed* curtain calls by opposing hitters.

Eleven months later, on June 9, 2000, Clemens and Piazza met again, this time at Yankee Stadium. With no score in the top of the third inning, Piazza walked to the plate with the bases loaded and Yankees fans in a panic. With his second pitch, Clemens threw a split-finger fastball that dipped, but not nearly far enough. *Crack!* The ball sailed over Bernie Williams' head in deep center, over the 408 sign. "There aren't many guys," Torre said later, "who hit the ball to the farthest point of this ballpark and flip their bat because they know it's gone."

Clemens was devastated—not simply because he had allowed a grand slam but because, at long last, an opponent had figured him out. Throughout his career, Clemens had been the one doing all the figuring. He knew to bust Albert Belle inside. He knew José Cruz Jr. couldn't hit a curveball. He knew Sal Fasano chased anything low and away. So how was it that Piazza, a *National League* player, could have Clemens so flummoxed?

On July 8, Clemens faced the Mets in the second game of a day-night doubleheader at Yankee Stadium. Riled up from the get-go, Clemens unleashed a series of high-and-tight pitches to the Mets' first three batters, Lenny Harris, Derek Bell and Edgardo Alfonzo, and got out of the inning unscathed. The Yankees failed to score off Glendon Rusch in the bottom of the frame, and Piazza, the Mets' designated hitter for the day, stepped into the batter's box. The first pitch, a fast-ball, was taken for strike one.

The second pitch was a 92-mph fastball straight at Piazza's head. The Met superstar ducked, but the ball still hit him on the front of his blue plastic helmet. As he crumbled to the ground, he looked as if he had been shot.

Piazza lay in the dirt, dazed. He blinked, then blinked again and again. Mets trainer Fred Hina and manager Bobby Valentine rushed to his side, as his teammates angrily stormed the field. John Stearns, the Mets' flammable bench coach, unleashed a string of obscenities toward the mound, where Clemens stood, head down, seemingly non-chalant. It was later announced that Piazza had suffered a concussion and would be forced to miss the All-Star Game.

In the home dugout, Yankee players were speechless. On the one hand, they were supposed to defend a teammate, and would do so later in postgame interviews. But many were disgusted. It was one thing to brush a guy back, even to hit a thigh or leg or elbow. But headhunting crossed the line. "I hope we're bigger than that," Torre said in a rare moment of meekness. "To hit somebody in the head . . . you don't do that."

In the visitors' dugout, there was a single emotion: rage. "I've seen him hit guys in the head," Valentine said. "I saw him hit Robbie Alomar in the head after he tried to bunt on him once. It's bullshit. It's terrible. I hope someday he pitches in a National League ballpark when we're playing against him. That's all I've got to say."

"They better watch out," added a player. "This is not over."

After the game, Clemens tried to call Piazza from the clubhouse—not to apologize but to make certain he was OK. When Piazza was told who was on the line, he refused to pick up.

"Fuck him," he said. "I don't wanna talk to that guy."

•   •   •

AS THE METS AND Yankees now prepared to face one another in the World Series, a familiar storyline was being offered of good versus evil, right versus wrong, and decent versus immoral. It was the tale of Mike Piazza versus Roger Clemens, and, as is often the case in the mainstream media, it was presented in an overly simplistic manner.

Unlike Clemens, who had blazed through the minor leagues, Piazza had discovered major league greatness only following a lifetime of mediocrity. Growing up in the Philadelphia suburb of Phoenixville, Pennsylvania, Piazza had spent much of his life behind his house, where his father, Vince, had installed a big-league pitching machine and a makeshift batting cage. "I was out there every day," he said. "I would come home from school, get a snack, watch cartoons and then hit. Every spring I would see that I was hitting the ball farther and farther." Despite the doggedness, nobody considered Piazza to be anything beyond a solid local talent. As a senior in 1986, he broke Phoenixville High's home-run record while hitting .400 as a first baseman. He was, however, defensively inept and unusually slow. If men like Bo Jackson and Deion Sanders were 100s on the athleticism scale, Piazza was a −6. Thanks to some help from Dodgers manager Tommy Lasorda, who was the boy's godfather, Piazza was allowed to walk on at the University of Miami, where he had one hit in nine at-bats as a freshman. He dropped out after the season, and played the following year at Miami-Dade North Community College. He batted .364 for the Sharks, but, really, who cared? Trying to draw the attention of a four-year college to his godson, Lasorda had Los Angeles select Piazza with the 1,389th pick in the 1988 amateur draft.

When the Dodgers called Piazza to find out what school he would be attending, he puzzled the club by asking for a tryout. With Ben Wade, the team's scouting director, looking on at Dodger Stadium, Piazza hammered one ball after another into the blue seats. He was presented a $15,000 signing bonus, then shipped out to Class A Salem, where he was ordered to learn to catch. When the season ended, he requested that the Dodgers send him to Camp Las Palmas, the organization's Dominican Republic–based academy for Latin prospects. He was the only American player ever to crave such an assignment, and he soon learned why: beans, rice and sugarcane juice for dinner and tarantulas in his bed.

By 1992, Piazza was in the big leagues, a strapping 23-year-old man who had defied long odds. Over the next eight years, he established himself as one of the great all-time offensive catchers, right up there with Yogi Berra, Johnny Bench and Gary Carter. It hardly hurt that he was bright, articulate, witty and accessible. In the same way reporters avoided Clemens when a good quotation was required, they dashed toward Piazza.

As the hundreds of major league ballplayers who turned to performance-enhancing drugs throughout the 1990s did their absolute best to keep the media at arm's length, Piazza took the opposite approach. According to several sources, when the subject of performance enhancing was broached with reporters he especially trusted, Piazza fessed up. "Sure, I use," he told one. "But in limited doses, and not all that often." (Piazza has denied using performance-enhancing drugs, but there has always been speculation.) Whether or not it was Piazza's intent, the tactic was brilliant: By letting the media know, off the record, Piazza made the information that much harder to report. Writers saw his bulging muscles, his acne-covered back. They certainly heard the under-the-breath comments from other major league players, some who considered Piazza's success to be 100 percent chemically delivered. "He's a guy who did it, and everybody knows it," says Reggie Jefferson, the longtime major league first baseman. "It's amazing how all these names, like Roger Clemens, are brought up, yet Mike Piazza goes untouched."

"There was nothing more obvious than Mike on steroids," says another major league veteran who played against Piazza for years. "Everyone talked about it, everyone knew it. Guys on my team, guys on the Mets. A lot of us came up playing against Mike, so we knew what he looked like back in the day. Frankly, he sucked on the field. Just sucked. After his body changed, he was entirely different. 'Power from nowhere,' we called it."

When asked, on a scale of 1 to 10, to grade the odds that Piazza had used performance enhancers, the player doesn't pause.

"A 12," he says. "Maybe even a 13."

SO THAT WAS THE juicy subtext to the Subway Series: the pending confrontation of the two New York superstars—presumptive Hall of Famers with questionable characters who happened to hate each other.

On the strength of his 15-strikeout gem against Seattle, Clemens was tabbed by Torre to start game two at Yankee Stadium, a nod to his lengthy résumé and recent success. The Yankees took the series opener in dramatic style, coming back from a 3-2 deficit to win on a 12th-inning single by little-used Jose Vizcaino.

Clemens spent his days prior to the start trying to lower the expectations of an inevitable brawl. Yes, he had thrown inside. But he certainly hadn't meant to injure Piazza. "I've revisited it the last couple of days a little bit," he said in a soft, humble tone, "and everybody just wants to push it behind and let it go."

When Clemens took the mound, however, those words rang hollow. In his two years with the Yankees, Clemens often frustrated Torre with a surprising lack of feistiness. At times, it had looked as if he wanted to be somewhere else, as if pitching were more chore than passion. On this night, however, Clemens was nearly as fired up as he had been 10 years earlier, when he had been ejected by umpire Terry Cooney during a play-off game and needed to be carried from the field. His cap pulled low, his scruff two days old, his stare icy, Clemens delivered his warm-up pitches with a robotic precision—*Pop! Pop! Pop! Pop!* It was his first start in seven days, and he was pumped.

When Timo Perez, the Mets' leadoff hitter, stepped to the plate, he was greeted by a 97-mph fastball for strike one, followed by a 96-mph heater that ran high and inside. Three pitches later, he swung through another 97-mph fastball for strike three. The next batter, Alfonzo, suffered the same fate—a series of high-90s fastballs, culminating in a 94-mph splitter that he swung through for strike three.

Up stepped Mike Piazza.

With the wind blowing and the temperatures hovering in the mid-40s, Piazza wiped both sides of his face on a long sleeve, then walked toward the plate. He took a half swing. Another half swing. Another. Clemens' first pitch, a 97-mph fastball, soared over the plate for strike one. Piazza took a step back, blew into his right hand and returned to the box. The next pitch was another 97-mph blazer on the inside corner. Strike two. Clemens missed with a splitter, running the count to 1-and-2.

With the fans standing and clapping, Clemens reared back and threw another 97-mph fastball. As the pitch tailed inside, Piazza swung, the wood and ball meeting near his grip. The bat cracked, with the handle remaining in Piazza's hands and the barrel of the bat bouncing toward Clemens. As the ball headed foul, Clemens fielded the sawed-off bat head, turned and whipped it toward Piazza, who was jogging up the first base line. The stunned Mets catcher slowed down, stopped, then began walking toward Clemens.

"What's your problem?" Piazza barked. "What is your problem?"

"I thought it was the ball," replied Clemens.

The Mets stormed onto the field. The Yankees stormed onto the field. Clemens turned toward Charlie Reliford, the home plate umpire. "I thought it was the ball," he repeated. "I thought it was the ball."

Was Clemens kidding? He thought a piece of wood, with a splintered end, was the ball? "I like Roger, but I have no idea where that statement came from in his head," says Tyler Kepner, who covered Clemens for *The New York Times*. "As far as unwise things to say, it's right up there with 'Brownie, you're doing a heck of a job.'"

Lenny Harris, the veteran Met utility player, was screaming at Clemens, trying to reach him through a crowd of players. Hamilton, the Mets outfielder, was furious—but not at the Yankees. "I wanted to know why Mike wasn't going after him," says Hamilton. "When he was hit in the head I understood, because he was shaken up. But in the World Series, why were you still confused? This guy threw a bat at you, and you do absolutely nothing? You don't stand up for yourself? You don't defend your manhood? Baseball is a game of pride, and we were all getting on Mike. 'Where's your pride, man? Where's your pride?'" (David Wells wrote in his autobiography, "Trust me, if I were Mike Piazza, that broken bat would still be shoved up Roger's ass.")

In the broadcast booth, Tim McCarver, who had past run-ins with Clemens, was incredulous. "There were a lot of people who defended Roger Clemens when he hit Mike Piazza in the head, and I was one of them," he said. "In my view right now, Roger Clemens is dead wrong. That's a blatant act. Foolish. Foolish."

Amazingly, Reliford and his fellow umpires neither ejected Clemens nor issued a warning. They simply got players back into their respective dugouts and guided Piazza to the plate. On the next pitch, he grounded out to second. With the inning over, Clemens approached Reliford, tapped himself on the chest and said, "That's my fault. That's my fault." Then he ran into the clubhouse and cried.

THE YANKEES WENT ON to win 6-5, taking a commanding lead in a series they would capture in five games. But in the immediate aftermath, nobody cared about Tino Martinez's three RBIs or Clemens' nine strikeouts over eight innings or even Piazza's ninth-inning homer off Jeff Nelson. No, in the dank bowels of Yankee Stadium, 80 to 100 reporters squeezed into a conference room to grill the greatest right-handed pitcher of his era. An electric current seemed to shoot through the gathering of notepad holders and TV pretty boys, as reporters congregated in groups of six and seven to replay what they had just witnessed, to express their disbelief and, in some corners, outrage (mock or otherwise). When Clemens finally entered, everything went silent. The scene was akin to watching a death-row inmate approach the noose. It was clear something horrible was about to go down—yet no one was 100 percent sure how it would transpire. As Clemens sat at a table and leaned into a microphone, looking more like a sullen eight-year-old than a mound legend, Yankee Stadium turned into a courtroom.

REPORTER: "Some of the Mets said that they thought it did look like there was intent."

CLEMENS: "No."

REPORTER: "But because they thought that . . ."

CLEMENS: "Not at all."

REPORTER: "Are you glad you're not pitching at Shea?"

CLEMENS: "I'm not going to answer that. Again, there was no intent."

REPORTER: "Would there be any fear batting against him?"

CLEMENS: "There was no intent."

REPORTER: "The amateur lip-readers among us, it looked like you said, 'I thought it was the ball.'"

CLEMENS: "I might have said that. Some of my guys said that, too."

REPORTER: "What did you mean by that?"

CLEMENS: "My emotions. I'm telling you, my feet were off the ground. I'm trying to let you all know. I went right to either Charlie or to the umpires, it was great that they just said, 'Hey, just relax a little bit.' And I said, 'Give me another ball. Let me get back up on the mound here.'"

REPORTER: "Could you explain or clarify a little bit the source of those emotions and why you were so sky-high?"

CLEMENS: "It's not too hard to figure it out. I don't think it's hard to figure it out."

REPORTER: "Is it because of what you've been reading and hearing?"

CLEMENS: "I haven't been reading it. I've been hearing it. Everybody in the clubhouse, leading up to today, was continually trying to keep me pumped up. They thought I might have been a little bit down. I was trying not to let it get me down. So, to be honest with you, if I didn't have the stuff I did tonight, it would have been hard work. I mean, I was fortunate. I had similar stuff that I had in Seattle. And I have seen many times late on TV how these guys have made rallies late and came back in games. So once they got the two runs and got some momentum, it wasn't comfortable."

REPORTER: "Piazza said that he had said to you after the bat had gone in his direction, he had said to you a couple of times, 'What's your problem? Do you have a problem?' You didn't answer at all. Was there a reason why you didn't answer at all?"

CLEMENS: "Because I didn't hear him, to be honest with you."

REPORTER: "You didn't hear him?"

CLEMENS: "I wasn't hearing much there, to be honest with you."

Yankee Stadium had never hosted such banal nonsense. In typical Clemens fashion, the pitcher simply brushed aside the questions he preferred not to answer. Reporters seemingly numbed by a lifetime of baseball's clichéd platitudes were trying—and failing—to evoke their inner Bob Woodwards. At one point Mike Lupica, the oft-ridiculed *Daily News* columnist, stood up and bellowed, "Roger, what I think the people here want to know is, *why did you do this?*" Clemens brushed the question aside, staring down his inquisitors as if they were a part of the stadium's cockroach infestation.

Moments late, Torre entered the room, sat down and, for one of the few times in his illustrious career with the Yankees, berated the media. The same manager who had lambasted Clemens as a headhunter when he was with Toronto was now defending the indefensible.

"I think we have to ask one other question: 'Why would he throw it at him?'" Torre said. "I mean that, to me, is the simple question. . . . So he could get thrown out of the game in the second game of the World Series? Does that make any sense to anybody? Somebody answer me. Somebody answer my question. . . ."

The room, loud as a playground moments earlier, was dead silent.

What was Roger Clemens thinking?

Nobody had the slightest idea.

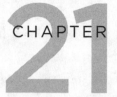

Greatness by Any Means Necessary

T hroughout the winter and spring of 2000–01, after Piazza-gate had died down (with little fuss, Clemens paid a $50,000 fine for the bat-throwing incident), New York baseball fans came to appreciate that Roger Clemens' final two play-off starts had been spectacular. He had struck out 15 Mariners. He had held the Mets to two hits. After going 15 years without a World Series ring, he now owned two. Clemens was 38 years old, well past the prime of an average pitcher, throwing 98 mph to start a game and 97 eight innings later.

Nolan Ryan was evoked, only Nolan Ryan hadn't been nearly as dominant.

Phil Niekro was evoked, only he threw a 70-mph knuckleball.

Really, there was no apt comparison.

Roger Clemens was an ageless marvel.

Looking back, it is unfortunate how easily the fable was lapped up by the mainstream media, fed to reporters in a gold-plated bowl with sparkling diamonds along the rim. If Roger Clemens said he worked hard, Roger Clemens worked hard. If Roger Clemens said he ate bumblebee stew for breakfast, Roger Clemens ate bumblebee stew for breakfast. For the nation's sportswriters, primarily white males in their late 30s and early 40s, Clemens' success mirrored what they desired in their own lives. *You can continue to perform at a high level! You can continue to beat the odds!* They wanted to believe in Roger Clemens, because it said as much about them as it did about him.

So what if his achievements were physically impossible?

In a glowing *Sports Illustrated* profile titled "Rocket Science," Tom Verducci, arguably America's best baseball writer, observed, "Fathers of teenagers aren't supposed to be blowing 96-mph heaters past Gen X batters and taking Wite-Out to the record book. They're supposed to be standing on the sideline at their kid's first high school football practice." In a *New York Times* piece titled "A Wonder of the Pitching World," Buster Olney broke down the three keys to Clemens' longevity: mechanics, genetics and training. "A few [pitchers] might learn how to nick the ball a bit or use a little moisture—cheat a little—to get some extra movement," Olney explained. "But Clemens still throws very hard, in spite of his age, for a variety of reasons."

Clemens was terrific at slinging fastballs and just as good at slinging mythology. He would take writers through his daily regimen, letting them see the sweat and pain that went into the making of the Rocket. He allowed them into his gym, into his home. He let them speak with Brian McNamee, who knew damn well he could broach any topic *but* performance enhancers. The access served two purposes, reinforcing the splendor of his greatness and turning many media members into giddy fan-club members.

"The whole I-work-out-harder-than-anyone-else thing was utterly ridiculous," says Pat Jordan, the veteran writer who profiled

Clemens for a 2001 *New York Times Magazine* cover piece. "Clemens enjoys working out. It's fun for him. It's a comfort zone. So when the media raves about his work ethic, there needs to be some perspective. Work is something you don't want to do, but do anyway. Exercising was what he *wanted* to do. It was a mindless activity for a mindless person."

Following two up-and-down years in New York, the 2001 season was a happy one for Clemens. This wasn't Boston, where the fans booed more than they cheered. This wasn't Toronto, where indifference reigned. This was New York, a city eager to love its stars. From game one through game 162, Clemens performed brilliantly. He beat the Royals on Opening Day, allowing three runs over eight and a third innings while bypassing Walter Johnson for the all-time American League strikeout lead. (He took the ball home to his mother, Bess, who had recently emerged from an intensive care unit while battling emphysema.) He pitched courageously against Pedro Martinez and the Red Sox on April 14, fighting through poor command and a tidal wave of Fenway Park boos to hold Boston to two runs over six innings in a 3-2 New York triumph. He passed Gaylord Perry for sixth place on the all-time strikeout list with a 3-1 win over Oakland on April 29, then one month later moved past Don Sutton into fifth. "He was just so darn good," says Brian Boehringer, a Yankees reliever. "Every time he was on the mound there was one thing he was focused on—getting the guy out. Was he well liked when he pitched? Definitely not. But that's fantastic. He was out there to win, not make friends."

Clemens entered the All-Star break with a 12-1 record and was selected to start the game by Joe Torre, the AL manager. With his sons Koby (14), Kory (13), Kacy (6) and Kody (5) in tow, Clemens strutted into a hotel ballroom from the All-Star press conference in Seattle the day before the game, grabbed a chair behind a table, leaned into the microphone and proceeded to field one question after another concerning his dazzling longevity, his dazzling stamina and his dazzling longevity and stamina.

"Considering his age," added Torre, "it's been a remarkable run."

REMARKABLE, OF COURSE, IS RELATIVE.

Roger Clemens going 20-3, winning his sixth Cy Young Award and reaching 98 mph on the radar gun at age 38—remarkable.

Roger Clemens going 20-3, winning his sixth Cy Young Award and reaching 98 mph on the radar gun at age 38 while being injected with performance-enhancing drugs—not so remarkable.

In the summer of 2001, with the Yankees rolling to 95 victories and yet another AL East crown, Clemens depended heavily on steroids. McNamee made weekly trips to Clemens' apartment on 98th Street and First Avenue. He would leave his car out front with the doorman, Carlos, and take the elevator up to the 10th floor. Clemens would retrieve the steroids and needle kit from a walk-in closet. The two would enter the master bedroom, and on the king-sized bed Clemens would carefully lay out a hand towel, on top of which he placed the ampoule, the needle, the gauze and a bottle of rubbing alcohol.

Clemens would then drop his pants, bend over and have McNamee inject him. He would alternate anabolic steroids—Sustanon 250 one visit, Deca-Durabolin the next.

Of the one dozen or so times McNamee injected Clemens in 2001, all but one took place inside the apartment. The lone exception was a July injection in the clubhouse at Yankee Stadium, immediately prior to the final game of a home stand. The two retreated to a side area beside the team's Jacuzzi, where McNamee plunged the needle into Clemens' buttocks and pushed down the ampoule. When he dressed after the game, Clemens followed his precise routine—deodorant, shirt pulled over head, underwear pulled up, pants pulled up, left boot on first, right boot on second. Good-bye, out the door.

To his dismay, however, this time a nickel-sized circle of blood had oozed from his rear end onto the back of his fancy dress slacks. The person who first noticed the stain was Mike Stanton, a loudmouth Yankee relief pitcher who sat behind Clemens on team flights. Though not especially close to his journeyman teammate, Clemens felt compelled to answer when Stanton quietly asked whether he had turned to drugs.

"Hey, man," Clemens replied, "whatever I can do to get an edge."

Clemens' usage of performance enhancers directly contradicted his oft-stated respect for baseball history. Whenever Clemens was closing in on the next pitcher on the all-time strikeout list, Rick Cerrone, the team's media relations director, would find a photograph of the player and hang it in the Rocket's locker. "Maybe Roger wouldn't know who, say, Rube Marquard is," says Cerrone of the legendary New York Giants pitcher. "Well, I'd hang him up so Roger had a frame of reference."

Early on, when Clemens passed Walter Johnson on the all-time strikeout list, Johnson's grandson, Hank Thomas, praised the Rocket as a worthy man to do so. "I'm just thrilled," he said. "I see Roger Clemens as a modern-day Walter Johnson. There's something magical about a power pitcher who can blow 'em by you whenever he wants." By the time Johnson was Clemens' age, he was a sub-.500 hack in the second-to-last year of his career. There were no steroids or growth hormones available then. Johnson pitched, and when the magic petered out, he retired. "That's how it's supposed to happen," says Dave Fleming, a Seattle Mariners left-hander in the early to mid-1990s whose career was cut short because of injuries. "You play, your body naturally breaks down with age and you move on with life. But once guys started cheating, you had to ask whether what you were seeing out of older pitchers was real or phony."

On September 5, one month removed from his 39th birthday, Clemens won his Yankee-record 15th straight decision, limiting Toronto to six hits and two runs over seven and a third innings in a 4-3 win at the

SkyDome. In front of 29,235 fans, Clemens became the first pitcher since Marquard in 1912 to start a season with a 19-1 mark. "Rocket is incredible," Torre said afterward. "At 39 and to be the pitcher that he is is remarkable." The win was a big one for Clemens, who saved the lineup card and cherished the baseball used for the final out, which was handed to him by closer Mariano Rivera.

Normally, it was the type of evening that would have Clemens floating on air for a week.

Normally, however, was no longer about to apply.

IF ONE WERE TO rank all 47 men who played for the New York Yankees in 2001 on the probability of embracing the Manhattan life-style, Roger Clemens would almost certainly place last.

He was an unabashed Texas country boy, a man who had never felt especially comfortable in Boston. But Clemens didn't simply enjoy living in Manhattan—he loved it.

Residing on the Upper East Side of Manhattan, Clemens lived it up. He and Debbie (when she wasn't at home with the children in Texas) attended the theater, ate at the fanciest restaurants, walked the streets of their neighborhood for the sheer joy of being surrounded by a vibrant urban environment. Clemens loved how New Yorkers would shout his name as he passed—"Go get 'em, Rog!" He couldn't understand why so many of his teammates moved to the suburbs of Westchester County or Long Island. "You don't know what you're missing," he would tell them. "This city is alive!"

On the morning of September 11, 2001, Clemens woke up assuming he would spend most of the day preparing for the chance to win his 20th game against the Red Sox at Yankee Stadium later that night. An early riser, Clemens was awake to answer the door when Carlos, his building's doorman, came knocking. He advised Clemens to turn on the television.

Debbie, who was in town for the evening's game, sat next to Roger on the couch.

"We see little planes flying down the Hudson River all the time and just thought somebody messed up," Clemens said. "I put on a shirt and some shorts and went up to the roof of our building. We could see the smoke from the [North Tower]." After a couple of minutes, Roger and Debbie listened in horror as they heard that a second airplane had hit the South Tower. "We went to watch television," Clemens said, "and by the time we got back on the roof, it was like being in Beirut or some-place like that. There were F-16s all over the place. It was like being in a different world. Everything had changed."

With the phone lines jammed, Clemens struggled to place a call to his sons in Texas. When he got through, he heard panic in their voices. *Yes, he and Debbie were OK. No, they didn't have to worry.* Carlos knocked again a few minutes later and warned that there was word of chemical leaks in the city. Roger and Debbie rushed to their SUV and drove to Connecticut, where they stayed for two days before making the 22-hour drive to Houston.

When Clemens returned to the city a few days later, he set out on a personal goodwill tour. He made repeated trips to Ground Zero, visiting with the rescue workers, signing autographs, posing for pictures, talking to the relatives of workers via cell phones. When Sotheby's announced an auction to raise money for 9/11 charities, he donated two of his cars—a Porsche Strosek wide-body 928S and a Mercedes custom AMG 500SL. He attended several benefits for fallen firefighters.

On one particular day Clemens and a friend decided to take Yankee memorabilia to a fire station close to his apartment. Upon pulling up in his car, he noticed that many of the firemen were returning from a funeral. "We just sat there and [thought about leaving]," said Clemens. "Finally, one of them noticed me in the car and came over. He said, 'It's a great time; get out.'" Besieged by the firefighters, Clemens wept.

After five days away from baseball, the Yankees congregated at the stadium on Saturday, September 15, for a brief workout. Before picking up so much as a ball, the players knelt on the grass around the pitching mound, removed their caps and bowed their heads for a prolonged moment of silence.

Read a piece in *Sports Illustrated:*

Some held hands. Others draped comforting arms around teammates' shoulders. Three family members of club employees are among the missing. For two somber hours they fielded balls and took batting practice. Lapses in concentration were not only tolerated but also expected. Afterward most of the players piled into vans and headed to Manhattan to visit hospitalized victims. "This is an enormous, heavy time," said manager Joe Torre.

The Yankees returned to action on September 18, in Chicago against the White Sox. For Clemens, it felt all wrong. He wanted to be with the people in his adopted city, not 790 miles away at Comiskey Park. Before the game, he entered the dugout wearing not his normal warmup jacket but one from his local firehouse, which he later signed and donated to charity.

Clemens finally won his 20th game with a 6-3 victory over the White Sox on September 19 but felt little thrill in victory. In the hours before the game, he sat in front of the clubhouse television with his teammates and listened to President Bush warn Osama bin Laden that he was "on notice." Afterward, he stood by his locker and answered questions with a raw candor that had been missing for years. "I know this is what we do and it is what I do, but it is not who I am," he said. "Right now, it doesn't have the same feeling it would have a couple of weeks ago. Maybe someday . . ."

Clemens and his teammates returned to New York City on September 25, with a chance to clinch the AL East against the Tampa Bay

Devil Rays. Since this was the club's first home game since the terrorist attacks, George Steinbrenner invited dozens of firefighters, police officers and emergency workers to attend. As Clemens prepared for the start, he walked past the uniformed public servants, all of whom were lined up along the hallways in the stadium's bowels.

"Go get 'em, Roger!"

"Give 'em hell, Rocket!"

"Clemens, do it for New York!"

"They're in their uniforms, and you can tell they've been crying," Clemens said. "You walk down the line, and almost all of them had lost loved ones or friends. You reach to shake their hand, and they want to hug you. After that, the game didn't mean a thing."

That Clemens went out and pitched one of his weakest efforts of the year in a 4-0 setback mattered little. The fact that a Red Sox loss to Baltimore that same evening clinched the title for New York mattered little as well.

"Roger Clemens is a Yankee now," said Kurt Englehardt, a Port Authority Police officer. "You've got to respect that."

FOR SOME MAJOR LEAGUE teams, the pressure of the play-offs is almost too much to bear.

Now try carrying the weight of a devastated city.

Although in hindsight it seems melodramatic, much was made of how baseball could "save" New York, how the Yankees were healing deep wounds. "[With baseball back]," wrote Tracy McDannald in *The Daily 49er,* "order and normalcy had taken a giant step toward being restored." Win a World Series, the thinking went, and people could rejoice again.

More than any Yankee, Clemens took this to heart. He wanted to heal New Yorkers, to make everything right, to throw the ball 200 mph and scale tall buildings in a single bound. Unfortunately for the

Yankees, the Roger Clemens who wanted to bean Osama bin Laden's skull with a fastball was also the Roger Clemens who regularly imploded come play-off time. With a crowd of 56,697 anticipating another magical fall moment and Clemens' heart pounding at 10,000 beats per minute, the A's came to Yankee Stadium for game one of the ALDS and battered New York's ace for four hits and two runs in four innings of work. The Roger Clemens who snarled like Dirty Harry was nowhere to be found, replaced by a meek impersonator who was mercifully pulled with a tight right hamstring. New York lost, 5-3.

The Yankees dropped the next contest as well and survived game three in Oakland thanks only to Derek Jeter, who saved the season with a miraculous flip to home plate to nail Jeremy Giambi. When the Yankees won game four behind Bernie Williams' five RBIs, it was back to New York for game five—and back to Clemens.

With his hamstring throbbing, Clemens again took the Yankee Stadium mound and again stared down Oakland's vaunted lineup. He surrendered five hits and three runs in four and a third innings. The Yankees won the game 5-3, and Clemens had delivered yet another adequate—if not gutsy—showing. "If I was not able to make this start because of this leg," he said afterward, "I would have felt I let a lot of guys down in this clubhouse."

The Yankees advanced to face Seattle in the ALCS. The Mariners had won 116 regular-season games but seemed overmatched in this series. The Yankees won the first two games at Seattle, lost the third at home, then handed the ball to Clemens, who was hampered by his tweaked hamstring. In a press conference leading up to the game, the desperate Clemens tried his best to lower expectations, explaining that, thanks to the injury, he still had little control over his pitches. "It's fairly amusing for people that are not in the know," he said, "but I really don't have any idea when I'm going in or out on pitches right now."

Clemens pitched courageously in game four, allowing but a single hit through five innings, before leaving with more hamstring pain. In the bottom of the ninth, second baseman Alfonso Soriano hit a two-run homer for the 3-1 victory.

The Yankees won again the next day, eliminating the Mariners in five games.

Another Fall Classic awaited.

WERE THERE EVER A World Series that the Yankees seemed pre-destined to win, this was it.

In only their fourth year as a major league team, the Arizona Diamondbacks were, in many ways, New York's polar opposite. Unlike the Yankees, who wore classic blue-and-white pin-striped uniforms, the Diamondbacks had their players dress in cartoonish outfits colored turquoise, copper, black and purple. Unlike the Yankees, whose "House That Ruth Built" was steeped in tradition, at Arizona's Bank One Ballpark, fans could dive into an outfield swimming pool.

The greatest contrast, however, was on the field. Unlike the Yankees, who had a powerful lineup, a deep rotation and, in Mariano Rivera, baseball's best closer, the Diamondbacks were thin. In 20-game winners Randy Johnson and Curt Schilling, Arizona boasted the best one-two pitching punch in baseball. But with the exception of left fielder Luis Gonzalez, whose 57 home runs and 142 RBIs made him a strong MVP candidate, the Diamondbacks didn't have much pop in their lineup. "If you looked on paper, New York was definitely the better all-around team," says Dave Buscema, who covered the Yankees for the *Times Herald-Record*. "Plus, they were playing for something bigger."

Not that this mattered to Arizona. "Obviously, we felt for New York," said catcher Damian Miller, "but we didn't feel for the Yankees." The Series opened at Bank One Ballpark on October 27, and Arizona torched New York starter Mike Mussina, who allowed five runs in three innings of a 9-1 laugher. (Schilling, meanwhile, allowed but a single run in seven innings.) The following night's game wasn't nearly as embarrassing but just as bad for New York—a 4-0 whitewashing at the hands of Johnson, who tossed a complete-game three-hitter.

It was a bad spot for the Yanks, who returned to New York and handed the ball to the man who rarely stepped up in big moments. "Roger is the key," said Torre. "Roger needs to go out and he needs to dominate."

For anyone who was at Yankee Stadium that night, well, it was unlike any baseball game ever played before. It started with the long, winding stretches of humanity that had to patiently pass through a metal detector and a security wand. There were bomb-sniffing dogs outside the stadium and sharpshooters on the roof. From the left of the speakers above the scoreboard facade waved an American flag that had been recovered from the World Trade Center site. Joey Navas, wide-eyed and nine years old, had lost his father at the Trade Center, and now he was being shown around the Yankee clubhouse, having his ball signed by Clemens and Bernie Williams.

President George W. Bush arrived to toss the first pitch. Minutes before he was called to take the field, Bush practiced throwing in an indoor batting cage below the stadium. When Jeter spotted the president, he asked whether he was going to stand on the rubber or in front of the mound. "If you throw from the base of the mound," he said, "they are going to boo you. You really need to take the rubber."

"Will they really boo me?" Bush asked.

"Yeah," said Jeter, flashing a sly grin. "It's New York."

With that bit of advice, Bush—clad in an FDNY pullover—strode onto the field, waved to the crowd, looked toward home plate and threw a perfect strike to backup catcher Todd Greene—from the rubber. He was escorted off by one of the loudest roars in modern Yankee Stadium history.

Moments later, Roger Clemens—the ace of America's baseball team—stood on that same mound and proceeded to pick Arizona apart. Was it a more masterful performance than his two 20-strikeout classics? No. Did it equal the 15-strikeout outing against Seattle? Probably not. But in a game the Yankees had to win, on a night their fans and their city *required* a win, Clemens went seven dazzling innings, striking out nine and allowing just one run in a 2-1 triumph. "Roger was awesome," said Jeter. "That's exactly what we needed."

Over the next two nights, the Yankees seemed to take control of the series, winning back-to-back games in dramatic fashion. Yet upon returning to Arizona, they collapsed. New York was pulverized in game six, losing to Johnson, 15-2. That left things up to Clemens and Schilling, who would start against each other in the series finale.

Though Schilling tended to be animated and brash (when asked about the Yankees' "mystique and aura," he famously replied, "Those are dancers in a nightclub"), he was humble in giving Clemens credit for his success in baseball. In the winter of 1991, Clemens, a hotshot with the Red Sox, had received permission from the Houston Astros to work out in the Astrodome weight room. One day, he had spotted Schilling, who was with the Astros, and asked him for a moment alone. "What I thought was going to be kind of a sit-down talk about pitching experience," said Schilling, "turned out to be an hour-and-a-half butt-chewing."

Clemens ripped into Schilling, demanding that he work harder, condition better, study more, take the game seriously and, for God's sake, get a haircut. He raised his voice, jabbed his finger in Schilling's chest. "I was hoping I was not going to waste my time," Clemens said. "It got pretty heated."

Schilling, who had finished 3-5 with Houston in 1991, went home and looked himself in the mirror. "I walked away saying to myself, 'You know, number one, why would he care as much as he did? And, number two, if he did care, there must be something there.' I began to turn a corner at that point in my career, both on and off the field."

As a member of the Phillies the following season, Schilling went

14-11, emerging as one of baseball's preeminent starters. Through the '01 postseason he was 4-0 with a 0.88 ERA. "I owe it to Roger," he said. "I really do."

At age 34, Schilling was now in the prime of his career. Clemens, at age 39, was the oldest game seven World Series starter in history. On the day before the game, Schilling received a full-body massage from Russell Nua, a Hawaiian massage therapist. On the day of the game, Clemens lathered himself in Icy Hot and wrapped much of his body like a mummy in athletic tape. For five innings, the men dispatched hitters with scorching velocity and pinpoint control. Clemens would hit 94 mph on the radar, Schilling would hit 94. Clemens would strike someone out with a nasty splitter, Schilling would strike someone out with a nasty change. The Diamondbacks finally broke through with a run in the bottom of the sixth. The Yankees answered the following inning on an RBI single by Tino Martinez.

Then, in the bottom of the seventh, Torre walked to the mound and, with one out and a runner on first, replaced Clemens with Mike Stanton. The Rocket had thrown 113 pitches, and his velocity was starting to fade. As he walked to the dugout, his eyes glued to the ground, he felt vindicated. "For a pitcher as great as Roger has been, he's really had to defend himself a lot," said Torre. "And after this game tonight, I don't think he will have to defend himself again."

The Yankees entered the bottom of the ninth leading 2-1, then watched as Rivera, an unparalleled postseason closer, blew it. With the bases loaded and one out, Luis Gonzalez singled up the middle, scoring Jay Bell with the winning run of a wondrous 3-2 game. Unlike some of the other Yankees, who couldn't bear to watch, Clemens never looked away from the field. When Bell touched home plate and euphoria broke out, he casually stood up, gathered his belongings and retreated to the clubhouse.

A few minutes later, beneath the stands, Clemens sought out Schilling and embraced him in a long, powerful hug.

"Awesome game," he said. "Just awesome."

Schilling was overwhelmed. "Thanks, Roger," he said. "That means a lot."

He paused.

"Here's a thought—let's do it again next year."

Clemens nodded. It sounded like a helluva idea.

22

Ignorance and Bliss

n the insular world of professional baseball, there exists a code of honor that, in any other sector of society, would make no sense whatsoever.

On the diamonds and inside the clubhouses, loyalty means standing up for your teammates, no matter the circumstance. Boston outfielder Wil Cordero is arrested for beating his wife in 1997? He's welcomed back with hugs and open arms. Mets pitcher David Cone allegedly exposes himself to female fans in the Shea Stadium bullpen in 1989? Most Mets laugh it off as wacky hijinks.

This so-called code faced one of its greatest tests in the winter of 2002, when the Yankees opted not to renew Brian McNamee's contract. In his two years with the organization, McNamee had become popular with a handful of players. Although his most notable work had been done with Clemens and Andy Pettitte, both of whom had hired him on their own in the off-season, several Yankees considered McNamee a vital piece of the puzzle. Throughout the league, many strength coaches came and went without much notice. But McNamee brought an unparalleled intensity to Yankee workouts.

So, the question must be asked, where were McNamee's supporters in February 2002, when the Yankees unceremoniously dumped him? Though team officials wouldn't officially comment on the trainer's departure, the justification behind the move was no secret: On October 6, 2001, while the Yankee were in Florida to play the Devil Rays, McNamee was allegedly involved in a sexual assault. According to police, a hotel manager found McNamee, another Yankee employee and a 40-year-old woman naked at 4 A.M. in the outdoor pool at the Renaissance Vinoy Resort in St. Petersburg. The woman had ingested gamma hydroxybutyrate, the so-called date-rape drug.

"The manager said it looked like [McNamee] was having sex with the woman," said Rick Stelljes, a police spokesman. "That's when the manager questioned McNamee and the woman cried out, 'Help me.'"

What was not said—and what has gone unsaid for years—is that McNamee was made the fall guy by the organization, which later launched an internal investigation that showed the trainer to be innocent. Earlier in the evening, the woman had been seen with one of New York's coaches, a married man with children who had paraded her around as if she were a trophy. Later on, she had been partying with a Yankee player—also a married man with children. Though McNamee was indeed in the swimming pool, he was there only at the player's behest. He was not naked and had neither raped the woman nor supplied her with any drugs or alcohol. In fact, according to someone with detailed knowledge of the incident, McNamee aided the woman when she passed out and began to drown. He was in the wrong place at the wrong time—but not in the wrong.

To McNamee, though, loyalty meant occasionally taking one for the team. He was, one must remember, the former police officer who accepted a 30-day suspension from the force so that a partner's bid for a promotion would not be damaged. "Brian was being the good soldier," says one person with detailed knowledge of the incident. "He didn't want any of the Yankees to get in trouble, so he took the heat." (Though a suspect of the St. Petersburg Police Department's investigation, McNamee was never charged.)

As word of the incident spread throughout the Yankee clubhouse, Clemens certainly learned of the details. This was, after all, a man Clemens had not only brought to the franchise, but trusted. Yet he never stepped up as a character witness for McNamee. He never told Brian Cashman, the team's general manager, or Joe Torre, the manager, that McNamee was likely being falsely accused. *The right thing,* after all, was relative. There was the code. And in Clemens' universe, the code came first. So although he continued to use McNamee as his personal fitness guru, the trainer was persona non grata in Yankee Stadium. If he wanted to attend a game, he damn well better purchase a ticket. "Needless to say, Roger didn't treat Mac very well," says a friend of McNamee. "It was callous. He sort of threw him out into the cold."

Even without McNamee around on a daily basis, Clemens remained one of baseball's better pitchers in 2002, compiling a 13-6 record and 4.35 ERA for a club that won its fifth straight divisional title with 103 wins. Yet much had changed in Yankee Land. A team that had specialized in continuity throughout its glorious late-1990s run was going through a seismic shift. Third baseman Scott Brosius and right fielder Paul O'Neill had retired, and erratic second baseman–outfielder Chuck Knoblauch had been allowed to walk. In came Robin Ventura from the Mets to play third, along with San Francisco's John Vander Wal and the Cubs' Rondell White as outfielders. David Wells was brought back to join the rotation.

The biggest switch involved first base, for which New York signed Oakland's Jason Giambi to a seven-year, $120 million free-agent deal and allowed Tino Martinez to depart. A six-year member of the club, Martinez had arrived via a trade from Seattle in 1996 as the beloved

Don Mattingly's replacement. Within months, though, Martinez had endeared himself to New York's fans. He played hard, manned his position well, hit for power and was unfailingly polite. By the time Torre's Yankees won their fourth title in 2000, Martinez was—with the exception of Derek Jeter—the team's most popular player.

So when Martinez learned that, following the '01 season, Clemens was placing recruiting calls to Giambi, he seethed—and with good reason. By the time New York had signed Giambi, it was widely assumed throughout major league front offices that he was powered by steroids, not spinach. How else to explain a one-time 190-pound third baseman who was selected in the 43rd round of the 1989 amateur draft now weighing 240 pounds and hitting monstrous shots to the northern pole of Pluto?

Were the Yankees in the know? Before Giambi signed with the team, officials agreed to delete references to steroids in the guarantee language of his mammoth contract. The commissioner's office, which reviews all contracts, was well aware of the omissions. Later in the season, when Giambi was going through a mild slump (it didn't last long—he hit .314 with 41 home runs), one New York player recalls Cashman standing in the Yankee Stadium clubhouse, looking up at the television during a game and screaming, "Jason, whatever you were taking in Oakland, get back fucking on it! Please!"

When the 2002 season ended with a dispiriting four-game loss to Anaheim in the Division Series, Clemens, now 40 years old, came to the conclusion that he was *almost* ready to retire. For the 2003 season he agreed to a one-year, $10.1 million contract, hoping to grab a final World Series title on the way out the door. "I'm going to be 41 this year, but I plan on leading this staff," he said. "I don't anticipate playing past this year. I plan on going out the right way, like I always have, full throttle."

It was the ninth or tenth time Clemens had insisted his retirement was on the horizon. The reasons offered had always varied. He wanted to retire to spend more time with his kids. He wanted to retire to be with his wife. He wanted to retire to try his hand at other things. He wanted to retire to let the young guys take over. He wanted to retire because he was too old. Despite the many previous teases, his teammates and the media seemed to take this one seriously. With 293 career wins, Clemens needed seven more to reach 300. Back at his home in the Memorial Park section of Houston, his prized possession was a Nolan Ryan Texas Rangers jersey signed by every 300-game winner. He desperately craved to add his signature to the garment.

Thanks to his imminent departure, as well as his proximity to 300, Clemens was much in demand heading into the 2003 season. Red Sox officials (yes, *Red Sox officials*) debated whether to retire his uniform number 21. *Sports Illustrated* featured Roger and Debbie in its annual swimsuit issue. Clemens was given a standing ovation at the University of Texas alumni baseball game, and *60 Minutes* planned a lengthy segment on his life and career. Gen. Richard Myers, the chairman of the Joint Chiefs of Staff, had Clemens and the comedian Drew Carey join him on a four-day goodwill tour of military bases in Afghanistan and the Persian Gulf. (Clemens was particularly moved by a soldier who was so convinced that his death was imminent, he asked the Yankee to write his family after it happened. "I told him sure," Clemens said, "but I wasn't prepared for that. How do you respond to something like that?")

Suddenly, every newspaper was writing pieces lamenting the end of a brilliant run; every TV sports reporter wanted to discuss Clemens' legacy. On January 13, shortly after news of his retirement plans broke, Clemens was the grand prize in "Take a Reebok Athlete to School Day." The winner, a Dyker Heights, New York, second-grader named Erin Cullen (who had filled out three entry forms at the local shoe store), couldn't believe her eyes when *the* Roger Clemens arrived at her house. The two hung out for 20 minutes, then rode together to the St. Ephrem School in Brooklyn, where Clemens spoke to the students in an assembly. "I was the third best pitcher on my high school baseball team," he told them. "Believe in yourself. If you put your mind to it, you can do it."

"After that," says John Cullen, Erin's father, "he told the kids that they should stay away from drugs."

IN TERMS OF PITCHING, 2003 probably ranks 10th or 11th among Roger Clemens' all-time best seasons.

In terms of strangeness, it was easily number one.

Early on in spring training, excerpts from David Wells' upcoming autobiography, *Perfect I'm Not*, were leaked to the New York media. Among the many intriguing tidbits, Wells wrote that he had been drunk during his 1998 perfect game, that 40 percent of major leaguers use steroids and amphetamines (in hindsight, that figure was far too low) and that Clemens deserved a Louisville Slugger up his buttocks after the 2000 Mike Piazza bat incident. Wells held a closed-door club-house meeting to explain the passages to teammates, but Clemens wasn't in a forgiving mood. "I guess you have to accept Boomer for who he is," Clemens said. "He's lied throughout this entire book. I'm not a jealous person, and I know Boomer is. But we're going to need him, and we need to put these distractions behind us."

A staunch supporter of the Iraq War, in mid-March Clemens was invited to speak at the send-off for two Tampa-based units of the military police. "This is a time when you want to rally and get behind people," he said. "I wonder if all these people protesting had anybody in that building, in either one of our twin towers, if they'd really be out there doing that." The line evoked loud applause, but Clemens was taken aback when he was slammed by a group called September Eleventh Families for Peaceful Tomorrows. "I am a patriot," said Rita Lasar, whose brother died in the North Tower, "and I can't believe Roger Clemens would make such a statement."

On the field, Clemens got off to a hot start, blowing away the Blue Jays on Opening Day and winning his first four decisions. Clemens had 299 wins going into his May 26 outing against the Red Sox at Yankee Stadium and invited some 25 ex-teammates and 55 family members and friends to witness the magic. Even Bess, now 73 years old, would attend, although she had recently been hospitalized yet again for her emphysema. Comedian Billy Crystal and Mayor Rudolph Giuliani showed up as well. Before the game, Clemens said he would enter the Hall of Fame only wearing a Yankees cap—and should that not be possible, he'd skip the induction ceremony. "To me, it's a no-brainer," he said, even though a mere 66 of his 299 career wins had come as a Yankee. "Reggie [Jackson] played here for five years. He went in as one."

Living up to his big-game reputation, Clemens came out overly amped against the Red Sox and was pounded. Over five and two-thirds humiliating innings, Clemens surrendered 10 hits and eight runs in an 8-4 loss. He also failed in his second attempt to win number 300, blowing a six-run lead against lowly Detroit in a game the Yankees wound up winning, 10-9, in 17 innings. He missed his third, chance, too, by falling to Kerry Wood and the Chicago Cubs at Wrigley Field before 480 members of the media. (Clemens actually departed leading 1-0, but reliever Juan Acevedo blew the game.)

Finally, on June 13, with Tino Martinez and the St. Louis Cardinals in town, Clemens reached one of his greatest goals. Over six and two-thirds innings in a cold, rain-drenched Yankee Stadium, he held St. Louis to six hits and two runs and even fanned Edgar Renteria for his 4,000th career strikeout. He then retreated to the clubhouse, shaved and watched nervously on a TV as relievers Chris Hammond, Antonio Osuna and Mariano Rivera wrapped up the 5-2 victory. Clemens had been saluted with a standing ovation from the 52,214 fans when Torre removed him midway through the seventh, and as Rivera got Miguel Cairo to ground out to end the game, the stadium erupted. Clemens received hugs from Torre and pitching coach Mel Stottlemyre, then bounded onto the field for a buffet of backslaps and and high fives from his teammates.

It had taken longer than anticipated, but, at long last, Clemens could sign the jersey.

OVER THE SEASON'S REMAINING months, Clemens told everyone he was retiring. "He never said he *might* retire, or he was *possibly* retiring, or he was 99 percent certain," says Rick Cerrone, the Yankees' media relations head. "He was retiring. Period."

- June 2, 2003, to *Sports Illustrated*'s Tom Verducci: "They're ready for me to come home, and I'm ready."
- September 27, 2003, to the Associated Press: "I'm at peace with [the decision] because I didn't leave anything behind."
- October 22, 2003, to Gordon Wittenmyer of the Saint Paul *Pioneer Press:* "I'm dead set on what I'm doing. This is it."

Just in case Clemens wasn't clear, Torre stepped up. "The best thing about it is, this is his choice, because the way he's pitching, he could still help people, obviously," the manager said. "His intention of leaving has everything to do with his family. There's not a day that goes by when he doesn't tell you a story about one of his boys. So the reason he's walking away has nothing to do with baseball, other than baseball takes him away from his family too much."

But Clemens didn't want to retire. He knew he was *supposed* to retire because, well, there were a wife and four children back home in Texas. But how could sitting around the house, hitting golf balls and watching Little League compare to the major league life? The once-bashful kid now lived for the attention. He didn't merely want it—he *needed* it. "You're talking about the ultimate narcissist," says Pat Jordan, the writer and former minor league pitcher. "Actors are fearful—their narcissism is a product of their fear. But an athlete's narcissism doesn't spring from fear, it springs from arrested development. A person like Roger Clemens has never cultivated anything but himself. Everything is about the arm, about maintaining the arm. The longer it goes on, the easier it is to become a Roger Clemens. You constantly call attention upon yourself, because you're all you know. I used to be like that when I played, and I wasn't one one-thousandth of the pitcher Roger was. It took me a long time to get out of the idea that if it rains on my parade, I'm the only one getting wet."

Clemens finished the regular season with a 17-9 record and 3.91 ERA, and New York won yet another American League East crown with a 101-61 mark. On September 27, in what was presumed to be his final regular season start at Yankee Stadium, Clemens pitched well through six innings, holding the Baltimore Orioles to two runs before a crowd of 42,702 fans. As had long been the norm, he walked to the mound to pitch the seventh inning against Baltimore, took his eight warmup pitches, then looked toward the New York dugout, from which Torre emerged with a wide smile. As the fans realized what was happening, they stood and saluted a parting legend. Taking the ball from Clemens, Torre said, "Congratulations," while patting him gently on the backside. In Baltimore's dugout, manager Mike Hargrove stood and applauded, along with most of his players. Clemens waved to the crowd, entered the dugout, then returned for a curtain call.

What does it all mean? he was asked afterward.

"It means I play for a great team," he said. "It's the stuff you dream about, and hopefully this dream isn't over."

It wasn't. The Yankees cruised past overmatched Minnesota in four games to win the AL Division Series. Clemens helped the Yanks to a 3-1 game three triumph by allowing a single run over seven innings.

And now they'd face the Boston Red Sox.

Having vanquished Oakland in five games, the Sox entered the

ALCS believing they were finally better than the Yankees. With an explosive lineup featuring shortstop Nomar Garciaparra, left fielder Manny Ramirez and DH David Ortiz, as well as an unparalleled ace in Pedro Martinez (and a very good number two starter in Derek Lowe), the Sox were more dangerous than they had been at any point since 1986, when a young stud named Clemens had guided them to the World Series.

The Red Sox came to Yankee Stadium and split the first two contests, but anyone covering the series knew it was all about game three, when Clemens and Martinez would square off on a Saturday evening at Fenway. "Clemens vs. Martinez is more than a baseball game," wrote Ronald Blum of the Associated Press. "It's the star who left Boston against the pitcher who replaced him as the ace of the Red Sox. It's the New York Yankees' warrior against an equally fierce but publicity-shy leader, a pair of prideful pitchers not afraid to leave batters sprawling."

For those who had closely followed Clemens' career, the accompanying pizzazz was not a good omen. Some pitchers are allergic to eating before playing. Others can't handle too much bullpen work. Clemens' kryptonite was hype. Motivated enough without the media attention and fan energy, he became Hulk Hogan on Jolt when the game became bigger than the game. Such was the case now, in Boston. "Saturday," said Kevin Millar, Boston's first baseman, "is going to be as electric as Fenway Park has ever been."

Millar was right. It was electric. And weird. Neither man pitched wonderfully, and neither pitched terribly. But in the top of the fourth inning, Martinez pitched . . . *oddly*. After Jorge Posada led off with a walk, Nick Johnson singled and Hideki Matsui doubled to drive in a run, Martinez fired a pitch that hit the back of Karim Garcia, New York's right fielder. "He can throw a pitch where he wants to," Garcia said later. "And he threw it right behind my head." Sitting in the dugout, Clemens immediately looked at Boston's lineup and selected which hitter he would bean in the bottom of the inning. But when umpire Tim McClelland warned both benches, the Yankee ace calmed down. Were he to hit someone, he would be automatically ejected.

Instead, Clemens returned to the mound focused on winning. While facing Ramirez, he threw his fourth pitch *sort of* high and *sort of* inside. Yet the Red Sox slugger flipped, charging toward Clemens with bat in hand. Both teams stormed onto the field, as did several Boston police officers. In the fray, Don Zimmer, New York's 72-year-old bench coach, charged toward Martinez and tried to throw a punch. Much like a bullfighter facing a three-legged boar, Boston's starter gently tossed Zimmer aside, then watched in shock as he stumbled to the grass. "I was just trying to dodge him," Martinez said later, "and his body fell." Calm was restored, Zimmer was taken to Beth Israel Deaconess Medical Center for observation, beer sales were immediately halted and the game resumed after a 13-minute delay. Ramirez struck out.

Despite the drama, Clemens pitched magnificently. Save for the first inning, when he gave up two runs, he held Boston scoreless through six, and New York triumphed, 4-3.

Ever resilient, Boston fought back to win two of the next three games, setting up another showdown between Clemens and Martinez, only now at Yankee Stadium.

This time out, Clemens lasted just three innings, giving up six hits and four runs. Luckily for the Yankees, Boston's reputation as historic play-off chokers continued. Leading 5-2 midway through the eighth inning, Grady Little, Boston's manager, left the 32-year-old Martinez in the game well past his expiration point. The Yankees rallied for three runs, then won the game on a dramatic 11th-inning home run from Aaron Boone.

In his last season, Clemens would have the chance to play in one last World Series.

"This is amazing," he said afterward. "I mean, since I'll definitely be retiring, it's a great way to go out."

• • • •

SIMILAR TO THE WORLD Series against Arizona two years earlier, the Yankees entered the 2003 Fall Classic all but guaranteed a win.

The reason: Roger Clemens.

For the Rocket, this was it. There would be no more "last game pitched in Anaheim" or "last game pitched on Yom Kippur" or "last game pitched on the same day as the *Friends* season finale." Clemens would make one World Series start, maybe two, and walk off into the sunset. Next stop, Cooperstown.

The Florida Marlins—the National League Wild Card entrant—were mere extras, bit players hired by the hour to sort of blend into the background and provide color. What with their aqua uniforms and largely obscure roster and a manager, Jack McKeon, who was thought more adept at telling stories than running a game, who could possibly consider the Marlins (*the Marlins!?*) serious threats to the throne?

Yet there was Florida, trailing two games to one on the night of October 22, when Clemens was scheduled to start game four against Carl Pavano, the Marlins' 27-year-old right-hander. At 41 years, two months and 18 days, Clemens was about to become the third oldest man to ever start a World Series game, trailing only Jack Quinn, who had been 45 with the 1929 Philadelphia Athletics, and Grover Cleveland Alexander, 41 years and seven months as a Cardinal in 1928. "This is it," Clemens said on the afternoon before the game. "My emotions will be happy and sad. Happy that I know it's over and I'm healthy. I did it right. I put in the time to be successful at this level. I'll be sad because it's my last game and that to go out there and compete—I won't have that. I won't be able to do that."

As far as settings go, Florida's Pro Player Stadium was a far cry from the House that Ruth Built. Constructed in the mid-1980s, the multisport facility lacked charm and uniqueness. Because this was the

World Series, 65,934 "loyal" Marlins fans would pack the building. On a normal night, that figure would read, oh, 6,000. Yet the setting was strangely appropriate. Twenty years earlier, Clemens had started his career in the Sunshine State as a member of the Winter Haven Red Sox. Now he would be ending it.

The Yankees lost 4-3 in a 12-inning thriller, but Clemens performed relatively well. He allowed eight hits and three runs over seven innings, and when he struck out Luis Castillo to end the seventh, everyone knew Clemens' night was done. The fans stood and clapped, as did the Yankees and Marlins. Clemens tipped his cap and proceeded into the darkness of the visitors' dugout.

Behind the pitching of Josh Beckett and Brad Penny, the Marlins won the series in six games. As for Clemens, his legacy was sealed: 310 career wins, six Cy Young trophies, the admiration and respect of his peers.

"I was sad to see him go," says Cerrone. "But I understood. Roger wanted to try a new adventure. He'd been a baseball player since childhood, and he wanted to take a look at the real world."

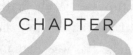

CHAPTER

23

Retirement

R etirement proved fantastic for Roger Clemens.

Truly fantastic.

Shortly after the World Series defeat, he was asked by Jose de Jesus Ortiz of *The Houston Chronicle* how he'd spend his remaining days on Earth. Clemens pointed to a nearby golf cart. "You're looking at it," he said. "Playing in golf tournaments and having some fun!"

Oh, Clemens had plans. Like playing golf. And eating food and stuff. Maybe a trip to Hawaii. Or Greece. Yeah, Greece seemed nice. Why, he might even read a book or two. *Harry Potter. Tuesdays with Morrie* . . .

"There's no scenario where I'd come back," he said. "I'm retired."

Those words were uttered on November 5, 2003.

One Mississippi . . .

Two Mississippi . . .

Three Mississippi . . .

One month later, on December 12, Clemens appeared on KKRW

Radio in Houston. Speaking with morning show hosts Dean and Rog, the Rocket was asked about the shocking news from a day earlier, when the Astros and left-hander Andy Pettitte, his former Yankees teammate and close pal, had agreed to a three-year, $31.5 million contract. "I'm gonna take the weekend to decide some things," Clemens said.

When he proceeded to concede that he might have to return the Hummer the Yankees had presented him as a retirement gift, Dean and Rog asked their listeners for assistance. Within minutes, Lee De-Montrond, a local automobile dealer, called the show and offered up a car should Clemens pitch for Houston in 2004. One hour later, a new Hummer arrived outside of Clemens' house in Memorial.

"This is getting very interesting," Clemens told the hosts. "I didn't know making a comment like that, you guys would show up in my front driveway with a burnt-orange H2."

So would he be in an Astros uniform come spring training?

"Maybe," said Clemens. "Maybe."

As soon as the Dean and Rog interview concluded, Clemens was once again the talk of the town—and he *loved* it. His face was everywhere. The buzz flew from one water-cooler conversation to another. The NFL invited Clemens to appear on stage at an event leading up to Houston's Super Bowl XXXVIII. Even Tiger Woods had an opinion, snidely asking, "When people retire, do they ever stay retired?" Soon enough Clemens was telling reporters that, having played golf with Astros first baseman Jeff Bagwell, he found the idea of a return "definitely" tempting.

Some who knew Clemens watched suspiciously from afar. While he would often brag of his kinship with Pettitte, the relationship was more older brother–younger brother than friend-friend. Having also grown up in Texas and attended San Jacinto, Pettitte would have jumped through fiery hoops to impress Clemens, his role model and mentor. When Roger spoke, Andy listened. So why was it that Clemens had to do his all to upstage his peer? "He couldn't just let Andy enjoy the excitement of signing with the Astros," says one person who knows both pitchers. "He had to steal the spotlight and make it his own. That's very typical Roger behavior. The attention belongs to him, or it belongs to no one."

His retirement lasted a whopping 78 days. On January 12, he agreed to a one-year, $5 million contract that also included a $3 million personal services clause and nearly $3.5 million more in attendance bonuses. The best part? Houston owner Drayton McLane told Clemens he would be allowed to leave the team and take care of personal matters whenever need be. Translation: Clemens could spend a lot of time at home watching his oldest son, Koby, now 17 and a highly regarded junior catcher and third baseman at Houston's Memorial High, play his games. "You have to remember, Roger was the most revered player in all of baseball," says McLane. "And we wanted someone to show us how to win. Who better than Roger Clemens?"

Since joining the major leagues as an expansion club in 1962 (they were known as the Colt 45s for three years), the Astros had always struggled to garner attention in a football-obsessed sports market. Despite having had numerous superstars through the years, from J. R. Richard and Nolan Ryan to Bagwell and Craig Biggio, the team had failed to truly become part of the city's fabric. "They'd been here 40 years, but the Astros couldn't capture Houston," says Fred Faour, a former sports editor of *The Houston Chronicle*. "Roger lit a fuse. He was the greatest pitcher anyone had ever seen, and he was making the choice to play here. We felt relevant."

Clemens' introductory news conference was covered as if President George W. Bush had come to town to name Houston America's new capital. In the days after the announcement, phone lines were jammed with fans anxious to snag tickets. McLane had the team hire temporary employees to assist in fielding calls. "I've never had anything like this in my 18 seasons with the franchise," said John Sorrentino, the team's ticket manager. CLEMENS 22 jerseys sold at team merchandising stores as fast as they were unpacked.

In New York City, however, the news wasn't greeted with equal elation. George Steinbrenner, for one, was beyond livid. The Yankees had treated Clemens like royalty. *This* was their thanks? "[Roger] told us he was retiring," Steinbrenner said, "and we had no choice but to believe him." WHAT AN ASSTRO! screamed the back page of the *New York Post*, and columnist Mike Vaccaro's piece reflected the mood of the city's Yankee loyalists. "Let him go," Vaccaro wrote. "Let him go home. Let him try to figure out the National League, and let the fans of Houston fall prey to his wicked charms. We're done. We've been there. Don't let the door of the Hummer hit you on your way out of the Yankees' pantheon of legends, Rog."

ROGER CLEMENS EXCEEDED THE hype in 2004, winning his seventh Cy Young trophy by going 18-4 with a 2.98 ERA. In his first regular-season start, an April 7 game at Minute Maid Park, Clemens pitched seven innings of shutout ball against the Giants, striking out Barry Bonds twice in a 10-1 win. A record 42,863 fans attended. "If you loved baseball, you wanted to be there," says Jose de Jesus Ortiz. "My daughter Kathleen was six months old at the time, and we wouldn't let her near anybody. But I told my wife, 'This is an event,' and we bought tickets for her to be there when Roger Clemens pitched the first time." Thrilled to be home, the Rocket proved to be worth every cent of the $5 million he was being paid. He worked with the Astros' young pitchers, made a number of visits to see children in the local hospital, began the season 9-0, started for the NL in the All-Star Game, landed a semifat endorsement deal with SuperPretzel (Clemens: "I couldn't be happier to be associated with the high-quality, great-tasting SuperPretzel!"), rarely turned down a promotional appearance and sold out start after start. Most important, he made people excited about Houston baseball. In 2003, the Astros drew 2,454,241 fans. With Clemens and Pettitte, that total soared to a franchise-record 3,087,872. "When he was around, there was always a hush in the room as he entered, because of the amount of respect we had," says Brandon Backe, an Astros pitcher. "We didn't initially care if he didn't show up every day, because Roger's aura alone was pretty impressive. He had something special."

Yet while the Houston media covered Clemens as if he were Pope John Paul II, the cracks in his performance-enhancing plaster were slowly starting to show. Through the previous two years, much of the focus had been on San Francisco's Barry Bonds, a suspiciously large, powerful outfielder accused of cheating by seemingly everyone. In 2001 Bonds had hit 73 home runs to break the single-season record, and very few non–Bay Area residents took his achievement seriously. He was the name and face of drugs in baseball, and as a result, men like the Rocket were largely able to hide in his shadow.

The first official evocation of Clemens' drug use in the media came on March 2, when Chris "Mad Dog" Russo of New York's WFAN sports radio listed the players he suspected of cheating. After naming Sammy Sosa and Jeff Bagwell, he turned to his partner, Mike Francesa, and said, "Have you ever seen the size of Roger Clemens' head?" The inference: The Rocket was surely using human growth hormone—one of the major side effects being an expanded skull.

The most pointed accusation came on July 18, when Yankees right fielder Gary Sheffield, who would soon face daily questions about his friendship with Bonds, fingered Clemens as a ballplayer who was receiving a free pass. "I get sick and tired of everyone wanting to flaunt their training method, to show that they're the biggest and strongest and baddest," Sheffield told Anthony McCarron of the New York *Daily News*. "All of that is a big hoax. Nobody trains harder than anybody else. It's a bunch of garbage and I'm sick and tired of hearing it.

"Roger Clemens, what makes him so different, because he's able to pitch? Longevity? I can tell you one thing, and I'm not accusing him of anything, but I bet you he's not just drinking soda water."

Much of the media greeted Sheffield's words with a dismissive shrug. Just another crazy rant from the king of crazy. "If Sheffield had any shame," Ortiz wrote in *The Houston Chronicle,* "[he'd] keep [his] stupid mouth shut." Yet, inside major league clubhouses, many ballplayers nodded in agreement and were thankful somebody was willing to speak out. "Sheff said a lot of stupid things over the years," says a former teammate. "But in that case, he was just stating what a lot of guys were thinking. Only he had the guts to stand up."

Although Clemens was no longer working with Brian McNamee, there were few places in baseball more hospitable to drug users than Minute Maid Park. The Astros were known throughout the league to have lots of players benefiting from performance enhancers. "It was a joke," says one opponent. "All you had to do was look at them. It was beyond obvious." From the ballplayer's standpoint, the beauty of Houston was the close proximity to Mexico, where most of the steroids originated. In Detroit or Chicago or Pittsburgh, one needed to go through an elongated process. With its border only 353 miles from Houston, Mexico served as a 24-hour CVS where $50 was accepted in lieu of a prescription.

How in the world could a soon-to-be 42-year-old man be throwing 96 mph while working out four, five hours per day? Beginning in their mid-30s, athletes' bodies break down. It's an undeniable certainty of human nature. A 42-year-old man cannot exercise with the same intensity as he did 10 years earlier. Yet Clemens' off-day routines had never really changed. "I was 100 percent suspicious of Roger and 90 percent convinced," says Howard Bryant, an ESPN.com writer and author of the groundbreaking book *Juicing the Game: Drugs, Power, and the Fight for the Soul of Major League Baseball.* "He fit the profile. Every argument you could make about Bonds you could make about Roger." Specifically, Bryant recalls Clemens' grooming patterns. "A lot of my steroid people had told me that a lot of users grew beards and goatees because they didn't want people to see the structure of their faces changing," he says. "The other thing with Roger was he was the first player I ever saw who shaved his entire body from toe to waist. He shaved his calves like a swimmer, and I'd never seen that in baseball. People told me that was a bright red flag, because when you take all that testosterone it makes you look like a werewolf. Think about it—a pitcher shaving his body does nothing to help his performance. The best way to not look like a Wookiee is to shave every day.

"To his credit," Bryant adds, "Roger never looked like a Wookiee."

As the *San Francisco Chronicle* poured money, resources and time into its groundbreaking BALCO investigation of Victor Conte and Barry Bonds (among others), *The Houston Chronicle* considered launching its own probe. "I had it all planned," says Faour. "We all had suspicions about Roger and some other guys, and we did a lot of digging. But that kind of thing takes a lot of time and costs a lot of money. I had an investigative reporter I had planned on hiring just for the task, but I was not allowed to bring him in.

"There was no commitment from management to go after it. So we let it die. If the players wanted to live a lie, we wouldn't stand in their way."

THE ASTROS STRUGGLED THROUGHOUT the first half of the season, going 44-44; manager Jimmy Williams was fired at the All-Star break and replaced by Phil Garner. No matter how the team performed, Clemens was a god. He never had to pay for a meal or a round of golf. Powered by his exceptional pitching, the Astros made the greatest second-half run in franchise history, riding a 36-10 streak (the second best winning percentage down the stretch for any National League team since 1945) to qualify for the play-offs as a wild-card entry. On the final day of the regular season, with Clemens missing the start with a stomach virus, Backe shut down the Colorado Rockies at Minute Maid. The moment the game ended, 43,082 fans stood and cheered for a solid five-minute stretch.

"That's what Roger meant to Houston baseball," says McLane. "That excitement."

Though the Astros eventually fell to St. Louis in a seven-game National League Championship Series (Clemens started game seven, surrendering four runs over six innings in a 5-2 defeat), the season was viewed as a huge success.

"I was very thankful to have the opportunity to come back and pitch here in front of my family," Clemens said in the Busch Stadium visitors' clubhouse after game seven. "And [I was happy to] leave a little something behind for some of the young guys on this team."

Wait. Was Clemens retiring? Again?

"He said the words," says Alyson Footer, the team's MLB.com beat writer. "But this time, nobody believed it."

SIX DAYS INTO 2005, Clifton Brown of *The New York Times* asked Clemens if he was going to return to the Astros for the upcoming season.

"I've pretty much painted myself into a corner," Clemens said of his verbal commitment to his hometown. "But I've talked to Joe Torre, and I get e-mails from Jorge Posada."

Like the Blue Jays and Yankees before them, the Astros had given Clemens as much power, authority and leeway as any American ballplayer since Babe Ruth's heyday. The Astros had taken Clemens at his word: That he was coming out of retirement only because he could pitch close to home. That it was playing for Houston or sitting in a rocking chair. That he was here to give back to the community.

So why was he even broaching the possibility *of a possibility* of a Yankee reunion?

Had George Steinbrenner been running the Astros, Clemens' fate would have been sealed. *You want to dance with another partner after all we've done for you? Then bug off.* But McLane was no Steinbrenner. He saw the power Clemens wielded over the city and feared that without the Rocket, the Astros would immediately revert to the dark, sub-.500 1970s days of Denis Menke and Wade Blasingame. Hence, when Clemens filed for a record $22 million in arbitration, the Astros quickly agreed to pay him $18 million. It was the highest salary for a pitcher in baseball history, a seemingly ludicrous amount to hand a man born during the Kennedy administration. Wrote Gorden Edes of *The Boston Globe*, "Of this we can be certain: Clemens is out of the business of giving any hometown discounts."

"Roger can make more of a difference for the Houston Astros than any player in baseball," McLane said. "There is only one Roger Clemens. We have some magnificent players here who have played great. But it was his personality, his championship attitude that lifted us last season."

In his post-signing press interviews, Clemens once again cited his need to be close to home—an odd utterance for a man who had spent his winter speaking at Notre Dame's annual baseball banquet, participating in the Bob Hope Chrysler Classic Golf Tournament in Bermuda Dunes, California, filming a commercial for the H-E-B supermarket chain in Dallas, having dinner at the White House and addressing Florida Atlantic University's baseball fund-raising dinner in Boca Raton. Not long after Clemens agreed to the $18 million deal, Randy Hendricks, his agent, told *The Houston Chronicle*, "This year proves his commitment to the city and the team. I know he basically wanted to retire, but . . . he wanted to do it for the city."

The one development that seemed to interrupt Clemens' airplane-hopping adventures was the February news of Jose Canseco's forthcoming tell-all, *Juiced: Wild Times, Rampant 'Roids, Smash Hits, and How Baseball Got Big*. Even though the text only coyly hints that the Rocket might have used steroids, Clemens' reaction to his old chum's literary effort was fierce. "When you're under house arrest and you have ankle bracelets on, you have a lot of time to write a book," he said, referring to Canseco's recent legal troubles. "I went to bat for Josey for a long time—and many times for different teams. I knew him when he was arrogant and wouldn't sign autographs even for us, but I also knew his softer side. Now don't ask me any more questions about steroids or Canseco. I think his book is doing well enough."

IF ONE WERE TO believe his Houston-based press clippings, Roger Clemens was just as dedicated to baseball in 2005 as he had been a year earlier. He was the leader, the hard worker, the spiritual guru, the man who showed the team how to win.

Much of this was garbage.

Although Houston's players—fearful of angering a legend—fed the local media what it wanted to hear about Clemens, inside the clubhouse there was mounting resentment toward their part-time teammate. On the days he pitched, he would arrive early, change at his locker, then—poof!—vanish. On the days he didn't pitch, well, one never knew. He came. He didn't come. The advice Clemens was supposedly dispensing to Houston's young players didn't exist. His rah-rah speeches and inspirational banter were fictitious. Nobody seemed to outwardly dislike Clemens—he was a nice guy who never turned down an autograph request. "But he kind of had it easy around here," says Backe. "I didn't resent it, but I noticed it. He might have missed 35, 40 games in the course of a season. It was different. But it was his right."

"The older players were the ones who resented it the most, and it's hard to blame them," says Mike Lamb, Houston's backup corner infielder. "I'm an old-school guy myself, and I'd rather have my teammates in the clubhouse or on the flights. But if you need a pitcher like Roger Clemens and his thinking is 'I don't need you, but I want to play,' you can make concessions. You would never do that for a rookie. But he was the Rocket. Such is life."

Had the Astros struggled, many might have found Clemens' absences troubling. But behind the Clemens–Pettitte–Roy Oswalt starting trio and an offense powered by Lance Berkman and Morgan Ensberg, the Astros staged another late-season surge to close in on a play-off spot. "We were good enough when it counted," says Lamb, "that nobody was going to give Roger much grief." With his private jet on standby, Clemens did his best to be in a thousand places at once. Koby, now 18 and a senior at Memorial High, had signed a letter of intent to attend Texas and was being scouted heavily by major league clubs. (He would be selected by the Astros in the eighth round of the June draft and spent the summer of '05 playing rookie ball in Greenville, Tennessee.) Clemens attended as many of the boy's games as possible, as well as son Kory's Friday-night prep football contests. As the Astros hit the road for Los Angeles or San Diego or Milwaukee, Clemens could often be found in the empty Minute Maid Park, throwing in the bullpen, sprinting from foul pole to foul pole, fielding grounders.

Did the special treatment and the many absences impair Clemens' ability to produce come game day? Hardly. Entering September, he was 11-6 with a 1.51 ERA. Did the special treatment hurt the Astros? Hardly. On September 1, the team was 71-62, one game behind Philadelphia in the Wild Card hunt.

"We were talented," says Garner. "Talent makes up for a lot of possible issues."

CHAPTER 24

Bess

Of the people Roger Clemens cared about deeply, no one could rival his mother, Bess, in the love he held for her. She was, in his mind, the perfect parent—compassionate but strict, driven but available. After her second husband, Woody Booher, had died when Roger was a young boy, she worked three jobs to support the family. When teachers called to say one of her children had been acting up, she was quick with the belt and a stern word. "She taught me my values," he said. "She gave me discipline, and she gave me great direction.

"I think that's all hogwash when I hear a single parent can't raise kids. My mom kept my butt in line. She taught me to respect other people and to apologize when I'm wrong and to stick to my guns when I'm right."

Whenever Clemens looked toward future accomplishments, he always mentioned the joy they would bring his mother. He had thought about his Hall of Fame induction speech countless times, about pointing to Bess in the audience and having her rise for a round of applause. "I wanted her to hang around," he said, "just so I could thank her properly."

On the night of September 9, 2005, Clemens endured perhaps his worst start of the season, allowing five runs over three innings in a 7-4 loss at Milwaukee. The following morning, he received word from his sisters that Bess, who had long suffered from emphysema related to a lifetime of smoking, was not doing well. It was a call Clemens had feared for years.

Clemens left his teammates in Milwaukee and took his private jet to Georgetown, Texas, to be with Bess. He sat by her bedside for much of the next few days, talking about old times and the current season. Even on her deathbed, Bess wanted to know about the Astros—who was playing well, who was struggling, what were their play-off chances.

Four nights later, Bess made her son promise that he would take the mound for his scheduled start the following day against the Florida Marlins at Minute Maid Park. At 4:30 A.M. she died in her sleep. She was 75. "I feel very blessed she's at peace now," Clemens said later in the day. "The last 10 years were hard on her. The last two or three days were grueling. She was very tough to the end. She didn't want to give up."

Here is the difference between Roger Clemens and 99 percent of other humans. Last wishes be damned, other humans do not pitch on the day their mother dies. They see a match-up against the Marlins as a game—one of 162 to be played in the course of a very long season. They take the time to cry and hurt and remember, to reflect on their own mortality and how they can best honor the loved one. They plan a funeral, call friends and family members.

But that's not the way Clemens was wired. His life was baseball, and baseball was his life. Over the course of decades the marketers inside Major League Baseball's offices had specialized in romanticizing what is—if one really considers it—a strikingly grimy, unromantic occupation. The triumphant music. The fireworks. The inevitable references to "the ghosts" of so-and-so stadium and the knowledge that so-and-so "is looking down on me today." Hitters crossing themselves as they approach home plate. Pitchers gazing skyward for divine intervention. Nobody is actually dead; they're floating on the nearest cloud, sitting alongside Ted Williams and the Babe. Like Jim Carrey's character in *The Truman Show,* Clemens was lost between the real and the make-believe. His emotions were not those of, in this case, a son losing his mother, but of a star baseball player losing his mother. *Everything* related to the sport. Perhaps that's why he had Bess buried wearing a necklace with 21 diamonds—signifying his longtime uniform number. He was Roger Clemens, and Roger Clemens did not compute unadulterated sadness. Skipping the start? Out of the question. Baseball was his grief counselor.

Roughly two hours before the 7:05 P.M. game between the Marlins and Astros, Clemens arrived at the stadium. Having just made the two-and-a-half-hour drive from Georgetown to Houston, he was exhausted and emotionally drained. Clemens walked the first hitter, second baseman Luis Castillo, on four pitches. "I was lost as soon as I climbed on the mound," he said afterward. "I knew I had to recover really quick so I could get through that."

Clemens somehow gathered himself, holding Florida to a single run before walking off the field at inning's end to a loud applause from the 30,911 spectators. Bess' passing had been big news in Houston, and everyone in the stadium was surely aware of what had transpired. Over six and a third innings, Clemens limited the Marlins to one run and five hits in a 10-2 triumph. When Phil Garner came to the mound to remove his starter, the reaction from the crowd was respectfully muted. Afterward, a tribute to Clemens' mother was played on the stadium Jumbotron.

"I'll never forget when that game ended," says Jose de Jesus Ortiz, the *Chronicle* beat writer. "His children are back in the media room, and they're in tears and they're hugging their mom. And I went to talk to Debbie and she said, '[Bess] would have been very proud of him today. She would have been very proud.' This was Roger's calling. He felt it was what he was meant to do."

In the days immediately following the game, Clemens returned to Ohio, where his mother was buried alongside Woody Booher at the Dayton Memorial Park Cemetery. Inside his wallet, Clemens placed a small photograph of Bess throwing out the first pitch during a Yankee game. "I went to the viewing," says Jean Crutcher, a family friend. "Bess had a hard life, and she looked better lying there than she ever had while living." While in town, Clemens knocked on the door of his childhood home, introduced himself and received a quick tour. He later sent the family some memorabilia and a kind note.

The remaining three weeks of the season proved joyful for Clemens and the Astros. Once considered long out of the race (on July 18 the Astros were a game under .500, fourteen and a half games behind St. Louis in the division and five games out of the Wild Card), Houston staged a thrilling comeback, wrestling the Wild Card spot away from Philadelphia, the Mets and the Marlins. On the second-to-last day of the season, Clemens took the mound for the first inning of a home game against the Cubs and turned to C.B. Bucknor, the home-plate umpire. "Don't pay attention to me today," he warned. "I woke up on the wrong side of the bed. I have a little fire in my belly." Clemens held Chicago to one run over seven innings in a 3-1 win. (He finished the year with a 13-8 record and league-leading 1.87 ERA.) With the win and a victory by Roy Oswalt the following day over the Cubs, the Astros were back in the postseason for a second straight year. "This time," says Oswalt, "we believed we could really make some noise."

Houston drew the Braves in the Division Series and for the second straight year beat them with relative ease, winning in four games. What would have otherwise been deemed a forgettable play-off round gained near-classic status in the fourth and deciding game, when— after 15 innings—the two teams were tied at 6.

Having started the second game of the series (a dispiriting 7-1 loss, during which he allowed five runs over five innings), Clemens wasn't even on the radar for a relief appearance. Yet as the game dragged on and on and the Astros burned through one pitcher after another, manager Phil Garner finally turned to Clemens and asked, casually, "So how are you feeling?" Through the season's final month, Clemens had pitched with two small tears in his back, a tender left hamstring and a sore groin. And he had thrown 92 pitches two days earlier. How was he feeling? Like he'd been run over by a Hess truck.

But Clemens didn't say so. Instead, he headed toward the indoor batting cages beneath the stadium. His oldest son, Koby, now an Astros minor leaguer, was called from the stands to help his old man loosen up. After approximately five minutes, Clemens returned to the dugout. "I'm good to go," he told Garner. "I'm ready."

Clemens warmed up in the bullpen during the top of the 15th, and the fans at Minute Maid Park let loose a sonic roar. This was the sort of drama Clemens lived for. He was alone in the bullpen, the Lone Ranger armed and ready to save the day. Having been through so many battles, Clemens was neither scared nor timid. "But he was very hungry," says Mark Bailey, Houston's bullpen coach. "He asked me to call down to the clubhouse and get him something to eat. So they brought us a thing of bananas, and he gobbled them up. He was starving.

"I don't think anyone could believe what they were seeing," says Bailey. "Was that really Roger Clemens, getting on his white horse and getting ready to come in? It sent chills down your spine."

Garner was handcuffed. He had already run out of position players, and Clemens was the last available arm. Were the game to go on even deeper into the night, the Astros would have moved right fielder Jason Lane—who had been a pitcher in college at the University of Southern California—to the mound. In the bottom of the 15th, Craig Biggio led off with a walk, and the crowd roared when Clemens pinch hit for reliever Dan Wheeler. "If Roger had homered," Lance Berkman later said, "they'd have just shut the game of baseball down. We wouldn't even have bothered to play the World Series, because you couldn't have topped it." Alas, the Fall Classic was safe. Clemens laid down a sacrifice bunt.

Over the next three innings, Clemens did some of the most memorable handy work of his 22-year career. He struck out four, relying on a mid-90s fastball that was cutting in hard on right-handed hitters. When outfielder Chris Burke ended the game with an 18th-inning home run off of Atlanta's Joey Devine, the euphoric reaction sounded as if someone had blown the top off the building. Upon reaching home plate, Burke was mobbed by teammates, equally relieved in finally being able to sleep as they were joyful for advancing to the NLCS. Combined, the two teams had used 42 players, a Division Series record. The game lasted five hours and 50 minutes, the longest in play-off history.

When ESPN's Erin Andrews collared Clemens on the field immediately after the game for an interview, he reached out and grabbed Burke by the right-shoulder sleeve, pulling him close in front of the camera.

Andrews: "Rocket, when you woke up this morning, did you ever think you'd be the winning pitcher?"

Clemens: "No, but I sure am proud of these guys. I think I said it a couple of days ago—it seems a lot longer than that now. It's been a lot of work for us."

Clemens paused briefly, then said, "How 'bout the kid?" turning toward Burke, a 25-year-old Kentuckian in his first full big-league season.

As Andrews asked Burke a few questions, Clemens walked off, content.

The win was the last transcendent moment of his career.

IN THE AFTERMATH OF one of the greatest games in Astros history, those who believed Roger Clemens to be a chemically enhanced ballplayer had something to laugh about. The idea of a 43-year-old man, having pitched two days earlier, returning to last three innings . . . while throwing mid-90s bullets? Preposterous. "Can't be done," says one major league peer of Clemens. "Not physically possible without help."

Yet as the Astros prepared to face St. Louis in the NLCS, manager Phil Garner remained clueless. A 16-year major league veteran known as "Scrap Iron" for his grittiness and determination, Garner admits to having taken creatine and androstenedione, both controversial yet legal supplements, to prolong his career. Whenever he suspected someone of using steroids or growth hormones, Garner insists, he pulled the player aside. "I would tell him that I considered taking drugs when I was playing," he says. "I had back problems and I wanted to get back on the field. But I decided against it because I knew the dangers. I didn't want to be 38 years old and have my heart blow out and my family left with nothing. So I told players about that and insisted that they don't listen to the guys in the gym or to the pushers. Health is more important than baseball."

Looking back, it's hard to see how Garner *didn't* know Clemens was using. Yet at the time, the last thing he was thinking about was cheating. "St. Louis was a big enough challenge," he says. "We had to win that series."

Houston went on to defeat the Cardinals in six games, advancing to its first-ever World Series, but the shadow of the 18-inning classic loomed large. What could top three relief innings from Clemens and Burke's homer and the raw thrill of the moment? Even when the Astros were swept by the Chicago White Sox in a forgettable Fall Classic, the city of Houston maintained its giddiness over what had transpired.

"As much as it hurt to lose to Chicago, the whole experience was just so thrilling," says Backe, the Astros pitcher. "We brought something special to Houston. I don't think anyone in that city will ever forget it."

•   •   •

IT SHOULD HAVE ENDED HERE.

In the feel-good sports biopic, Roger Clemens' baseball career ends after the 2005 season.

But instead, Clemens made a rather large mess of things. He told the *New York Post* that his mother's dying wish was that he retire after the season. So he retired. Then he unretired again. And retired again. Then he met with Boston GM Theo Epstein about coming back to pitch for the Red Sox. He spoke with Rangers GM Jon Daniels. He pitched for Team USA in the World Baseball Classic, where he lost to Mexico (*Mexico?!*) in an elimination game. He threw to minor league hitters at the Astros spring training facility in Kissimmee, Florida— just another batting-practice pitcher trying to earn his keep.

On April 3, he sat at home with his family and watched on TV as the Astros opened their season against Florida. "My little ones, they're putting their two cents in every night," he told the Associated Press. "I said, 'I'm playing for the home team right now.' We're going to go out and hit in the cage and do the things we love to do around the house."

Nobody bought it. Since the Astros hadn't offered him salary arbitration, Clemens was ineligible to re-sign with the team until May 1. Which was fine, because it only gave fans and sportswriters more time to speculate about what he'd do. Clemens *loved* speculation. "If I come back, it's not necessarily a team that's winning a division," he said. "It's a team that I still think can win and a team I can help in a big way. That's my approach."

The media ate from Clemens' palm. Every day someone different ran a story about the Roger Derby. Houston? Texas? New York? Boston? Retirement? CLEMENS GETS READY TO MAKE DECISION read a *Washington Post* headline, one day before *The Seattle Times* ran a piece titled "Don't Expect Clemens to Play Soon."

Finally, on May 31, Clemens agreed to a one-year, $22,000,022 deal to spend the remainder of the season with the Astros. Even in Houston, where Clemens once would have had a 50-50 shot had he run for mayor, the news was greeted with moderate exasperation. To many of the city's residents, the pitcher's delays and dalliances were mere ploys to keep the Clemens family's Q-rating at a high level. Since returning to Houston, Roger and Debbie had become the city's unofficial first couple, appearing seemingly anywhere—as long as the cameras were available to follow. Once reluctant to give the media more than a few seconds of time, Clemens, over the course of his time as an Astro, graced the covers of such powerhouse Houston-based magazines as *Houston Intown, Absolute Katy, Avid Golfer, Women's Golf Texas* and *Watch Aficionado* (a sampling of writer Barbara Green's probing interview: Q: "We hear you love watches." A: "I love watches"). Debbie, who in 2003 begged her husband to appear with her in *Sports Illustrated*'s swimsuit issue, was starting a clothing-jewelry line and desperately craved the publicity her last name allowed. "They were all over the place, to the point that it became really embarrassing," says a person who knows the family well. "They were always appearing at this party or that opening."

Wrote Stephen A. Smith in a *Philadelphia Inquirer* piece headlined "Roger Clemens' Phony Encore":

> It doesn't appear that Clemens cares much about anything, at least not with regard to the game's integrity. And he certainly does not care as much about that as he cared about the money, the publicity, and, more important than anything else, his insatiable need to feel wanted, no matter how phony he looks in the process.

Clemens' season didn't turn out all that badly. He pitched reasonably well, going 7-6 in 19 starts with a 2.30 ERA. Even though the Astros finished 82-80, the team stayed involved in the Wild Card race for most of the second half. On September 24, in what many assumed would be his final major league start, Clemens held the Cardinals to one run over five innings in a 7-3 win. Following the game, he was asked to leave the dugout and wave to the crowd of 43,704. He basked in a lengthy ovation.

Yet, come season's end, the Clemens '06 Experiment had to be deemed a failure. Players bashed his selfishness, off the record, to the media. Garner, a normally good-natured man, bristled at managing a player who made his own schedule. For $22 million (prorated to $12.4 million), the team deserved more. "There was this whole 'Roger's helping everyone' sort of thing, and it wasn't true anymore, because he wasn't there," says Alyson Footer, the Astros beat writer for MLB.com. "As a reporter you like to think you can find anyone. But Roger was unfindable."

That's because, save for when he pitched, Clemens rarely—if ever—showed up to games. He had his sons' Little League events to attend, a golf handicap to whittle down, a massive home with a pool. "I had hoped that he would be kind of a mentor," said Jason Hirsh, a rookie pitcher who debuted with the Astros in August. "But when I got there, he was pretty much nonexistent in terms of his presence in the clubhouse. You like to believe that nobody is above the game, and the kind of stuff he's granted, it almost seems like he is."

That, for Clemens, was the genius of the deal.

He wanted to retire.

He wanted to play.

So, in 2006, he did both.

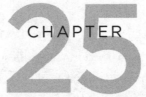

CHAPTER

25

Credibility Lost

B y the time the 2006 baseball season was coming to a close, Roger Clemens was no longer just fighting for one more contract. He was fighting his first pitched battle in what would be a long, ugly and, ultimately, losing war to protect his legacy.

On October 1, the *Los Angeles Times* reported that Clemens was among a handful of major leaguers accused of using performance-enhancing drugs by Jason Grimsley, a former Yankees relief pitcher who was now the subject of a federal investigation involving steroids and human growth hormone. Long suspected as a user of performance enhancers, Grimsley had begun cooperating with authorities after he was caught with a $3,200 shipment of growth hormone by an undercover postal inspector. Grimsley, who was looking at jail time, had agreed to name names and provide details in exchange for leniency from prosecutors.

Though those names were blacked out on the 20-page affidavit filed by government officials, an anonymous source informed the *Times* that Clemens, along with Andy Pettitte and a handful of Baltimore Orioles, had been fingered by Grimsley.

In a tone that expressed both agitation and disbelief, Clemens denied, denied, denied. "I just think it's incredibly dangerous to sit out there and just throw names out there," he said the following afternoon in Atlanta, where the Astros were wrapping up their season. "I haven't seen [the report], nor do I need to see it.

"Like I told you guys before, I've been tested plenty of times. My physicals that I've taken, they've taken my blood work. I've passed every test anybody wants. Again, I find it just amazing that you can just throw anybody out there. Like I was telling Andy [Pettitte] and some of the guys here today, I guess tomorrow they're going to accuse us of robbing a bank."

A few days later, the U.S. Attorney's Office said that the *Los Angeles Times* report contained "significant inaccuracies" and that Clemens wasn't one of the players Grimsley had named. The Rocket was on a golf course in Hawaii when reporters caught up to him for comment, and he played up his mock indignation with the brio of a Broadway stage veteran. "It's unfortunate that people don't really do thorough work before people drag people through the mud," he told them. "Really, it's sad."

Those "significant inaccuracies" were a gift to Clemens, just not for the reason he thought. Yes, they allowed him to dismiss any performance-enhancing rumors with a forceful rebuttal. But had he been blessed with more brains and less ego, Clemens would have viewed the Grimsley dust-up as a dire warning. Even though he'd skated this time, he should have known that reporters and investigators would be coming at him again. Thanks to a bevy of recent steroid scandals, ranging from Barry Bonds and BALCO to the March 17, 2005, congressional testimony on steroid use by Mark McGwire, Jose Canseco, Rafael Palmeiro, Curt Schilling and Sammy Sosa, performance enhancers were suddenly big news in baseball. An aging superstar whose recent performance seemed to defy nature was an obvious target.

With nothing left to accomplish or prove, Clemens easily could have hung up his glove and cleats and strolled off into the sunset. But he refused to let go. "I genuinely think that Roger started to believe his own lie," says a former major leaguer. "He convinced himself that he wasn't cheating."

When the Grimsley talk died down (Grimsley had been released by the Diamondbacks on July 7, 2006, and some of the information from his investigation would later prove useful in the Mitchell Report), Clemens once again debated aloud whether he would pitch another season. His sound bites in 2007 were eerily similar to ones from 2006, 2005 and 2004. Faux humility over "the honor" of being wooed. Faux doubt over his interest or readiness. He told MLB.com that getting back into playing shape could prove impossible. He told the *Hartford Courant* that he was "failing miserably at retirement." He told *The Desert Sun* of Palm Springs, California, that he wasn't even thinking about coming back. In the February 17 edition of the *Newark Star-Ledger,* he said flatly, "I don't want to play."

That didn't deter GMs. The Astros wanted him back but could pay only about $10 million for the year. The Red Sox, dreaming of a Rocket reunion, dangled $18 million, plus a chance at redemption. As soon as Boston's offer came in, Clemens' agents wisely called Yankees GM Brian Cashman. Within hours, New York blew away the competition with a $28 million prorated deal, plus the same perks Houston had offered: *Come when you want, go when you want.* "As I pledged just a few days ago," Yankees owner George Steinbrenner said in a statement, "I will do everything within my power to support Brian Cashman, Joe Torre and this team as we fight to bring a 27th championship to New York." How could Roger Clemens refuse?

On Sunday, May 6, a month into the season, the Yankees and Mariners were engaged in an afternoon game at the stadium—a yawn-inducing battle of two second-place teams awash in mediocrity. At the end of the seventh-inning stretch, with the Yankees holding a 3-0 lead, public address announcer Bob Sheppard asked the 52,553 spectators in attendance to turn their attention to Steinbrenner's private box high above the playing field. A buzz shot through the crowd, followed by an ear-shattering scream of recognition. There, standing with a microphone in his hand, was Clemens. Dressed in a dark business suit, sporting a *Happy Days* crew cut, the ageless ace leaned forward toward the crowd. "Thank you all!" he said, a familiar twang trailing his words. "Well, they came and got me out of Texas and I can tell you it's a privilege to be back! I'll be talking to y'all soon!"

Fans cheered wildly, Yankee players high-fived and Clemens, floating above it all, waved, Pope-like, down upon his devoted masses. From the nearby WCBS radio broadcast booth, Suzyn Waldman, a Yankee announcer and notorious homer, channeled the spirit of "Mean Gene" Okerlund. With her volume on maximum output and her voice sounding as if she had swallowed a swath of sandpaper, Waldman dove into what will likely go down as the most embarrassing monologue in New York sports radio history: "Roger Clemens is in George's box, and Roger Clemens is coming back! Oh! My! Goodness gracious! Of all the dramatic things! Of all the dramatic things I've ever seen! Roger Clemens standing right in George Steinbrenner's box, announcing he is back! Roger Clemens is a New York Yankee!"

In their ensuing three-minute interview with Clemens, Waldman and her partner, John Sterling, never broached performance-enhancing drugs, or the fact that Clemens had retired and unretired for the 12,471st time, or that he was older than Casey Stengel. They didn't find out about the $28 million prorated contract, or that his agreement featured the same show-up-when-you-feel-like-it perks as his Houston days. "Make no mistake about it," Clemens said. "I've come back to do what they only know how to do here with the Yankees, and that's win a championship. Anything else is a failure."

From New York, Clemens flew to Lexington, Kentucky, to work out with his son Koby, now a third baseman for the Class A Lexington Legends of the Astros orgainzation The dramatic, *after*-the-last-minute signing of Clemens was the biggest story in baseball for weeks. The local newspapers treated it like the second coming of, if not the Messiah, the Beatles. Oddly, nobody bothered to ask Yankee owner George Steinbrenner, general manager Brian Cashman or manager Joe Torre how they felt about adding a player now viewed suspiciously by much of the league. No one disputed that the Yankees, who were 14-15 at the time, desperately needed mound help—they had already used 18 pitchers, including five rookie starters—but were they *this* desperate? A $28 million contract—and nary a single steroid inquiry? "You know why, of course," says Howard Bryant, the author of *Juicing the Game.* "Because there are some answers you don't want to know. Never ask what you don't want to learn."

Of the three principles, it is Torre's indifference that remains most striking. Come day's end, Steinbrenner and Cashman are business-men. They wear suits and ties, ponder dollars and cents, fret over sala-ries. But Torre, beloved for his decency and understanding, had been a ballplayer himself. As Bob Gibson's friend, catcher and teammate with St. Louis from 1969 through 1974, he saw up close that even the best power pitchers die with advanced age. Exceptional even at age 36, when he won 19 games, Gibson was a 3-10 has-been just three years later. What Clemens was doing was not merely impossible but physi-cally dangerous to his health.

Although the traditional media failed to challenge the Clemens idolatry, the new media stepped up. In a piece titled "It's Important That You Remember That Roger Clemens Is Your Savior," Deadspin. com editor Will Leitch wrote what many were thinking:

> Roger Clemens . . . somehow conflated a Lou Gehrig moment
> for himself yesterday, a moment all the more pleasing for him
> because he didn't have to, you know, actually be dying. Clem-
> ens is the master of playing the prettiest girl at the prom, but

yesterday might have been the most egregious example yet: Clemens really did fancy himself a god.

And gods do not come cheaply. Darren Rovell at CNBC has calculated Clemens' ridiculous salary, and discovered it makes no financial sense at all for the Yankees, even if they do make the play-offs. Clemens, when you do all the salary math, will make $8,888 a pitch; no amount of play-off ticketing and extra Clemens-ecstatic last-minute sales can make up that amount.

But Roger Clemens gets to feel like the conquering savior, and he gets to do it live. That 45-year-old arm better still have tons of oomph left, because yesterday's masturbatory construction is going to look awfully silly if he doesn't turn the Yankees around. Or, say, if he forgets that baseball's still steroid testing. Let's hope it doesn't turn into his "Mission: Accomplished" moment.

As Leitch predicted, Clemens wasn't worth the money, and his come-and-go-as-you-please clause in his contract wasn't worth the damage it did to team morale. On May 17, weeks before Clemens even joined the club, Yankee reliever Kyle Farnsworth appeared as a guest on a Chicago radio station and warned that his new teammate's personalized schedule "might cause some friction. I think if you're going to be a part of the team, you should always be there."

After three minor league starts and a "fatigued" right groin that delayed his return, Clemens made his 2007 debut against the Pirates on June 9. He entered the clubhouse for the first time at approximately 10 A.M., shaking hands with new teammates such as Chris Basak and Brian Bruney, going over the signs with Torre, designing a game plan with veteran catcher Jorge Posada. After five innings of work against a lineup that ranked last in the NL in many offensive categories, Clemens led 4-3. He had thrown 96 pitches, and Torre assumed he would ask to be taken out. Instead, Clemens returned for the sixth, striking out Freddy Sanchez with two on to end a threat. When the 9-3 Yankee rout was in the books, Clemens had his 349th victory. "I'm going to savor this moment," he said afterward. "Because I don't know what's ahead of us."

He didn't know, but smart baseball people had a pretty good idea. When the Yankees agreed to spend nearly $30 million on a pitcher who'd be available for only half the season, they assumed they were acquiring a legitimate ace. But even with the help of steroids, Clemens was a 45-year-old man who'd pitched over 4,817 innings in the major leagues. Over 18 starts, he was wildly inconsistent, holding the Angels to a single run over eight innings one start, then permitting eight runs in one and two-thirds innings against the White Sox before being booed off the Yankee Stadium mound in another. "He never really got in a groove," says Tyler Kepner, the *New York Times* beat writer. "He wasn't the same pitcher he had been when he left New York the first time."

Clemens tried to help the team any way he could (the rare occasions he was with the team, that is). Joba Chamberlain, a hard-throwing 22-year-old rookie, had the locker next to Clemens' in the Yankees clubhouse, and the Rocket offered support and wisdom. "He's invaluable," Torre said. "He's a teacher and a great example." A good teacher, perhaps, but a mediocre pitcher. He went 6-6 with a 4.18 ERA in 2007; despite that underwhelming contribution, the Yankees won 94 games and reached the postseason as the wild-card entry.

Clemens was kept on the shelf for the final few games of the regular season, because Torre hoped that a fresh Rocket would dominate in the play-offs. Starting game three against Cleveland in the Division Series, the $28 million man lasted but two and a third innings before leaving with a hamstring injury. When asked in the immediate aftermath whether he would return for a 25th season, Clemens said with a smile, "You know I haven't been very good at [retirement]. I thought three or four years ago I was done."

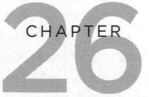

CHAPTER

Dead Pitcher Walking

O n December 13, 2007, Major League Baseball released a 409-page document officially titled "The Report to the Commissioner of Baseball of an Independent Investigation into the Illegal Use of Steroids and Other Performance Enhancing Substances by Players in Major League Baseball." The result of a 20-month, multimillion-dollar investigation spurred by baseball commissioner Bud Selig and conducted by former U.S. Senator George Mitchell, the so-called Mitchell Report examined the spiraling problem with performance-enhancing drugs and suggested ways to clean up the game. It was a detailed, scrupulously and mercilessly documented indictment of the profligate cheating that had radically changed baseball over the past decade.

The report mentioned 89 players by name, ranging from All-Stars such as Andy Pettitte, Eric Gagne and Troy Glaus to nobodies such as Chris Donnels and Paxton Crawford. The evidence it cited included telephone records, photocopies of canceled checks, and awkward-sounding denials that screamed "Guilty!" It was the juiciest baseball incident since the 1919 Black Sox scandal, and its leading man was Roger Clemens.

From pages 167 through 175, the portrait painted of Clemens is that of a desperate man eager to load up on steroids and human growth hormone in an attempt to prolong his career. Most of the evidence against him had been provided by Brian McNamee, who'd also told Mitchell about Pettitte's use of HGH. The minute the report became public, Clemens' already tattered reputation turned to mud. And yet, there were still ways to possibly preserve . . . *something*. Clemens could have hid behind the walls of his Houston estate. He could have asked for privacy in this difficult time. He could have admitted his wrongdoing; held a press conference from a hotel conference room with cookies and those little glass bottles of Coca-Cola; uttered words along the lines of, "Yes, I used performance-enhancing drugs. It wasn't smart, and I truly regret it. I am a role model, and I don't want kids to follow my stupid behavior. I believe in hard work, but at the end of my career my body wasn't recovering like it used to. So I made the wrong choice. I apologize to everyone, because nothing is more important to me than the integrity of the game I love."

"Man, I wish he had taken a different approach," says Bruce Hurst, his longtime teammate with the Red Sox. "Just come clean, say you did wrong and ask for forgiveness. Because America is a very forgiving place, and we want to love our heroes. That's all Roger had to do."

Instead, Clemens attacked.

How many times in his life had Clemens been called a bulldog? A fighter? Clemens was a high, tight 95-mph fastball to the head, a splintered bat whipping across the first-base line, a prize fighter in baseball garb. What was it he once told ESPN's Dan Patrick? "With me, I try to beat you three ways. Physically, I'm going to try and beat you. If that's failing, my mental game has to go to a new level. And if those two fail, I go to emotions. Whatever it takes to elevate my game." Was he really going to let a bureaucrat like George Mitchell crush his legacy? And what of McNamee? Where was the loyalty? The decency? Before Clemens came along, McNamee was a nobody. Now look at all the fame, all the clients, all the dough. And this . . . *backstabbing* was the thanks Clemens received? "I believe Roger's ego took over," says Joe Hesketh, his former Boston teammate. "He was backed in a corner, and instead of waving a white flag, he decided to throw a whole load of punches."

The day the Mitchell Report was released, Clemens' attorney, Rusty Hardin, issued a strongly worded denial: "He has not been charged with anything," Hardin said. "He will not be charged with anything and yet he is being tried in the court of public opinion with no recourse. That is totally wrong. There has never been one shred of tangible evidence that he ever used these substances and yet he is being slandered today." Hardin's premise was simple: Destroy the messenger (McNamee), and you destroy the message. He dismissed McNamee as a "troubled man" who'd been pressured by authorities to stay out of jail.

There were two fundamental flaws in this strategy: First, unbeknownst to Clemens and Hardin, McNamee had saved syringes, needles and gauze pads that had been used to administer the drugs to the Rocket (and that, according to McNamee's attorneys, contained samples of Clemens' DNA). Second, two days after Hardin's denunciation of McNamee, Pettitte, Roger Clemens' close friend and off-season training buddy, released a statement in which he admitted to twice having used human growth hormones to recover from an elbow injury in 2002. Pettitte, a quiet, religious man, had long felt guilty over this transgression. "I have tried to do things the right way in my entire life," Pettitte said, "and ask that you put those two days in the proper context."

This was a devastating blow for Clemens. As Gerry Callahan put it in the *Boston Herald*, "Are we supposed to believe McNamee is lying about Clemens but not about Andy Pettitte?"

There were other problems with Hardin's "destroy the messenger" gambit: McNamee had given Mitchell detailed information on steroid use by Pettitte and former Yankee second baseman Chuck Knoblauch—all of which was confirmed. Also, he had been granted immunity in exchange for his testimony, which meant that the only way he would go to jail was if he lied under oath. Why would he untruthfully rat out his star client? Money? The most money he ever made came from working with Clemens. Business? For most trainers, being associated with drug users isn't the best way to drum up new clients. Pride? What pride was there in being a part of a scandal? "There was nothing for Mac to gain," says C. J. Nitkowski, a former major league pitcher and McNamee client. "Absolutely nothing. What possible benefit comes from being an informant for the Mitchell Report? None."

Many major leaguers quietly celebrated the Mitchell Report. It brought out into the open a dirty secret they'd been whispering about—and fuming over—for years. The players who hadn't cheated were tired of competing against pumped-up freaks who could throw harder and hit the baseball farther than nature and time would normally allow. Curt Schilling, who had idolized Clemens for years, told the Associated Press that if the Rocket failed to clear his name, he should be forced to return the four Cy Young Award trophies he had won after he'd first picked up a hypodermic needle.

Back home in Houston, Clemens huddled with Hardin, scrambling to clear his name. They decided to stay the course, play up the contrasts between the beloved legend and his Judas-like accuser, who, they knew, had once been suspended by the New York Police Department. "I don't blame Rusty, because if you look at Brian's background and some of the things he's been implicated in, he has credibility problems," says Earl Ward, McNamee's attorney. "I'm sure that's what Rusty was thinking, that Brian was a defense attorney's dream." McNamee was a former cop who had later been accused of rape. Roger Clemens was a family man who regularly took time out of his hectic life to visit sick children. Brian McNamee was a hanger-on. Roger Clemens was a superstar.

On December 23, 2007, Clemens filmed a short, rambling, choppy, oft-incoherent statement that he then posted on YouTube. "Let me be clear, the answer is 'No,'" he said in an unemotional deep-voiced drawl. "I did not use steroids or human growth hormone, and I've never done so." Two weeks later, Clemens appeared on *60 Minutes* with Mike Wallace, who did little to hide his unabashed love of the Rocket. Despite the fact that Wallace tossed out repeated softballs, Clemens came off as confused, ornery, awkward, simple—and deceitful. "If I have these needles and these steroids and all these drugs, where did I get them?" he said in one of many non sequiturs. "Where is the person out there [who] gave them to me? Please come forward. . . . Why didn't I keep doing it if it was so good for me? Why didn't I break down? Why didn't my tendons turn to dust?"

When asked if McNamee had injected him with *any* drugs, Clemens said he had, but only "Lidocaine and B12. It's for my joints, and B12. I still take today." He said again that McNamee's accusation was "ridiculous," and "If he's doing that to me, I should have a third ear coming out of my forehead. I'd be pulling tractors with my teeth." Clemens insisted, again, that he'd never used steroids.

"Never a human growth hormone?" Wallace asked.

"Never," said Clemens.

"Never anabolic steroids?"

"Never."

"Swear?" Wallace asked.

"Swear," Clemens said.

In an article that appeared in the *Connecticut Post* shortly after Clemens' sitdown with Wallace, Dr. Jeff Anderson, the director of the University of Connecticut's sports medicine program, noted skeptically, "No one injects lidocaine intramuscularly. You use lidocaine all the time if you're stitching somebody up or things like that. There's certain injuries you can numb up with lidocaine and it's safe to do. But you're not getting a shot in the butt from your strength coach."

WITH HIS CLIENT GASPING for air, Hardin decided on two different tactics.

First, on January 6, Clemens filed a defamation suit against Mc-Namee, claiming the trainer was threatened with jail if he didn't tie the pitcher to steroids. Then, on January 7, he and Clemens alerted the media that they would be holding a press conference in a room at Houston's George R. Brown Convention Center. There would be, news outlets were assured, proof of Clemens' innocence.

Reporters were greeted by a smiling Hardin and a scowling Clemens, sitting side by side on the dais. "The first thing Roger said really pissed me off," says a reporter who covered the event. "It symbolizes what I don't like about him and what I don't like about his representatives. The son of his college coach had died, and the funeral was that day. So he gets up there and he blames us for him not being able to attend. I was like, 'Dude, I did not do this. Believe me, I'd rather not be working at 7 P.M. on a Monday.'" Clemens and Hardin proceeded to offer their "evidence"—a recording of a telephone conversation between Clemens and McNamee that had taken place just three days before. They played the tape for the reporters.

In the 17-minute recording, McNamee repeatedly asked Clemens, "What do you want me to do?"

> CLEMENS: "I need somebody to tell the truth, Mac. For the life of me, I'm trying to figure out why you told the guys I did steroids."
> MCNAMEE: "I understand that."
> CLEMENS: "I'm telling the truth and I want it out there."
> MCNAMEE: "Tell me what you want me to do. I will go to jail, I will

do whatever you want. I want it to go away. I'm with you, in your corner . . . but I also don't want to go to jail."

It was an excruciatingly embarrassing conversation for both men—McNamee came off whiny and clearly conflicted; Clemens sounded cold, detached and, in his clumsy way, manipulative. To most reporters, it seemed as though Clemens had been trying to trick McNamee into saying something incriminating.

When the tape ended, Clemens fielded 13 questions from reporters before testily storming out of the press conference *he* had called. At one point, Hardin slipped him a note reading "Lighten up." Clemens looked at the piece of paper and scoffed. "You want me to lighten up?" he said. "It's hard. Thank you."

Three weeks later, the Clemens camp offered up some more exculpatory "evidence." Clemens' agent, Randy Hendricks, released a 49-page statistical analysis (supplemented with 30 charts) that concluded the Rocket's career numbers were comparable to those of other accomplished longtime veterans, including Nolan Ryan and Randy Johnson. "Clemens' longevity," it stated, "was due to his ability to adjust his style of pitching as he got older, incorporating his very effective split-finger fastball to offset the decrease in the speed of his regular fastball caused by aging."

Adi Wyner, an associate professor of statistics at the Wharton School of the University of Pennsylvania, couldn't keep himself from laughing as he read Hendricks' "report." Yes, it was possible to have a lengthy pitching career. And yes, Roger Clemens had talent that would surely help him last longer than the average right-hander. "But," says Wyner, "they were very selective about the measures they used, and they were also selective about Roger Clemens in a way that I thought was funny."

Wyner and three colleagues then analyzed the career trajectories of successful starting major league pitchers who'd had long careers and found a startling commonality: "They all have this beautiful career trajectory that arcs," Wyner says. "They start off, they improve, then they get worse. They might bump around a tiny bit, but that's the overall trend." Clemens was the only pitcher they could find who had excelled early, then had fallen off for several years, then had bounced back to reach—and surpass—his previous best. "The guy was great, he got crappy, then he was great again," says Wyner. "It's incredibly rare."

Wyner and his colleagues published a piece about their survey— "Report Backing Clemens Chooses Its Facts Carefully"—in *The New York Times* on February 10. The next day, Hendricks' agency began to barrage Wyner with e-mails and phone calls, threatening to sue for libel. "We're academics, and it's our job to speak out about things," says Wyner. "There's no way on earth I'm going to be intimidated by this [suit]. This is what I've been placed on this earth to do—research. They were bullies, and they were trying to bully us. But we wouldn't have it."

FEBRUARY WAS ANOTHER CRUEL month for Clemens. First, word leaked that Pettitte was about to confirm that Clemens had received HGH injections from McNamee. Then, Clemens was summoned to testify—along with McNamee—before Congress in a nationally televised hearing. Clemens got to D.C. early and spent three days working Capitol Hill like a seasoned politician, holding private meetings with 25 committee members, signing autographs, telling old stories about this game and that game, all the while insisting he had never cheated. Some members of Congress called him "Mr. Clemens"; others called him "Rocket." Edolphus Towns, a New York congressman, asked for an autograph. Even former president George H. Bush contacted Clemens on the day before the hearing to wish him good luck.

"That made us really nervous," says Ward, McNamee's attorney, who was sitting beside his client as he was sworn in. "This was a body that was going to make a decision about what this controversy was all about, and here you have them treating Clemens like their hero."

In his opening statement, committee chairman Harry Waxman confirmed that Pettitte had already given sworn testimony that implicated Clemens. "During his deposition," Waxman said, "Mr. Pettitte told the committee that in 1999 or 2000 that 'Mr. Clemens told me he had taken HGH.'" Waxman said that when Pettitte was asked whether he had any doubts, he replied, "I mean, no. He told me that."

"That," says Ward, "was big. Really, really, really big."

For Clemens the four-hour hearing proved a disaster. Sitting at the same table as McNamee, the Rocket—wearing a dark pinstriped suit and red tie, his brown hair cut short—stumbled and groped for words. In his opening statement, he spoke of achieving all through hard work, then focused his attention on McNamee. Though he never turned to face his former trainer, Clemens' words served as a fierce stare down. "There were times over the years in which I wondered about what kind of person he was and what he was doing when he was not around me," Clemens said. "I questioned McNamee about these things, and at the end of the day, I was willing to take him at his word and give him the benefit of the doubt."

He added: "I had no idea that this man would exploit the trust I gave him to try to save his own skin by making up lies that have devastated me and my family."

Once again, neither man looked good. Clemens came off as arrogant, confused and dishonest. (One could almost hear the nation snicker as Clemens denied knowing his wife, Debbie, had used McNamee-supplied HGH leading up to the couple's spread in the 2003 *Sports Illustrated* swimsuit issue.) McNamee came off as naive, dumb, and dishonest. With rare exceptions, the members of the congressional committee came off as fawning fans. Virginia Foxx, Republican of North Carolina, posted a series of four photographs of Clemens taken between 1996 and 2006, the period of time during which he allegedly received injections. "Mr. Clemens," she said, "you know I am not an expert in any of these issues, but you appear to me to be about the same size in all of those photos." William Lacy Clay, Democrat of Missouri, asked Clemens, "What uniform you will wear into the Hall of Fame?"

A few committee members comported themselves with dignity. When Congressman Elijah Cummings, Democrat of Maryland, asked Clemens whether he thought Pettitte had not told the truth in his testimony, Clemens paused.

"Mr. Clemens," Cummings said, "I'm reminding you that you are under oath."

"Mr. Congressman," Clemens replied at last, "Andy Pettitte is my friend. He was my friend before this. He will be my friend after this. I think Andy has, uh, misheard. I think he misremembers our conversation."

Cummings sighed. "It's hard to believe you," he said. "It's hard to believe you, sir. You're one of my heroes, but it's hard to believe you."

In his closing remarks, Waxman issued what could be interpreted only as a fierce repudiation of Clemens. "This is what I've learned," he said. "Chuck Knoblauch and Andy Pettitte confirmed what Brian McNamee told Senator Mitchell. We learned of conversations that Andy Pettitte believed he had with Roger Clemens about HGH—even though Clemens says his relationship with Mr. Pettitte was so close that they would know and share information with each other. Evidently Mr. Pettitte didn't believe what Mr. Clemens said in that 2005 conversation. . . ."

Violating House rules, Clemens leaned into his microphone to interrupt. "It doesn't mean he was not mistaken, sir," he said.

"Doesn't mean that?" Waxman said.

"That does not mean that he was not mistaken, sir." Clemens replied.

Waxman pounded his gavel and flashed a stern look. "Excuse me," he said, "but this is not your time to argue with me."

IN THE AFTERMATH OF the highly publicized hearing, the national reaction was relatively universal.

Brian McNamee may well have been a sleaze—but he was a sleaze telling the truth. According to a *USA Today*/Gallop Poll, 57 percent of fans said they believed Clemens had lied under oath. "The only surprise," cracked Richard Emery, one of McNamee's attorneys, "is that 31 percent of the fans were duped by Roger Clemens."

Wrote Richard Justice in Clemens' hometown *Houston Chronicle*:

> To believe Clemens is to believe that McNamee manufactured evidence and risked jail to make up an outrageous story.
>
> To believe Clemens is to believe that Andy Pettitte is a liar. . . .
>
> To believe Clemens is to believe an affidavit in which he admits to discussing HGH with McNamee, then denies discussing HGH, is no inconsistency.

Despite the obvious contradictions, Clemens forged ahead with his defamation suit, a move that stunned and bewildered the trainer's legal team. "At any point, Roger could have admitted wrongdoing, and everything probably would have gone away," says Ward. "But he kept digging a deeper and deeper grave. I don't know if he was getting bad advice from his attorneys, or just not listening to them."

McNamee and his team opted to mount a dirty but very effective counteroffensive. They too decided to "kill the messenger"—in this case, Clemens—and his reputation. New York's *Daily News* had assigned an investigative team to uncover all there was to know about Clemens and steroids. McNamee's attorneys reached out to the newspaper and, day by day, released one piece of damaging information about Clemens after another. It was not merely details about steroids. They leaked news of his affair with Mindy McCready, the former country starlet who was now a has-been recovering drug addict. (Says a McCready friend, "When this whole thing with Roger came down, she was immediately thinking how she could score some publicity for herself.") They offered details on the many other women Clemens had slept with while married to Debbie. "We slowly let the information out, in a very deliberate manner," says Ward. "We gave Clemens and his attorneys advance warning. We never wanted it to go down this road. We said to them, 'Let's end this thing. Don't go before Congress. Don't sue Brian.' But that's not how Roger Clemens thinks. He wanted a fight. So we gave him one." Though some of the scurrilous and often salacious claims in the *Daily News* were wrong (Clemens, for example, did not meet McCready when she was 15, as many *Daily News* stories claimed), and the arrangement the newspaper made with McNamee's team seemed grossly unethical (McNamee's attorneys provided the newspaper with anonymous details and were then quoted on the record expressing shock and anger about those facts), the *Daily News* series blew a hole in Clemens' reputation the size of Texas. "You can get away with the performance-enhancing stuff," says Ward. "But he was a liar. That's hard to overcome."

IT WAS OVER FOR Roger Clemens. He was, finally, done. Or, more accurately, baseball was done with him. The Astros discussed rescinding his 10-year personal service deal and requested that he stay away from the team and its facilities. Plans for a Clemens-themed restaurant in Houston were flushed. Memorial Hermann, a Houston-based health system, chose to rename its Clemens Institute for Sports Medicine and

Human Performance. Gifford Nielsen, a former Houston Oilers quarterback who now worked as a local sports TV anchor, asked Clemens to stop helping with a charity golf tournament they had cohosted for four years. Clemens was now a recluse. During the 2008 season, he attended just one Astros game, sitting a handful of rows behind home plate with a ticket he had purchased. Once staples of the Houston restaurant and arts scenes, he and Debbie turned invisible. A local rap artist named Paul Wall paid for two billboards, both reading HOUSTON SUPPORTS ROGER CLEMENS, to be placed along I-45. "I've always loved the Rocket, and I wanted to show my affection," says Wall. "But I'll be honest—around here, he's been left to decay in the dirt."

On the evening of Sunday, September 21, 2008, before their final home game of the season, the Yankees held a ceremony to bid farewell to Yankee Stadium, which would be replaced come the 2009 season. Dozens of former stars were on hand—including Yogi Berra, Whitey Ford, Don Larsen, Don Mattingly, Paul O'Neill and Bernie Williams. Even second-tier Yankee standouts such as Knoblauch and Jimmy Key appeared in a video montage saluting the many great Yankees who'd performed on baseball's grandest stage. It was a stirring ceremony and a magnificent night, a potent reminder of why the New York Yankees engender so much passion in their fans.

One former star, however, was not invited.

Once, not so long before, Roger Clemens had insisted he would wear a Yankees cap into the Baseball Hall of Fame.

Now he couldn't even wear one into Yankee Stadium.

Epilogue

On the evening of November 5, 2008, less than 24 hours after Barack Obama had been elected the 44th president of the United States, a reporter pulled up to the Georgian Apartments complex on South Austin Avenue in Georgetown, Texas.

Armed with nothing more than a pen, a notepad and a promising tip, he headed upstairs and knocked on the door of apartment number 223. While waiting, he took inventory of his surroundings: Two stories high and constructed of beige brick, the Georgian looked as if it could have been a halfway passable Days Inn 20 or 30 years ago. There was a railing with small rust spots peeking through. A rectangular pool surrounded by garage sale–quality furniture. Above each apartment door was an old plastic light emitting a glow that had the brownish tint of a smoker's front teeth.

When no one answered, the reporter knocked again, a bit louder. This time, the door opened.

There, at long last, stood the ghost.

He was approximately 5-foot-10 and 180 pounds. He had a blue tattoo on one of his wrists, and his skin was badly weathered, much like that of an old seaman. He had a wiry build and sunken eyes.

"Mr. Clemens?" the reporter asked.

A lengthy pause.

"No," he replied, scowling.

As the door began to shut, the reporter quickly explained that he was doing research for a book on Roger Clemens, the baseball player, and he was eager to talk to his older brother. He wasn't looking to invade anyone's privacy, but . . .

"Yeah, well, I'm not interested," the ghost said. "So you keep moving."

With that, Randy Clemens vanished behind his closed door.

APPROXIMATELY 170 MILES AWAY, in the tony Memorial Park section of Houston, as Roger Clemens sat in his 13,000-square-foot palace, he surely must have been wondering how his life had come to this. The man who had once ruled the city was now scorned. No longer in demand as a charity spokesperson, no longer asked to endorse products, no longer invited to red-carpet events, no longer offered fat contracts to pitch half a season, Clemens was Houston's baseball version of Enron—an embarrassment most people wanted to forget.

Having earned hundreds of millions of dollars through the years, Clemens will likely never have to worry about money. He has myriad investments and a fleet of fancy automobiles, and his home includes a 7,000-square-foot gymnasium, an indoor batting cage, a weight room and enough baseball memorabilia to fill a Costco warehouse.

It is what Clemens does not have—and what he will almost certainly never have—that torments him.

In Major League Baseball's long history, few players have craved induction into the Hall of Fame with greater intensity than Clemens. It was his destiny—he just *knew* it. Having accomplished every one of his other professional goals, all that remained for the Rocket was a sunny July day on a stage in Cooperstown. Why, the entire scene had played out in his mind thousands of times. The audience would be filled with teammates and coaches and friends and family members from all the stages of his life. Jim Rice over here. Derek Jeter over there. *I'd like to point out for all of y'all that my high school coach, Charlie Maiorana, is in attendance. A funny thing about Coach. One time we were* . . . Clemens would tell the audience about a fat boy from Ohio who, through love, grit and hard work, had become *the man standing before you today.* He would talk about Woody Booher's whiskers, his brother Richard's service in Vietnam, the unstinting love and generosity of his sisters. Clemens would point toward the sky. A tear would stream down his cheek. He'd get choked up. From the front row, Debbie would offer a reassuring nod. 'You can do this, honey. You can do this.' *I'd like to talk about my mom, Bess, who raised all of us while working three jobs. Without her, there would be no Rocket.*

Lastly, he would use the occasion to make peace with Randy. He would reserve a front-row seat for his boyhood hero, buy him a new suit, put him up in the Otesaga Resort Hotel. *Many of you might not know this, but Randy was a helluva athlete back at* . . . Randy would stand. Take an awkward bow. Then, at his brother's urging, he would approach the stage, climb its handful of steps. There, in the heart of baseball's historic district, Roger Clemens and Randy Clemens would hug. *That's my hero right there,* Roger would say. *That's my hero.*

It would go down as the best speech in Hall of Fame history.

Roger Clemens knew it. He just knew it.

BUT NOW EVEN CLEMENS must realize that he will never stand on that stage.

After ignoring its steroid problem for far too long, Major League

Baseball has drastically reversed course. Those who are caught are punished and forever stigmatized to the point that, when it comes to Cooperstown, even the gaudiest of statistics have no value. All Clemens has to do is look at the pitiful plight of Mark McGwire, the man many credited with saving baseball with his eclipse of Roger Maris' single-season home-run mark in 1998. Less than a decade ago, McGwire was one of baseball's biggest—and most beloved—stars, a Paul Bunyan–esque slugger who would unquestionably be voted into the Hall of Fame in his first year of eligibility. Now, however, he is a leper. McGwire's self-immolation came on March 17, 2005, with his painful attempt at pleading the Fifth when he was called before Congress to discuss steroids. He has been shunned by baseball writers who vote on Hall of Fame ballots, drawing less and less support with each succeeding year.

ON JANUARY 12, 2009, it was announced that a federal grand jury would examine Roger Clemens' testimony before Congress to determine whether he should be indicted for perjury.

In other words, being shunned by the Hall of Fame might not be the worst of it.

When Clemens agreed to appear before Congress in 2008, few outside of his small circle of advisers deemed the move wise. "Even if he wasn't cheating," says Earl Ward, one of McNamee's attorneys, "what was there for him to gain? It was a really, really, really big gamble. The dumbest part about it was, we knew he was lying, and he surely knew he was lying. If I were his lawyer, I would have begged him not to do it."

The result of that gamble: Clemens now faces the very real possibility of jail time. Daniel P. Butler, an assistant United States attorney, is leading the government's inquiry into whether Clemens lied under oath. As of mid-January he had already met at length with McNamee and Kirk Radomski, the man who sold steroids to dozens of major leaguers. Both have stated repeatedly that Clemens was a customer, and Radomski—who was promoting his new book at the time—went even further, telling Jeremy Schapp in an ESPN interview that he had shipped HGH to Clemens' home in Houston. "If Brian was such a bad person, why did Andy Pettitte back him?" Radomski asked Schapp. "Why did Chuck Knoblauch back him? You let a guy you don't trust and you don't respect stay in your house and be around your family? And be around your kids? He admits his wife got a shot [of human growth hormone] in the bedroom. Think about this—he let someone go in a bedroom with his wife and inject his wife. And you didn't trust the guy? If he didn't trust the guy, he would have knocked the guy out. That would have been it. But he let him do it. What does that tell you?"

It tells you Clemens is in deep trouble.

"I think Clemens lied before Congress," Katherine Darmer, a former federal prosecutor, told the New York *Daily News*. "I think he will be indicted, and I think he will be convicted. This is not a complicated case. An indictment could come at any time."

Once upon a time, Roger Clemens stood beside men like Christy Mathewson, Warren Spahn and Sandy Koufax as one of the greatest pitchers in baseball history. He was a hero, an icon. Now, however, it appears that he will be grouped with others, shackled to a group that includes not merely McGwire, Sosa and Bonds but also Shoeless Joe Jackson and Pete Rose.

The legacy of each of those players can be summed in two words: He cheated.

ACKNOWLEDGMENTS

On November 28, 2008, Brian Hickey, the former managing editor of Philadelphia's *City Paper*, was walking along Atlantic Avenue in Collingswood, New Jersey, when he was hit by a car and left for dead. His skull cracked open, his back broken, Hickey was taken to nearby Cooper University Hospital, where he underwent bilateral decompression to relieve the pressure on his brain.

I first met Hickey (few call him by his first name) some 15 years earlier, when we worked together as editors on the University of Delaware's student newspaper, *The Review*. He is a dogged, scrappy, hard-nosed reporter whose dream is to one day win a Pulitzer Prize. In fact, before the accident, he was planning on helping with the reporting for this book. I have little doubt he would have done a spectacular job.

Thankfully, my friend has made a startling recovery. Comatose for more than a week, he is now home with his wonderful wife, Angie, playing Wii, enduring physical therapy, jamming to Ween and plotting a journalistic comeback that, I believe, will inevitably result in the fruition of his long-pursued goal.

Hence, I'd like to corrupt these final pages with a plea for assistance. If, by some chance, you know of any details from the night of November 28, please contact the Collingswood Police Department at (856) 854-1900. Your anonymity will be respected.

Hickey, this book is for you.

• • •

I OWE MANY PEOPLE a great deal of gratitude. David Hirshey, my friend and editor, is a giant in the book business and a man whose takes are almost always dead on; George Quraishi, whose Zen-like demeanor and silky smooth stylings remind me of a young Shannon Hoon; Bob Roe, the mismatched two-shoe wonder and, for my money, America's best content editor; Kate Hamill, a cool-rhyming hip-hop diva who brings the funk à la Grandmaster Flash; David Black, my agent, who combines Ari Gold's tenacity and Grandma Mollie's compassion into one incomparable package; Nick Trautwein, whose wisdom will eternally be sought (and appreciated); Art Haviland, the best publicist this side of Dave Kolberg.

For this endeavor, I surrounded myself with a dream team of aides: Michael Lewis of the *Daytona Beach News-Journal,* who—*Moneyball* be damned—reigns as *the* Michael Lewis; Paul Duer, whose advice is as reliable as his one-handed, middle-of-nowhere, over-the-shoulder jumper; Casey Angle, the fact-checking Oates to my spotlight-hogging Hall; Stephen Cannella, president and CEO of the Gar Finnvold Fan Club; L. Jon Wertheim, author of the remarkable *Blood in the Cage;* and Doug Donovan, my former boss at the Delaware *Review* and a man who sides with Karen Levinson on most issues.

A huge helping of gratitude goes to Thomas Repicci, the world's biggest Roger Clemens fan and a good and trusting friend. Tom has followed the Rocket's career for decades. He was understandably conflicted about contributing to a project that would examine Clemens in an honest, unfiltered light. Tom, I hope you know how vital your input proved to be and that it does not diminish your loyalty to your hero.

I would like to note the excellent reporting of Sam Cook of the Fort Myers *News-Press,* who was open to sharing details of the Mindy McCready story, which—despite his good work—the *New York Daily News* stubbornly refused to acknowledge. Also, a big nod to Dan Shaughnessy of *The Boston Globe.* Nobody has covered Roger Clemens better. Alyson Footer, Houston's MLB.com writer, is as classy as they come. A special thumbs-up to Joy Birdsong and Natasha Simon of the *Sports Illustrated* library.

There were many other key contributors, including Martha Reagan of the *Boston Herald*'s library, Rob Massimi (for the Rob Nichols reference), Marci Moschetti (for watching my stuff in Starbucks), the Dean Martin–esque Peter Karten of Così, Amy Frishberg (who, via Facebook, kept me sane during a week of isolation) and Prime Minister Peter Nicc (aka "Pete Nash"), whose new CD, *Songs in the Key of Luis Aponte,* drops later this year. Big props to Jordan and Isaiah Williams, Lisa and Michael Jude Duer, C. J. Nitkowski, Donna Massaro, Jonathan Mayo, Joseph Kuppinger, Norma Pearlman, Brian Johnson, Stanley Herz, Joan Pearlman, David Pearlman, Laura Fasbach Donovan, Adrienne Lewin, Robyn Furman, Kevin Clark, Kim Lionetti, Laura and Rodney Cole, Bev Oden, Richard and Susan Guggenheimer, Ed Stewart, Rich Green, Carol Atwood and the entire Herz, Stewart & Co. wrecking crew. A special holla to Norma "Thug Life" Shapiro, the Tupac Shakur of Palm Beach.

On my visit to San Jacinto Junior College, I was blessed to meet Martha Hood of the Lee Davis Library, who marched me into the student newspaper offices and bellowed, "He's a writer, he's from New York and he's only here for a few hours! Let's get going!" From there, I was introduced to the wonderful Rikki Saldivar, editor in chief of the San Jacinto *Times,* who offered up a mound of priceless yellowed newspapers.

Another outstanding future star, David Henry of the University of Texas' student newspaper, *The Daily Texan,* took great care in digging through the archives for all things '80s Longhorn baseball. Steven Silver, pride of Northwestern and a *Tennessean* intern, burrowed through Mindy McCready clips with a starved gopher's tenacity. Thanks to Maureen M. Honeycutt for the photographs, *Golf Digest*'s Matt Rudy for the digits, Ronnie Kirschbaum for the *Lakeview Echoes* assignments, Jen Scharer-Katz and Richard Scharer for the Tri-Delta love, Laurel Turnbull for unparalleled goodness and Wes Eichenwald for his guts. A big hug for Martha Frankel, author of *Hats and Eyeglasses,* a spectacular book. And Jeannine McTigue, Brewster High's famed English teacher—thanks for the perspicacity.

We are an odd bunch, the sports book writers of America, and I have been aided greatly by conversations with such talents as Mark Kriegel, Jonathan Eig, Howard Bryant, Ian O'Connor, Leigh Montville and Mike Vaccaro.

My children, Casey Marta and Emmett Leo, know nothing of Roger Clemens, steroids or Yankee–Red Sox. But, with a smile or laugh or hug or Blind Melon sing-along, they always make my day. Daddy loves you.

I traditionally end the acknowledgments by praising my wife, and with good reason. When Catherine and I married seven years ago, I knew a few things: She could cook, she was short, she liked sushi and I loved her. But now, having gone through the grinder yet again, I appreciate more than ever how fortunate I am. Earlie, this has been the roughest one yet, and your compassion, guidance, editing and spot-on Sue Simmons impersonation have pulled me through the darkest depths of literary hell. The book you're holding is not mine.

It's ours.

NOTES

Note: Full references for books quoted in the notes appear in the bibliography.

Chapter 2: Fat Boy from Ohio

8 "It was one of those impossible things": Bruce Newman, "The Fireball Express," *Sports Illustrated,* June 6, 1988.

8 "My father had called my mother and was irritating": Michael P. Geffner, "Roger, Over and Out?" *Texas Monthly,* August 2000.

9 "I had a tremendous amount of fun playing": Dan Shaughnessy, *One Strike Away,* pp. 67–78.

9 Woody was an even-tempered man: Bruce Newman, "The Fireball Express," *Sports Illustrated,* June 6, 1988.

9 We would watch *Bonanza* on TV every week: Greg Cote, "Notorious but Happy, Clemens Keeps Firing Away," *The Miami Herald,* April 1, 2001.

11 "I'm a Christian": Marian Christy, "Clemens: 'I Have Been Misunderstood.'" *The Boston Globe,* April 19, 1990.

12 "I can remember [Grandma] twisting off a chicken's neck": Joe Donnelly, "Bigger . . . Better . . . Best?" *Newsday,* May 22, 1988.

14 He even promised those around him that: *60 Minutes,* interview with Mike Wallace, CBS, August 26, 2001

15 Four years earlier, to much ridicule: Jim Nichols, "Cute Batter Up," *Dayton Daily News,* 1973.

Chapter 3: Houston Bound

22 "I was dazzling [at Dulles)]": Dan Shaughnessy, *One Strike Away,* p. 69.

22 "We'll watch this seven-inning game": Roger Clemens and Peter Gammons, *Rocket Man,* p. 29.

24 "I'd never heard of Roger": Ian O'Connor, "Clemens Never Tires of Making History," *Journal News,* September 11, 2001.

24 To allow her son to attend the school: Shaughnessy, *One Strike Away,* p. 69.

26 Sprinting down Gessner Road, Clemens would pass: Dan Shaughnessy, "Family Pride," *The Boston Globe,* May 23, 1986.

29 In his autobiography, *Rocket Man,* Clemens writes: Clemens and Gammons, *Rocket Man,* p. 32.

Chapter 4: College

33 "The people at work have gotten used to me": Mickie Lawson, "Maroon Spots Plague Woman Who Wants Some Answers," *North Star,* June 11, 1981.

34 "The mental aspect means a great deal": Adrian Garcia, "Gators Closer to Becoming a Team," *North Star,* December 5, 1980.

35 "He's capable of pitching better than that": Mike Simmons, "Two Approaches, Two Wins for Gators," *The Pasadena Citizen,* March 19, 1981.

39 Clemens could now point to a statistical line: Roger Clemens and Peter Gammons, *Rocket Man,* p. 36.

39 "On the junior college level . . . you have to": Mike Simmons, "Graham's First Season as SJC's Coach Successful," *The Pasadena Citizen,* May 30, 1981.

39 When the Mets traveled to Houston to face: Clemens and Gammons, *Rocket Man,* pp. 36–40.

Chapter 5: A Legendary Longhorn

45 "It was so intimidating, so overwhelming": Michael P. Geffner, "Roger, Over and Out?" *Texas Monthly,* August 2000.

45 The primary cause of Clemens' early insecurities: Wilbur Evans and Bill Little, *Texas Longhorn Baseball: Kings of the Diamond,* pp. 398–402.

47 "If football has the Bear": Roger Campbell, "Texas Will Win Again with Gus," *The Daily Texan,* February 19, 1982.

47 For more than 20 years, the coach: Roger Clemens and Peter Gammons, *Rocket Man,* p. 37.

47 The Longhorns began mandatory: Susie Woodhams, "Longhorns' Machin Signs with Phillies," *The Daily Texan*, January 21, 1982.

48 "They call me 'Goose'": Charlie McCoy, "Texas Defeats Shockers Twice," *Daily Texan*, March 2, 1982.

51 "Clemens, owner of a 93 mph fastball": Steve Campbell, "Gustafson's Pitching Aces Ponder Problems in Sliding Season," *The Daily Texan*, May 7, 1982.

55 "Never mind that I was pitching nine innings": Clemens and Gammons, *Rocket Man*, p. 45.

57 "The word was that he lacked the heart": Peter Gammons, "Striking Out Toward Cooperstown," *Sports Illustrated*, May 12, 1986.

57 "As far as I was concerned": Clemens and Gammons, *Rocket Man*, p. 46.

57 With a weight off his shoulders: Ed Combs, "Texas Beats OSU in 11 Innings, 6–5," *The Daily Texan*, June 7, 1983.

58 Catcher Jeff Hearron, the team's resident cutup: Allan Ryan, "Clemens Ready to 'Pick up Slack,'" *Toronto Star*, June 10, 1986.

58 "You tested me, you motherfucker!": Bruce Buschel, "Fastballs from the Edge," *The New York Times*, June 2, 1991.

59 That evening, Texas' conquering heroes: Debbie Fetterman, "Austin Applauds No. 1 Longhorns," *The Daily Texan*, June 13, 1983.

Chapter 6: Going Pro

67 Entering the small, no-frills Red Sox clubhouse: Roger Clemens and Peter Gammons, *Rocket Man*, p. 54.

68 "We have a lot in common . . . We both grew up": Marian Christy, "Clemens: 'I Have Been Misunderstood.'" *The Boston Globe*, April 19, 1990.

69 "My first impression of Roger was": Ibid.

70 "Our workouts consisted of something": Clemens and Gammons, *Rocket Man*, p. 55.

70 "He's got good poise": Joe Giuliotti, "No. 21 Confident He'll Make BoSox," *Sporting News*, March 26, 1984.

71 "I felt going down for a month": Dan Shaughnessy, "Houk Recalls a Clemens Move," *The Boston Globe*, March 12, 1987.

Chapter 7: Rah-jah in Beantown

73 For Roger, here, at last, was the realization: Roger Clemens and Peter Gammons, *Rocket Man*, p. 58.

76 "I remember it being real cold": Mike Peticca, "Clemens' Career Began at Stadium," Cleveland *Plain Dealer,* July 10, 2003.

76 "What really impresses me about [Roger] is his poise": Peter Gammons, "Not Too Bad for Starters," *The Boston Globe,* May 16, 2003.

79 "Whatever Jim Rice wants": No byline, "They Said It," *Sports Illustrated,* October 20, 1986.

82 After the game, Clemens told the media: Ben Walker, no headline, Associated Press, August 22, 1984.

Chapter 8: The Can

84 Born and raised in the poorest part of Meridian: Peter Gammons, "One Woe After Another," *Sports Illustrated,* August 4, 1986.

86 "I'm all right": No byline, "Sports News," United Press International, March 5, 1985.

87 "Boston," wrote John Franks: John Franks, "Sports News," United Press International, March 14, 1985.

87 He had been scheduled to start the day: Roger Clemens and Peter Gammons, *Rocket Man*, pp. 72–73.

88 "I couldn't stand the idea": Peter Gammons, "Striking Out Toward Cooperstown," *Sports Illustrated,* May 12, 1986.

88 "I just want to know what is wrong": Joe Giuliotti, "Clemens Probably Out for the Season," *Sporting News,* September 2, 1985.

89 On February 23, 1986, newspapers across the country: Dave O'Hara, no headline, Associated Press, February 23, 1986.

89 "I haven't had any setbacks yet": No byline, no headline, United Press International, February 26, 1986.

90 In his exhibition season debut against Detroit: Dave O'Hara, no headline, Associated Press, March 9, 1986.

90 His next start was little better: Dave O'Hara, no headline, Associated Press, March 16, 1986.

90 Then there was the third start: Dave O'Hara, "Twins 8, Red Sox 1," Associated Press, March 21, 1986.

90 After Clemens was clubbed: Dave O'Hara, no headline, Associated Press, March 27, 1986.

90 "You're throwing all breaking stuff": Gammons, "Striking Out Toward Cooperstown."

91 "I felt great": Joe Mooshil, no headline, Associated Press, April 11, 1986.

Chapter 9: Dominance

93 The stadium photographer's well: Leigh Montville, "Roger Clemens—The King of Ks," *Sports Illustrated,* July 3, 2006.

93 He had woken up that morning with a severe headache: Roger Clemens and Peter Gammons, *Rocket Man,* p. 89.

93 On his drive to the ballpark: Steven Krasner, "Roger's 20 Still Stands," *Austin American-Statesman,* April 30, 1996.

94 One day earlier, Clemens had played 36 holes of golf: Ibid.

97 By this point, the local radio and TV: Dan Shaughnessy, " 'Sides Was One of a Kind," *The Boston Globe,* June 16, 2007.

98 "Roger's fastball was coming in at about 120": Bob Verdi, "Last Stop Becomes Toughest on Clemens' Glory Road," *Chicago Tribune,* October 26, 1986.

98 "Rocket, do you realize that you're one": Peter Gammons, "Striking Out Toward Cooperstown," *Sports Illustrated,* May 12, 1986.

99 The record was now one K away": Ibid.

99 A three-time All-Big Eight quarterback: Ivan Maisel, "Seattle's New Power Source," *Sports Illustrated,* July 1, 1985.

99 In the dugout, Moss told Hurst: Leigh Montville, "A Whiff of Immortality," *The Boston Globe,* April 30, 1986.

100 "Two things make Clemens unusual": Gammons, "Striking Out Toward Cooperstown."

100 If Clemens was the evening's most fortunate man: Michael Madden, "Set of Circumstances Clicked," *The Boston Globe,* May 11, 1986.

101 Late that night, Clemens tossed and turned: Leigh Montville, "A Whiff of Immortality."

101 With a smile peeking out from beneath his mustache: No byline, "Designated Collector," *Sports Illustrated,* May 12, 1986.

101 *People* magazine, ordinarily the terrain of Burt Reynolds: No byline, "What's 23 Years Old and Goes K-K-K-K-K-K-K-K-K-K-K-K-K-K-K-K-K-K-K-K? Red Sox Strikeout Ace Roger Clemens," *People,* May 19, 1986.

101 During a visit to Massachusetts, Corazon Aquino: Peter Gammons, "Playoff Preview," *Sports Illustrated,* October 6, 1986.

102 When, in the months following the 20-strikeout game: John Robertson, "Clemens Had Better Get Used to Losing," *Toronto Star,* October 12, 1986.

103 Raved Thomas Boswell of the *Washington Post:* Thomas Boswell, "Red Sox Hope Breathtaking Clemens Is the Answer," *The Washington Post,* June 6, 1986.

104 "For fastball aficionados, it's almost": Dave Anderson, "'Star Wars: Dueling K's," *The New York Times,* July 7, 1986.

105 "Roger Clemens," Mets outfielder Darryl Strawberry: Richard Justice, "American League Pitches in for 3-2 Victory," *The Washington Post,* July 16, 1986.

106 Not one to follow the pack, Clemens won: No byline, "Quotable Quotes," *The Christian Science Monitor,* July 30, 1986.

107 "When he's pitching and we get three or four runs": Ed Sherman, "How Do You Spell M-V-P? C-L-E-M-E-N-S," *Chicago Tribune,* August 10, 1986.

107 As the colt bucked, Clemens: Leigh Montville, "The high-riding hero has a storybook finale," *The Boston Globe,* September. 29, 1986.

109 "He could've been overstrong": Thomas Boswell, "Angels Batter Clemens, Win First Game, 8-1," *The Washington Post,* October 8, 1986.

109 "No . . . I love to be too strong": Murray Chass, "Angels Smother Clemens and Red Sox in Opener," *The New York Times,* October 8, 1986.

109 "What am I gonna do": Shaughnessy, *One Strike Away,* p. 193.

109–10 Clemens had experienced an allergic reaction: Don Aucion, "Clemens has New Pitch: Don't smoke," *The Boston Globe,* July 8, 1994.

110 Yet after Clemens gave up a leadoff home run: Ibid., pp. 203–4.

110 "It's like we were on our death bed": Michael Martinez, "The World Series '86: Game 2," *The New York Times,* October 18, 1986.

111 The following afternoon, a man spotted Angels slugger Reggie Jackson: Shaughnessy, *One Strike Away,* p. 218.

112 "This year has been grueling on me": Richard Justice, "Clemens Tries to End Mets' Dream Season," *The Washington Post,* October 25, 1986.

113 Having logged 254 innings during the regular season: Tony Kornheiser, "The Choke Lives On," *The Washington Post,* October 25, 1986.

115 Clemens couldn't leave New York soon enough: Shaughnessy, *One Strike Away,* p. 259.

Chapter 10: A Legend in Bloom

116 "I'm gonna tie the baby's right hand behind": No byline, "Insiders Say," *Sporting News,* January 5, 1987.

116 A few days later, Roger ordered 100 Koby Clemens baseball cards: Stan Isle, " 'Next Willie Mays' Talk Pressures Eric Davis," *Sporting News,* February 23, 1987.

117 "The decision was definitely all Mac's": Dan Shaughnessy, "Clemens' Times," *The Boston Globe Magazine,* July 24, 1988.

117 "Everybody thinks he can do your job": Larry Whiteside, "A Pair of Aces," *Street and Smith's Baseball,* Spring 1987.

118 "Starting tomorrow, our offer to the Red Sox": No byline, "Clemens Might Sit Out '87 Season," *The Washington Post,* March 11, 1987.

119 Of baseball's 33 free agents from 1985 and '86: John Helyar, *Lords of the Realm,* p. 360.

119 "Clubs are working together, making fewer dumb": Helyar, *Lords of the Realm,* p. 369.

119 Clemens was stung by Gorman's take-back: Dan Shaughnessy, "Clemens' Times."

119 On March 11, five days after he walked out: No byline, "Clemens Sends Family Packing," *Toronto Star,* March 12, 1987.

119 At a press conference from his Houston office: No byline, "Clemens' Agent Claims Red Sox in Conspiracy," *The Washington Post,* March 26, 1987.

120 "I guarantee you, everybody on this team agrees": Larry Whiteside, "Clemens Takes a Hike over Salary," *The Boston Globe,* March 7, 1987.

120 "When a baseball player talks about principle": Ross Newhan, "McCaskill and Joyner Voice Support for Clemens," *Los Angeles Times,* March 28, 1987.

121 "Would someone please tell this kid": Scott Ostler, "From the Real World, Here's One Sincere Plea for Clemens," *Los Angeles Times,* March 30, 1987.

121 Those Red Sox loyalists who hoped: Richard Justice, "Red Sox Still Smoking from Series Burnout," *The Washington Post,* March 24, 1987.

122 "He doesn't have the control he had": Dan Shaughnessy, "Numbers Down . . . How About Clemens?" *The Boston Globe,* June 11, 1986

122 McNamara, who was in charge of: No byline, "Clemens Accepts Decision," *Toronto Star,* July 11, 1987.

123 One of the few highlights (and oddest moments): No byline, "Roger Clemens to Make Appearance at Jordan Marsh," *PR Newswire,* August 27, 1987.

123 In his final start of the year at Milwaukee: No byline, "Clemens Wins 20th Game on Two-Hitter," *Los Angeles Times,* October 5, 1987.

123 "It's gratifying because it puts me in a class with people": No byline, "Sports News," United Press International, November 12, 1987.

124 Once, while preparing for a start in Oakland: Dan Shaughnessy, "Clemens' Times."

124–25 upon being asked whether anyone would match his 31-win: Bill Hageman and Rich Lorenz, "Clemens Impresses McClain," *Chicago Tribune,* June 9, 1988.

125 "It was the best of times, it was the worst of times": Richard Justice, "Clemens: Birth of a Legend," *The Washington Post,* June 1, 1988.

125 Immediately after the game Clemens' trip to the airport: Dave Strege, "With Wife in Labor, Clemens Delivers Victory over Angels," *Orange County Register,* May 31, 1988.

126 When a nurse asked Cindy Garvey: Pat Jordan, "Trouble in Paradise," *Inside Sports,* 1980.

126 Never a fan of Clemens, third baseman Wade Boggs: Murray Chass, "Gossip Is Latest Arrival at Red Sox Camp," *The New York Times,* February 17, 1988.

127 A French dilettante once said: Pat Jordan, "Roger Clemens Refuses to Grow Up," *The New York Times Magazine,* March 4, 2001.

128 Lee Smith, the team's new closer: Peter Gammons, "Inside Baseball," *Sports Illustrated,* July 25, 1988.

129 Yet at a time he should have been carrying his: Ben Walker, No headline, Associated Press, August 14, 1988.

129 "Strange as it sounds, Clemens has been": Dan Shaughnessy, "Will Clemens Get the Nod?" *The Boston Globe,* September 21, 1988.

130 For six innings, Clemens was the Rocket of old: Jackie MacMullan, "An Overpowering Sense of Loss for Clemens," *The Boston Globe,* October 7, 1988.

Chapter 11: Baggage

131   He wanted the families of players to be given: Dan Shaughnessy, "Clemens Airs Complaints," *The Boston Globe,* March 2, 1989.

132   "When I saw that Clemens on TV": Will McDonough, "Greed Is the Game," *The Boston Globe,* December 8, 1988.

132   "The average person does not think": Will McDonough, "Hurst Can't Kid Us," *The Boston Globe,* December 10, 1988.

133   The backlash stunned Clemens: Dan Shaughnessy, "Clemens Takes Aim at Reporters," *The Boston Globe,* January 12, 1989.

134   The *Boston Herald* fired him as a guest columnist: Dan Shaughnessy, "Image Problem," *The Boston Globe,* April 3, 1989.

134   Clemens even had it out with his boyhood idol: Buster Olney, "The Power of his Pitches and the Vigor of His Person," *The New York Times,* April 5, 1999.

137   "If Lou [Gorman] wants to get nasty about this": Dan Shaughnessy, "Clemens' Brother Warns of 'Knock-down' Fight," *The Boston Globe,* March 9, 1987.

138   "The same press that sat on my lawn": Marian Christy, "Clemens: 'I Have Been Misunderstood,'" *Boston Globe,* April 19, 1990.

138   Following a three-hitter at Milwaukee: Sean McAdam, "Off the Field, Clemens No Match for Ryan," *St. Louis Post-Dispatch,* July 31, 1990.

138   When Clemens demanded that: Ross Newhan, "For Once, Clemens Didn't Get His Way," *Los Angeles Times,* October 12, 1990.

139   Clemens captured his 20th win: Steve Fainaru, "Sure Thing," *The Boston Globe,* August 30, 1990.

140   "Your real estate taxes have been doubled": Dan Shaughnessy, "A Double Dose of Hardship Has Overtaken Boston's Team of Destiny," *The Boston Globe,* September 6, 1990.

140   During Clemens' time away, Jim Palmer: Nick Cafardo, "Clemens Story Line a Convoluted Tale," *The Boston Globe,* September 26, 1990.

140   "If Roger Clemens told me he could walk on water": Ross Newhan, "Clemens Makes Title Pitch," *Los Angeles Times,* September 30, 1990.

Chapter 12: Unraveling

143   After his game one start: Nicholas Dawidoff, "Control Problems," *Sports Illustrated,* October 22, 1990.

143   "What are you drinking now?": No byline, "Baseball's Latest Fall Guys," *The New York Times,* October 20, 1990.

143   "I worry about Roger": Newhan, "For Once, Clemens Didn't Get His Way."

143   Oakland's Harold Baines, an 11-year veteran: Leigh Montville, "A Moment of Madness," *Sports Illustrated,* November 26, 1990.

144   "What makes Dave Stewart so good": Bruce Buschel, "Fastballs from the Edge," *The New York Times,* June 2, 1991.

144   Later that afternoon, Clemens intentionally rammed: Ibid.

145   He decided every strikeout would be followed: Leigh Montville, "A Moment of Madness," *Sports Illustrated,* November 26, 1990.

145   Surrounding his mouth was a brown Fu Manchu: Ibid.

146   "I was looking down at the dirt": Michael Madden, "Umpire Ignited Explosion," *The Boston Globe,* October 11, 1990.

148   "The stenographer was a little lady straight out of *Little House*": Tom Verducci, "It's All About the Power," *Sports Illustrated,* June 2, 2003.

150   The Pressman Toy Corporation contacted: John Branch, "Toying with Roger," *Toronto Star,* May 6, 1991.

151   "It was an all-out brawl": Nick Cafardo, "No Hearing Date Yet in Clemens Assault Case," *The Boston Globe,* January 21, 1991.

151   "When I walk into a place": Buschel, "Fastballs from the Edge."

Chapter 13: The Ladies' Man

161   That's where Roger Clemens and a handful of his Boston teammates: Sam Cook, "Clearing the Air on McCready-Clemens Affair," Fort Myers *News-Press,* May 6, 2008

162   "There was a desperation to leave the life": Robert K. Oermann, "McCready Kisses the Glamour Girl Goodbye," *The Tennessean,* January 1, 1998.

162   Her life was, in many regards, a clichéd country song: Laurence Leamer, *Three Chords and the Truth,* pp. 181–208.

162   The oldest of three siblings, Mindy was 11: Brian Mansfield, "Guardian Angel," *New Country,* Spring 1997.

162   "I was given the choice to act like a child": Oermann, "McCready Kisses the Glamour Girl Goodbye."

164   One night, for example, Clemens went out with some fellow: Laurel J. Sweet, "Ex-waitress: Randy Rocket Once Made Pitch to Me, Too," *Boston Herald,* April 30, 2008.

164 Why, he had just built a 13,000-square-foot: Bruce Buschel, "Fast-balls from the Edge," *The New York Times*, June 2, 1991.

165 "I think once I shut it down in Beantown": Joe Giuliotti, "Rocket: No Liftoff," *Boston Herald*, March 27, 1993.

165 "I'd like to play until the year 2000": Mel Antonen, "Clemens Projects End of His Career in 2000," *USA Today*, May 23, 1993.

165 While on the disabled list in June with a strained right groin muscle: Desmond Conner, "Different Drive for Clemens," *Hartford Courant*, June 24, 1993.

166 When the team traveled to Minneapolis: Nick Cafardo, "Clemens Avoids Hobson's Doghouse," *The Boston Globe*, August 4, 1993.

166 He followed the path of thousands of poorly: Greg Krupa, "Clemens on the Bill," *The Boston Globe*, June 29, 1993.

166 On September 30, Jack O'Connell: Jack O'Connell, "Bargains n' Busts," *The Vancouver Sun*, September 30, 1993.

166 Five days later, in Mike Shalin's Red Sox report card: Mike Shalin, "Red Sox Report Card," *Boston Herald*, October 5, 1993.

Chapter 14: The Devil and Dan Duquette

168 As a fifth-grader he had been kicked out of class: Peter Gammons, "A Student of the Game," *The Boston Globe*, January 28, 1992.

169 now a 31-year-old veteran: Nick Cafardo, "Duquette at Home as Red Sox GM," *The Boston Globe*, January 28, 1994.

171 "His persona is so negative": No byline, "Stars Who Are Hard to Market," *The New York Times*, September 9, 1991.

171 With his mother Bess, a cigarette smoker for 35 years: Don Aucoin, "Clemens Has a New Pitch: Don't Smoke," *The Boston Globe*, July 8, 1994.

174–75 "Baseball is at a standstill": Jerry Greene, "Clemens: No Ball, Still Active," *Orlando Sentinel*, January 28, 1995.

175 First, he sported a new haircut that: Karen Guregian, "Rocket Steals the Show," *Boston Herald*, April 6, 1995.

176 This is prime time, when the true greats: Will McDonough, "All right, Clemens . . . Now's the Time," *The Boston Globe*, September 30, 1995.

177 "For one reason or another": Ken Rosenthal, "Always Something for Clemens in October," Baltimore *Sun*, October 4, 1996.

Chapter 15: War

178 CLEMENS PITCHES IN FOR KIDS: Seth Livingstone, "Clemens Pitches in for Kids," *Patriot Ledger,* April 1, 1996.

180 When asked by the *Boston Globe* to assess: Nick Cafardo, "Opening Act Still Worth Seeing," *The Boston Globe,* April 1, 1996.

180 "I'll tell you what Felipe Alou once told me": Michael Madden, "What, Boston Brass Worry?" *The Boston Globe,* September 27, 1996.

181 As Boston battled the Texas Rangers at Fenway Park: No byline, "Red Sox Pitcher Roger Clemens Bids on JFK's Golf Clubs," Associated Press, April 25, 1996.

183 "I've had some teammates in the past who just": Alex Griffin, "It Takes Teamwork to Win on and off the Field," *Houston Intown,* May 2005.

184 Wrote Mark Newman in the *Sporting News:* Mark Newman, "The Jose Way," *Sporting News,* September 11, 1995.

185 "I wanted to become faster, stronger, better": Jose Canseco, *Juiced: Wild Times, Rampant 'Roids, Smash Hits, and How Baseball Got Big,* p. 46.

186 "I don't know what the big deal is": Steve Krasner, "Clemens Is Balking at Final Appearance," *Providence Journal-Bulletin,* September 25, 1996.

187 In the visiting dugout, Yankee players": Phil O'Neill, "Yanks Join Tribute to Rocket," *Telegram & Gazette,* September 29, 1996.

187 "A guy walks off the mound after the way": Frank Dell'Apa, "The Final Bow?" *The Boston Globe,* September 29, 1996.

Chapter 16: Twilight

189 Toward the end of the 1996 season: Howard Ulman, "Boston Star Emotional About Last Start," Associated Press, September 27, 1996.

189 Face it: If Clemens had not once been able: Mike Barnicle, "Big-League Arm, Bush Heart," *The Boston Globe,* December 15, 1996.

189 Duquette offered a four-year, $22 million: No byline, "Potential Free Agents," Associated Press, October 4, 1996.

190 "If you check the book": Bryan Denbrock, "Clemens Exits with a Snarl for Sox GM," *Buffalo News,* December 14, 1996.

191 It had been a whirlwind month: Gerry Callahan, "Commanding Presence," *Sports Illustrated,* March 31, 1997.

191   Their season-ticket base slipped to 22,000: Ibid.

192   "I'm here to win a World Series": Jim Byers, "Clemens' Greatness Seen Early," *Toronto Star*, December 14, 1996.

192   "Good riddance!": Peter May, "It Was Blast Off Time for the Rocket Man," *The Boston Globe*, December 25, 1996.

192   Said Nicholas Burns, a State Department: Clint Cooper, "Sports People," *Chattanooga Free Press*, December 22, 1996.

192   In a fawning piece for *Toronto Life* magazine: Jay Teitel, "One Sensitive Guy," *Toronto Life*, August, 1997.

194   In exchange for uniform number 21: No byline, "It Took Time, but Delgado Rewarded by Clemens," Associated Press, February 16, 1997.

194   "It's just so blue!": Callahan, "Commanding Presence."

195   In a piece that appeared in *The Record:* No byline, "Jays Opener Won't Be Sold Out," Kitchener-Waterloo *Record*, April 1, 1997.

195   Now, as Clemens walked onto the field: Mike Rutsey, "Blue Jays Have Liftoff," *Toronto Sun*, April 3, 1997.

196   "The worst thing you can do": LaVelle E. Neal III, "Rocket's Ire Appears," *Kansas City Star*, April 29, 1997.

196   "It's not just that Roger pitches well": Jack O'Connell, "Clemens Is Worth It," *Hartford Courant*, May 21, 1997.

196–97   When confronted by Allan Ryan: Allan Ryan, "Blue Days!" *Toronto Star*, June 28, 1997.

197   "One of the reasons Roger ended up coming": Lorne Rubenstein, "Clemens Upset He Can't Golf for Free," *The Globe and Mail*, May 5, 1997.

199   Wrote Robert Rodriguez in *Avid Golfer:* Robert Rodriguez, "Ace in the Hole," *Avid Golfer*, August 2003.

199   "This is my sixth All-Star Game": Mike Zeisberger, "Jays' Season Not What Clemens Expected," *Toronto Sun*, July 8, 1997.

199   "It's a matter of channeling my emotions": Stephen Brunt, "Rocket Prepares for Return to Boston Launching Pad," *The Globe and Mail*, July 11, 1997.

200   Say this about Roger Clemens: Steve Buckley, "The Rocket Delivers a Night to Remember," *Boston Herald*, July 13, 1997.

201   Following Toronto's 3-1 victory: Bob Elliott, "Clemens Shows His Inner Fire," *Toronto Sun*, July 13, 1997.

Chapter 17: Under the Influence

203 "He got his velocity back": Murray Chass, "At 35, Clemens Rises to Top of His Game," *The New York Times,* September 2, 1997.

205 "I'll communicate with each of my players": Jim Proudfoot, "Johnson's Passion for Game Refreshing," *Toronto Star,* November 25, 1997.

205 "One of our complaints was that": Jeff Blair, "The Clemens-McNamee Story Began in Toronto," *The Globe and Mail,* February 13, 2008.

206 "He was a very good baseball player here": Ibid.

206 McNamee's greatest achievement occurred: John Valenti, "Redmen Win, Rams Eliminated," *Newsday,* May 28, 1988.

206 For three and a half years: Jon Heyman, "The Sixth Man," SI.com, November 14, 2006.

206 McNamee was called to the scene in 1991: Gabriel Grüner, "Perhaps It Will Be a Gigantic Flop," *Stern Magazine,* February 19, 1998.

206 The thing that Lyon couldn't get over was how hard: Jon Heyman, "The Sixth Man."

207 In the suspension's aftermath: Shaun Assael, Luke Cyphers and Amy K. Nelson, "McNamee Takes Center Stage with Bombshells About Clemens," ESPN.com, December 13, 2007.

208 "Baseball players often talk about their game": Mark Zwolinski, "Little Spring at This Camp," *Toronto Star,* February 8, 1998.

208 "I could care less about a no-hitter": Mark Zwolinski, "Clemens Close to Perfection," *Toronto Star,* May 3, 1998.

209 "He has this history and this aura": Dan Graziano, "An Exercise in Durability," *Newark Star-Ledger,* April 21, 2000.

210 Clemens knew that McNamee's one-year-old son: Committee on Oversight and Government Reform, U.S. House of Representatives: Deposition of: Brian Jerome McNamee, Sr., February 7, 2008, pages 10–20.

210 "Every other pitch I threw would be released differently": www.rocket-roger.com, Post Game Interview with K. K. Campbell, June 8, 1998.

210 "I noticed right away that I was": www.rocketroger.com, Post Game Interview with K. K. Campbell, June 19, 1998.

211 The pitcher who had been topping out at 92 mph: Thomas Hill, "Rocket Still Feels the Burn," New York *Daily News,* May 23, 1999.

211 "When Roger signed with Toronto": Laura Garraway, "After the Dust Settles, Clemens Still a Blue Jay," *Vancouver Sun,* August 1, 1998.

212 In an attempt to put baseball into perspective: Joel Sherman, "Blue Jays' Manager Haunted by Lies," *New York Post*, December 15, 1998.

Chapter 18: A (Not So) Yankee Doodle Dandy

215 "I like everything [Clemens] stands for": George King, "Won't Get Fooled Again," *New York Post*, December 5, 1998.

215 Clemens ranked alongside Baltimore second baseman Jerry Hairston: Buster Olney, *The Last Night of the Yankee Dynasty*, p. 82.

215 The loathing of the Rocket: Joe Donnelly, "Roger Dodges a Bullet," *Newsday*, September 16, 1991.

216 Finally, with spring training just days away: Verducci, "Booster Rocket," *Sports Illustrated*, March 1, 1999.

216 "If you liked Metallica, tattoos, Howard Stern": Jack Curry, "Stunned and Saddened, Wells Is No Longer a Yankee," *The New York Times*, February 19, 1999.

216 The pitcher earned his place in Yankee folklore: Olney, *The Last Night of the Yankee Dynasty*, p. 115.

217 A couple of hours after Ash: Tom Verducci, "Booster Rocket," *Sports Illustrated*, March 1, 1999.

219 "We had a great pitcher out there and he had a bad": Don Amore, "Clemens Fizzles . . . and Hears About It," *Hartford Courant*, April 16, 1999.

219–20 Teammates were intrigued by Clemens' unconventional rituals: Olney, *The Last Night of the Yankee Dynasty*, p. 67.

221 "I thought we were going to see the Clemens of old": Ken Davidoff, "Roger, Chuck Concern Boss," Bergen *Record*, September 9, 1999.

221 "[Clemens] is not a savior, I guarantee that": George King, "Clemens: I Won't Read It," *New York Post*, June 9, 1999.

221 He even switched his uniform number from 12 to 22: Ken Davidoff, "Rocket Changes Number," Bergen *Record*, July 25, 1999.

222 In his play-off preview, *Newsday*'s David Lennon: David Lennon, "Yankees Scouting Report," *Newsday*, October 5, 1999.

222 The *Daily News*' Mark Kriegel went one step: Mark Kriegel, "Roger Clemens Is One Who Can Live Up to His Reputation," New York *Daily News*, September 30, 1999.

223 "If you take a Koufax against Marichal": Ben Walker, "Clemens vs. Martinez—October Baseball at Its Best," Associated Press, October 15, 1999.

225 "Very much needed and deserved": Buster Olney, "They're Clemens's People Now," *The New York Times,* March 31, 2000.

225 "Tonight . . . I know what it's like": Ronald Blum, "The Moment Clemens Spent His Lfe Waiting For," Associated Press, October 27, 1999.

Chapter 19: Happiness

226 He was fitted for a three-carat diamond: Josh Dubow, "Clemens Rings in Championship Year," Associated Press, May 29, 2000.

226 (To placate Clemens): Joe Torre and Tom Verducci, *The Yankee Years,* p. 100.

229 "When we're right as a team swinging the bats": Josh Dubow, "Yankees 9, White Sox 4," Associated Press, May 18, 2000.

229 Not merely at the killers: Steve Brewer, "5 Indicted in Teacher's Slaying," *Houston Chronicle,* August 16, 2000.

231 With his wife and children back home in Texas: Brad Schmitt, "Mindy M's Got a New Label and a Brand-New Man," *The Tennessean,* November 29, 2000.

232 The question is getting closer to a naked cry: Bob Klapisch, "Clemens to Doom Yankees," New Orleans *Times-Picayune,* June 11, 2000.

232 So, like before, he began injecting Clemens: Mitchell Report, pp. 170–71.

233 THE ROCKET IS BACK! screamed a headline: Allen Barra, "The Rocket Is Back!," Salon.com, August 18, 2000.

233 "He's got the body language now": Bob Herzog, "Rocket's the Man," *Newsday,* September 14, 2000.

234 Though Torre told the media that Clemens: Tara Sullivan, "Rocket to Get Plenty of Rest," Bergen *Record,* October 10, 2000.

235 "Roger was as dominant as I have": Kerry Eggers, "Clemens the One for Yankees," *Oregonian,* October 15, 2000.

235 (Two days after that, Clemens sent . . .): Tom Verducci, "It's All About the Power," *Sports Illustrated,* June 2, 2003.

Chapter 20: Subway Crash

236 Yet leading up to the highly anticipated 2000 World Series: Stephen Borelli, "Torrez Can Relate to Clemens," *USA Today,* October 26, 2000.

237 The big moment came in the bottom of: Josh Dubow, "Mets 5, Yankees 2," Associated Press, July 9, 1999.

237 "There aren't many guys": Mike Lupica, "Real Apple Star's Drive Takes Clemens for a Subway Ride," New York *Daily News,* June 10, 2000.

238 "I hope we're bigger than that": Jon Heyman, "Shame on You, Roger Clemens," *Newsday,* July 9, 2000.

238 "I've seen him hit guys in the head": David Waldstein, "Mets Certain Clemens Pitched with a Purpose," Newark *Star-Ledger,* July 9, 2000.

239 Growing up in the Philadelphia suburb of Phoenixville: Kelly Whiteside, "A Piazza with Everything," *Sports Illustrated,* July 5, 1993.

241 "I've revisited it the last couple of days": Colin Stephenson, "Rocket Brushes Off Talk About Piazza," Newark *Star-Ledger,* October 22, 2000.

243 "Trust me, if I were Mike Piazza": David Wells with Chris Kreski, *Perfect I'm Not,* p. 377.

Chapter 21: Greatness by Any Means Necessary

248 In a glowing *Sports Illustrated* profile: Tom Verducci, "Rocket Science," *Sports Illustrated,* September 10, 2001.

248 In a *New York Times* piece titled "A Wonder of the Pitching World": Buster Olney, "A Wonder of the Pitching World," *The New York Times,* February 25, 2001.

249 (He took the ball home to his mother, Bess . . .): George King, "Rocket Did Pass Train," *New York Post,* April 4, 2001.

250 McNamee made weekly trips to Clemens: "Deposition of: Brian Jerome McNamee, Sr.," Committee on Oversight and Government Reform, U.S. House of Representatives, February 7, 2008.

251 "I'm just thrilled": Michael O'Keeffe and Peter Botte, "Clemens to Receive Honor in Wake of Legend Walter Johnson," *New York Post,* April 5, 2001.

251 On September 5, one month removed from his 39th birthday: Joan Susan Herz, "Clemens Racks up 15th Straight Win; now 19-1" Ontario *Sault Star,* September 6, 2001.

252 On the morning of September 11, 2001, Clemens woke up: Richard Justice, "Duty and Honor," *The Houston Chronicle,* January 19, 2003.

253 With the phone lines jammed, Clemens struggled to place: Buster Olney, *The Last Night of the Yankee Dynasty*, p. 10.

253 He attended several benefits for fallen firefighters: Anthony McCarron, "Clemens' Season Grades an A-plus," New York *Daily News*, October 10, 2001.

253 On one particular day Clemens and a friend decided: Tyler Kepner, "Clemens Pays Tribute as Yanks Sweep," *The New York Times*, September 12, 2003.

255 "They're in their uniforms, and you can tell": Richard Justice, "Duty and Honor," *The Houston Chronicle*, January 19, 2003.

255 "Roger Clemens is a Yankee now": Buster Olney, "He's Deep in the Heart of New York," *The New York Times*, September 25, 2001.

255 "[With baseball back]," wrote Tracy McDannald: Tracy McDannald, "Baseball Helped Heal Nation on Sept. 11," *The Daily 49er*, September 11, 2008.

256 "If I was not able to make this start because": Sam Donnellon, "'Rocket' Fizzles Once More," *Philadelphia Daily News*, October 16, 2001.

256 "It's fairly amusing for people that are": Chris Jenkins, "Rocket Claims He's Off Course," *The San Diego Union-Tribune*, October 21, 2001.

257 "Obviously, we felt for New York": Buster Olney, *The Last Night of the Yankee Dynasty*, p. 13.

258 "Roger is the key": Howard Bryant, "It's Showtime," Bergen *Record*, October 30, 2001.

258 Joey Navas, wide-eyed and 9 years old: Richard Cowen, "Boy Shines Among Stars," Bergen *Record*, November 1, 2001.

259 In the winter of 1991, Clemens, a hotshot with the Red Sox: Ben Walker, "Decade after discussion, Clemens vs. Schilling in Game 7," Associated Press, November 3, 2001.

260 On the day before the game, Schilling: Tom Verducci, "Desert Classic," *Sports Illustrated*, November 12, 2001.

Chapter 22: Ignorance and Bliss

263 On October 6, 2001, while the Yankees: George King, "McNamee Questioned in '01 Sexual Battery Incident," *New York Post*, December 13, 2007.

265 "I'm going to be 41 this year": Kevin Kernan, "Rocket Has Landed," *New York Post*, Decmber 31, 2002.

266 Gen. Richard Myers, the chairman of the Joint Chiefs of Staff: Richard Justice, "Duty and Honor," *The Houston Chronicle,* January 19, 2003.

267 "I was the third-best pitcher on my high school": Joyce Shelby, "Bombers Ace & School Fan Score Big Hit," New York *Daily News,* January 14, 2003.

267 "I guess you have to accept Boomer": George King, "Family Feud— Rocket: Wells' Book All Lies, My Sister's Out to Bop Boomer," *New York Post,* March 7, 2003.

268 "To me, it's a no-brainer": Richard Justice, "Clemens Goes for 300th," *The Houston Chronicle,* May 26, 2001.

269 "The best thing about it is, this is his choice": Dan Graziano, "Rocket Receives the Ultimate Send-off," Newark *Star-Ledger,* September 28, 2003.

270 On September 27, in what was presumed to be: Ibid.

271 "Clemens vs. Martinez is more than a baseball game": Ronald Blum, "Gods and Green Monsters," San Bernardino *Sun,* October 10, 2003.

271 "Saturday," said Kevin Millar: Dave Sheinin, "Clemens Brings His Own Energy," *The Washington Post,* October 11, 2003.

Chapter 23: Retirement

275 "You're looking at it . . . Playing in golf tournaments": Jose de Jesus Ortiz, "Clemens Stands Firm on Retirement Issue," *The Houston Chronicle,* November 6, 2003.

275 "There's no scenario where I'd come back . . . I'm retired": Connor Ennis, "With Olympics Out, Clemens Says He's Done," Associated Press, November 12, 2003.

275 One month later, on December 12, Clemens appeared: Richard Justice, "Astros Raise Bar to the Limit," *The Houston Chronicle,* December 13, 2003.

276 Even Tiger Woods had an opinion: Art Spander, "Clemens Ponders Birdies, Baseballs," *The Oakland Tribune,* January 9, 2004.

277 "I've never had anything like this in my 18 seasons": Richard Justice, "Hometown Signing," *The Houston Chronicle,* January 13, 2004.

278 "[Roger] told us he was retiring": Tyler Kepner, "Yankees Were Caught off Guard," *The New York Times,* January 13, 2004.

278 "Let him go . . . Let him go home": Mike Vaccaro, "Turncoat Roger Two-Times Yanks—Should Have Known Better than to Trust this Rat," *New York Post,* January 13, 2004.

279 "I get sick and tired of everyone wanting to flaunt their training method": Anthony McCarron, "Sheff in a Stew About Rocket," New York *Daily News,* July 18, 2004.

280 "If Sheffield had any shame": Jose de Jesus Ortiz, "Clemens Incident Unfairly Put Kid in Spotlight," *The Houston Chronicle,* August 8, 2004.

282 "I've pretty much painted myself into a corner": Clifton Brown, "Clemens Still Undecided," *The New York Times,* January 6, 2005.

283 "Roger can make more of a difference for the Houston": David Barron, "18 Million Reasons to Play," *The Houston Chronicle,* January 22, 2005.

283 Not long after Clemens agreed to the $18 million: Jose de Jesus Ortiz, "No. 22 Gunning for More," *The Houston Chronicle,* April 8, 2005.

283 "When you're under house arrest and you have ankle bracelets": Michael Morrissey, "Roger's Brushback," *New York Post,* February 19, 2005.

285 As the Astros hit the road: Tim Brown, "Special Case? Roger That," *Los Angeles Times,* August 28, 2005.

Chapter 24: Bess

286 "She taught me my values": Tony Massarotti, "Rog Close to His Mom," *The Boston Herald,* September 24, 1993.

287 "I wanted her to hang around": Jose de Jesus Ortiz, *Houston Astros: Armed and Dangerous,* p. 170.

287 On the night of September 9: Ortiz, *Houston Astros: Armed and Dangerous,* pp. 170–71.

289 On the second-to-last day of the season, Clemens took the mound: Gene Duffey, "Astros One Win Away from Playoffs," *Austin American-Statesman,* October 2, 2005.

290 Through the season's final month, Clemens: Ortiz, *Houston Astros: Armed and Dangerous,* p. 196.

293 He told the *New York Post* that his mother's dying wish: Michael Morrissey, "Roger May Heed Mom's Last Wish," *New York Post,* February 15, 2006.

293 On April 3, he sat at home with his family and watched: Chris Duncan, "Clemens Gets NLCS Ring, Future Uncertain," Associated Press Online, April 5, 2006.

294 It doesn't appear that Clemens cares much about anything: Stephen A. Smith, "Roger Clemens' Phony Encore," *The Philadelphia Inquirer,* June 1, 2006.

295 "I had hoped that he would be kind of a mentor": Troy E. Renck, "Clemens Backlash, Support," *The Denver Post,* May 9, 2007.

Chapter 25: Credibility Lost

297 "Like I told you guys before, I've been tested:" Jose de Jesus Ortiz, "Clemens, Pettitte Deny Grimsley's Allegations," *The Houston Chronicle,* October 2, 2006.

298 He told the *Hartford Courant* that: Dom Amore, "Clemens 'Failing at Retirement,'" *Hartford Courant,* February 1, 2007.

298 He told *The Desert Sun* of Palm Springs, California: Leighton Ginn, "Clemens Back in the Fold," *The Desert Sun,* January 18, 2007.

298 In the February 17 edition of the *Newark Star-Ledger:* No byline, "'I Don't Want to Play,'" Newark *Star Ledger,* February 17, 2007.

299 "Make no mistake about it": Kat O'Brien, "A Rocket Hits the Bronx," *Newsday,* May 7, 2007.

300 Roger Clemens . . . somehow conflated a Lou Gehrig: Will Leitch, "It's Important That You Remember That Roger Clemens Is Your Savior," Deadspin.com, May 7, 2007.

301 On May 17, weeks before Clemens even joined the club: Peter Abraham, "Farnsworth Speaks Out About Clemens," *Journal News,* May 18, 2007.

301 He entered the clubhouse for the first time at approximately 10 A.M.: Dave Sheinin, "In Return, Clemens Has Something Left," *The Washington Post,* June 10, 2007.

Chapter 26: Dead Pitcher Walking

305 The day the Mitchell Report was released, his attorney, Rusty Hardin: Steve Simmons, "Clemens Is the New Bonds," *Ottawa Sun,* December 14, 2007.

305 "I have tried to do things the right way": Ed Price, "Pettitte Admits He Used HGH," *The Times* (Trenton), December 16, 2007.

305 As Gerry Callahan put it in: Gerry Callahan, "True Fraud? Roger That," *The Boston Herald,* December 18, 2007.

306 Curt Schilling, who had idolized Clemens: Jimmy Golen, "Schil-

ling Calls on Clemens to Give Up Cy Youngs if Rocket Doesn't Clear Name," Associated Press, December 20, 2007.

307 "No one injects lidocaine intramuscularly": Neill Ostrout and Mike Pignataro, "UConn Doctor Questions Clemens' Story," *Connecticut Post*, January 5, 2008.

313 To believe Clemens is to believe that McNamee: Richard Justice, "In the End, Neither One Is Credible," *The Houston Chronicle*, February 14, 2008.

314 Plans for a Clemens-themed restaurant: Matthew Tresaugue, "Houston Sports Clinic Will Drop Clemens' Name," *The Houston Chronicle*, December 29, 2008.

BIBLIOGRAPHY

Boggs, Wade. *Boggs!* Chicago: Contemporary Books, 1986.

Bonazelli, Andrew. *Mechaniks.* Edwardsville, Pa.: McCarren Publishing, 2008.

Brenner, Richard J. *Roger Clemens, Darryl Strawberry.* New York: Lynx Books, 1989.

Brunt, Stephen. *Diamond Dreams: 20 Years of Blue Jays Baseball.* Toronto: Penguin Books, 1997.

Bryant, Howard. *Shut Out: A Story of Race and Baseball in Boston.* Boston: Beacon Press, 2002.

Canseco, Jose. *Juiced.* New York: Regan Books, 2005.

———. *Vindicated.* New York: Simon Spotlight Entertainment, 2008.

Clemens, Roger and Peter Gammons. *Rocket Man.* New York: Penguin Books, 1987.

Devaney, John. *Sports Great Roger Clemens.* Hillside, N.J.: Enslow Publishers, 1990.

Evans, Wilbur and Bill Little. *Texas Longhorn Baseball: Kings of the Diamond.* Huntsville, Ala.: Strode Publishers, 1983.

Giamatti, A. Bartlett. *A Great and Glorious Game.* Chapel Hill, N.C.: Algonquin Books, 1998.

Gille, Janean. *Airlog: 1971 Vandalia-Butler High School Yearbook.* Dayton, Ohio: Robert Wherry Press, 1971.

Gorman, Lou. *High and Inside: My Life in the Front Offices of Baseball.* Jefferson, N.C.: McFarland, 2008.

———. *One Pitch From Glory.* Champaign, Ill.: Sports Publishing, 2005.

Helyar, John. *Lords of the Realm: The Real History of Baseball.* New York: Random House, 1994.

Janczak, Joseph. *The Rocket: Baseball Legend Roger Clemens.* Washington, D.C.: Potomac Books, 2007.

Jordan, Pat and Alex Belth. *The Best Sports Writing of Pat Jordan*. New York: Persea Books, 2008.

Kahn, Roger. *The Head Game: Baseball Seen from the Pitcher's Mound*. New York: Harcourt, 2000.

Kernan, Kevin. *Rocket!* New York: Sports Publishing. 1999.

Kinslow, Gina and Quyen Vu. *Safari: 1985 Spring Woods High School Yearbook*. Dallas: Taylor Publishing, 1985.

Leamer, Laurence. *Three Chords and the Truth: Hope, Heartbreak, and Changing Fortunes in Nashville*. New York: HarperCollins, 1994.

Macht, Norman L. *Roger Clemens*. Philadelphia: Chelsea House Publishers, 1999.

Mayo, Jonathan. *Facing Clemens*. Guilford, Conn.: Lyons Press, 2008.

Morgan, Bill. *Roger Clemens*. New York: Scholastic, 1992.

Nowlin, Bill. *Fenway Lives: The Team Behind the Team*. Cambridge, Mass.: Rounder Books, 2004.

Nowlin, Bill and Jim Prime. *The Boston Red Sox World Series Encyclopedia*. Burlington, Mass.: Rounder Books, 2008.

Olney, Buster. *The Last Night of the Yankee Dynasty*. New York: HarperCollins, 2004.

Ortiz, Jr., Jose de Jesus. *Houston Astros: Armed and Dangerous*. Champaign, Ill.: Sports Publishing, 2006.

Patrick, Dan. *Outtakes*. New York: Hyperion, 2000.

Ryan, Nolan and Jerry Jenkins. *Miracle Man*. Dallas: Word Publishing, 1992.

Ryan, Nolan and Tom House. *Nolan Ryan's Pitcher's Bible*. New York: Simon & Schuster, 1991.

Shaughnessy, Dan. *The Curse of the Bambino*. New York: Penguin Books, 1990.

———. *One Strike Away: The Story of the 1986 Red Sox*. New York: Beaufort Books Publishers, 1990.

Shroyer, Sande. *Chargers: 1976–77 Smith Junior High School Yearbook*. Dayton, Ohio. Smith Junior High School, 1977.

Stottlemyre, Mel and John Harper. *Pride and Pinstripes*. New York: HarperCollins, 2007.

Torre, Joe and Tom Verducci. *The Yankee Years*. New York: Doubleday, 2009.

Wells, David and Chris Kreski. *Perfect I'm Not*. New York: HarperCollins, 2003.